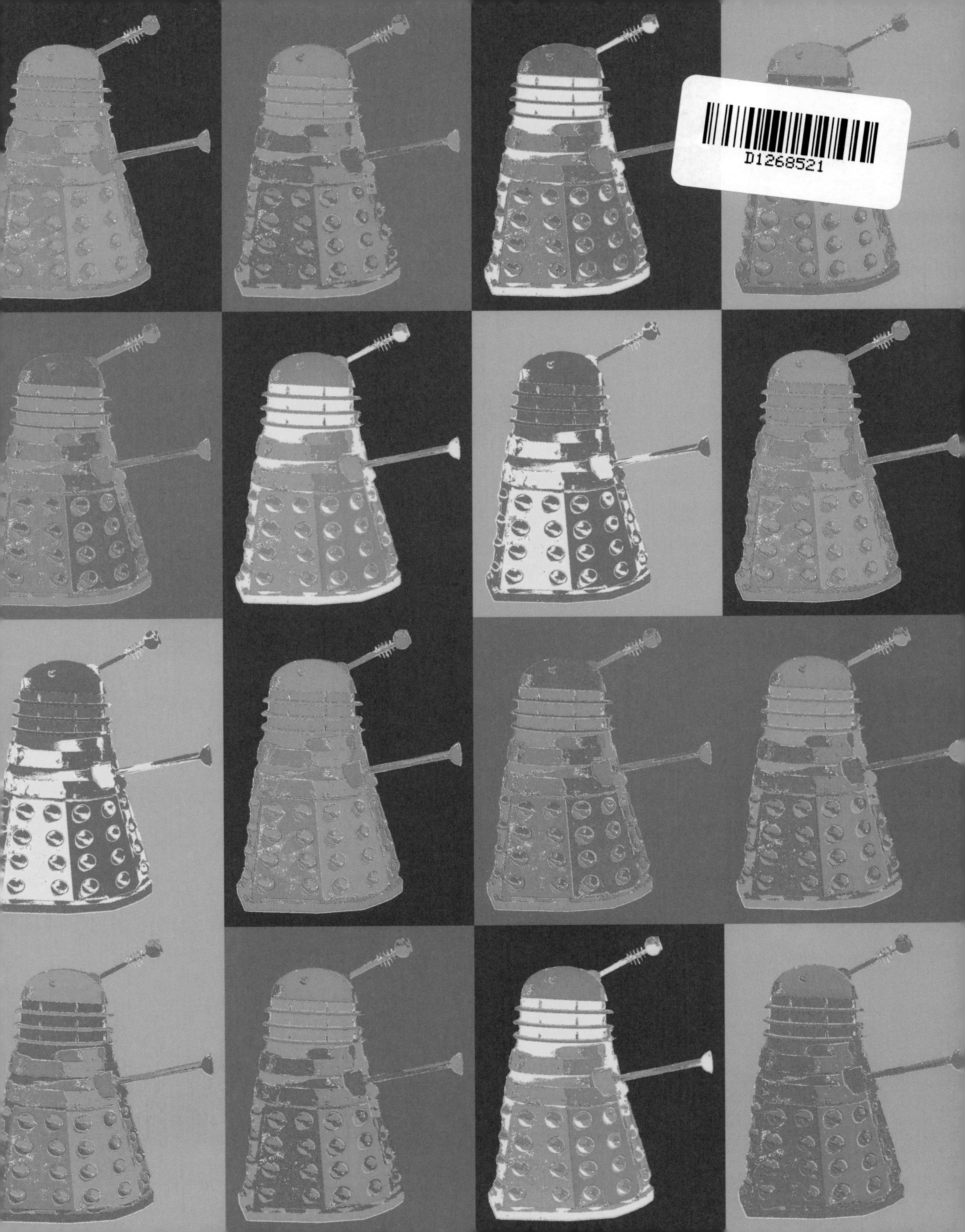

THE DOCTORS
30 YEARS OF TIME TRAVEL

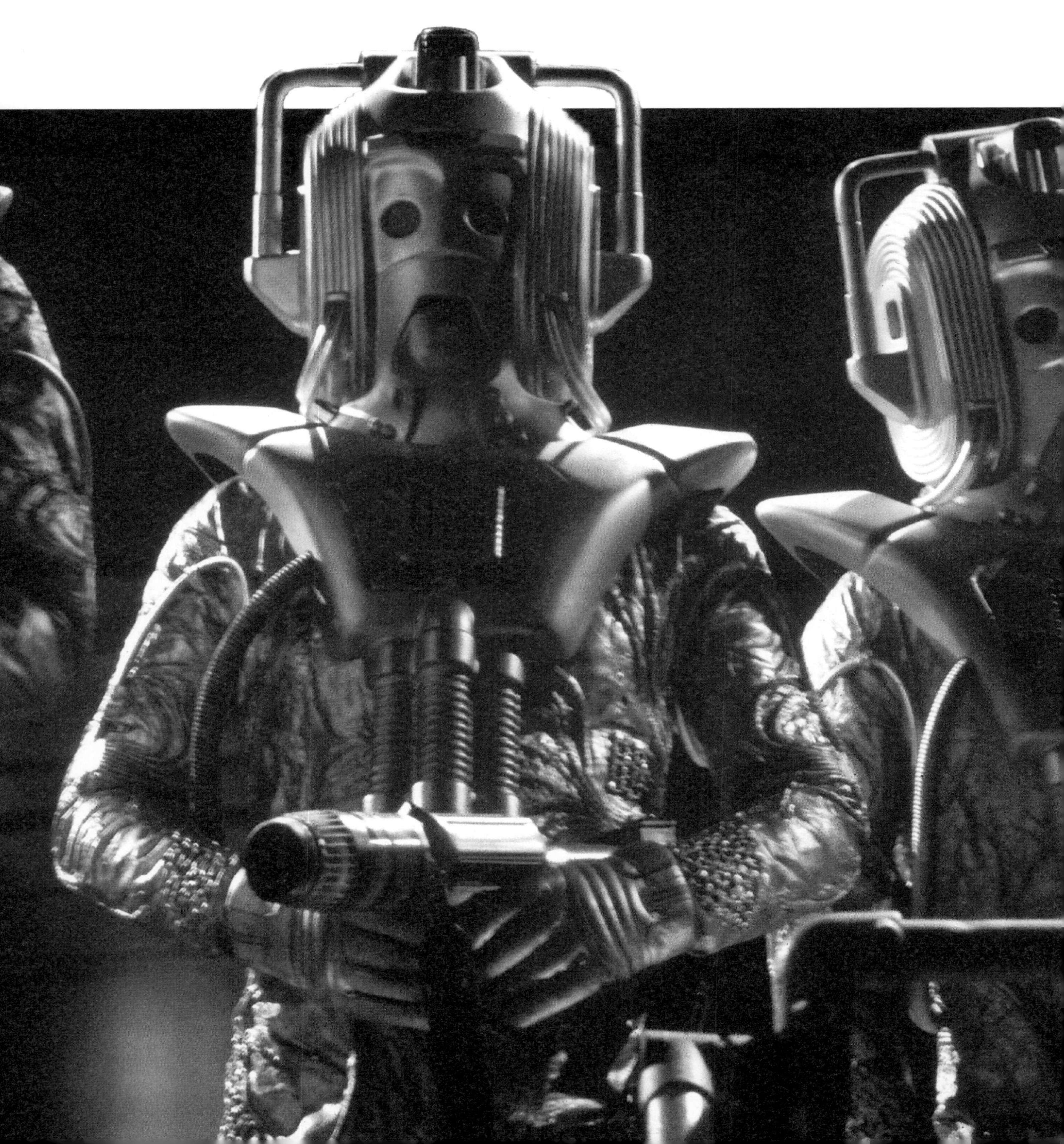

BOXTREE

THE DOCTORS

30 YEARS OF TIME TRAVEL

ADRIAN RIGELSFORD

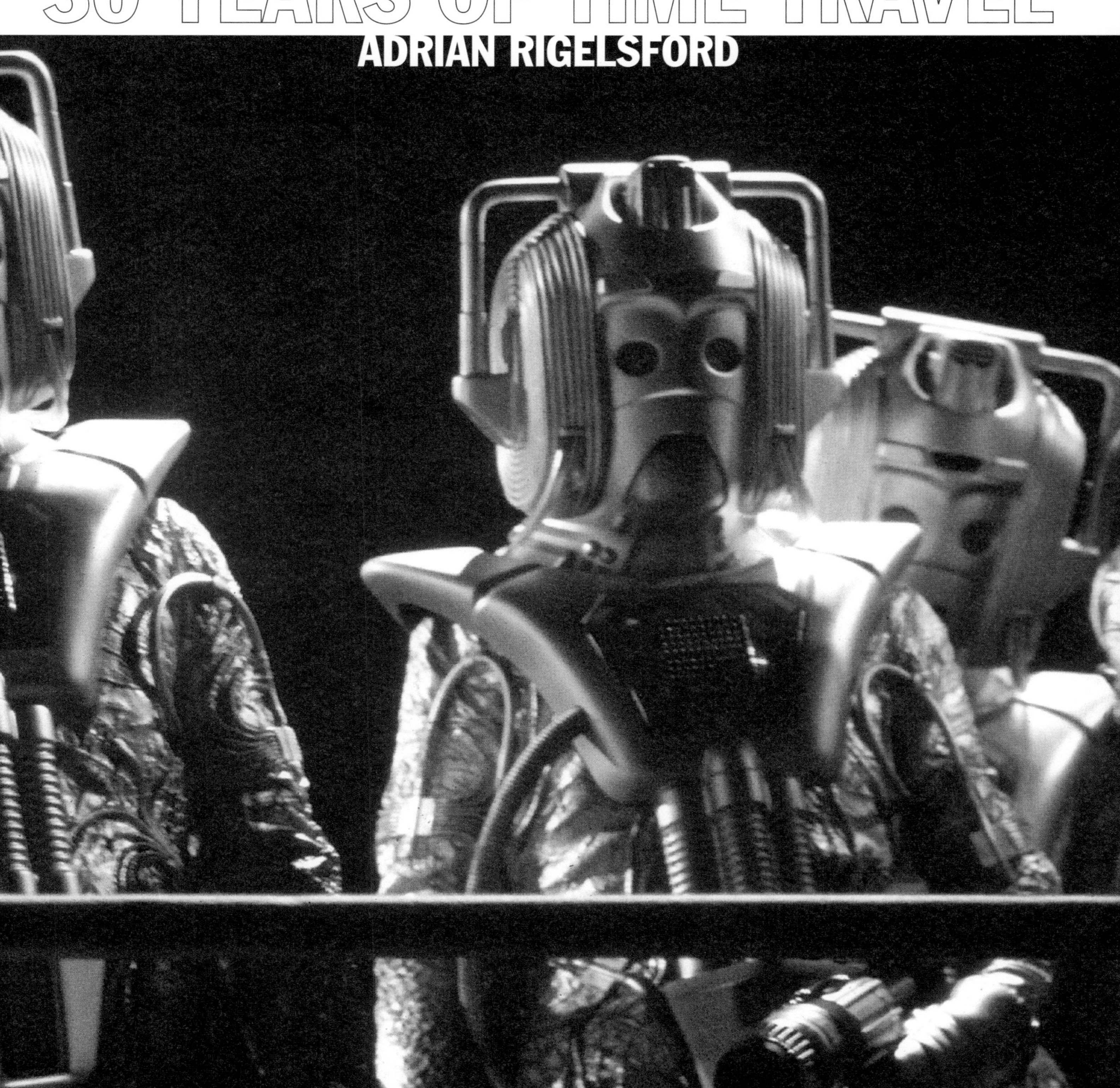

Author's Acknowledgments

There are countless people to thank for helping to bring this project together, and in no particular order, they are – Marcus Hearn, for leading the way in Doctor Who archivism and pointing me in the right direction. Gary Russell, for his sympathy and advice in all matters pictorial, Clive Banks, for his dedicated expertise in researching the past, Gary Leigh for further help in photographic matters and Dave Sheppard for unearthing some hidden gems.

Of the interviewees, I'm indebted to those who dredged their memory banks once again; Shaun Sutton, Barry Letts, Barry Newbery, Ray Cusick, Donald and Gilliam Baverstock, Rex Tucker, Graeme Harper and Michael E Briant.

From the past, thanks to several people who are all sadly missed; Patrick Troughton, Robert Holmes, Dennis Spooner, Innes Lloyd, Ian Marter, Ron Jones, Douglas Camfield. And thanks to Tony Jacobson for his material from William Hartnell, Roger Delgado, David Whitaker, Mervyn Pinfield, etc, etc... Any anyone else I might have forgotten....

Photographically, thanks to Ray Cusick, Barry Newbery, Colin Hargreaves, Clive Banks, Michael Briant, Tony Gaskell, Graeme Harper, David Maloney, Dave Sheppard, Peter Halliday, Chris Doyl John, Alexandra Tyson, John Bloomfield, Rod Chapman, Alan Keats, and the numerous others who were there with a camera at the right time. At 'Luke Book', on the first of many voyages, thanks to Gary Shoefield, Sharon Shoefield, Luke Shoefield and Paul Shoefield. Paul Laurence, Andy Granitt, Simon Carter and Sarah Brown. And thanks to all at Blackjacks with their trained panthers.

Finally, thanks to Richard Hollis, Rob Lewis, Ian MacClachlin, Jill Harris, Anthony Clark, Anthony Brown, Bobbie, Margaret, Ali and the gang in C' block, Alisdair Milne, Rod Morgan, Kevin Davies, Ness and Brian, Caroline Batten, Krystyna Zukowska, Jake Lingwood, Kathy Dawn and her guitar, Morris Barry, Chris Fitzgerald, Andrew Skilleter, Mr Waits, Neil Ingoe, Malcolm Chapman, Cliff Goodwin, Mum, Nicola and Midge. And perhaps the biggest thankyou of all to the Editor who survived it all, Rod Green.

First published in Great Britain in 1994 by Boxtree Limited,
Broadwall House, 21 Broadwall, London SE1 9PL

Designed by Blackjacks, London
Endpaper illustrations copyright © Blackjacks 1994
Colour Reproduction by Scanners
Printed and bound in Portugal by Printer Portuguesa Grafica LDA

A CIP catalogue entry for this book is available from the British Library.

12345678910

ISBN - 0 7522 0959 0

CONTENTS

CHAPTER 1

CURIOUS SOULS ASTRAY

CURIOUS SOULS ASTRAY

CURIOUS SOULS ASTRAY

"Doctor Who was never the kind of part I envisaged myself playing...never in a million years. Sergeants, villains and crooks – that kind of thing – they were my repertoire, but suddenly there I was, travelling through time, with the stars as my friends..."

WILLIAM HARTNELL unpublished interview – August 1967

"The traveller moves through time using his wondrous time machine, and arrives at a point in the far distant future..."

A publicity line that could so easily have been used to herald the arrival of *Doctor Who*, but not quite. This was some fourteen years before that particular event would take place, when one of the earliest post-war science fiction plays was broadcast. H.G. Wells' *The Time Machine* went out live from the BBC Television Studio high up on the hill at Alexandra Palace. The date was 25 January 1949 and little, other than a few faded memories, survives from it.

Television was only just coming back to life following the self-imposed shutdown during World War II and, as the 1950's began, so did talk of a second channel. Lord Reith and the BBC were far from amused by the prospect of such competition and dismissed it as being no more than a pipedream, but in 1954 it became a reality as Parliament passed the Independent Television Act and ITV was born.

Months of preparation and planning followed with work coming to a head on 22 September 1955, when after an hour of live coverage on ITV's formal opening ceremony, the screen suddenly went black. Seconds later, viewers were confronted with the image of a toothbrush frozen in a block of ice, as a dramatic announcement was made.

"It's Fresh, It's Tingling! It's Gibbs SR Toothpaste!"

Commercial television had arrived and the BBC knew they would have to fight to keep their viewers, so they decided to capitalise on their stock of reliable hits. *Dixon Of Dock Green* started earlier that year and was quickly brought back for a second series. The popularity of its star, Jack Warner, was such that it quickly became a national institution and ran for an incredible twenty-one years. Negotiations were underway to bring Tony Hancock's radio show, *Hancock's Half Hour*, to the small screen and hopefully bring its immense following with it, and the decision was made to revive the exploits of Professor Bernard Quatermass – A surefire way to guarantee huge viewing figures.

When the BBC started up television production again during the mid-1940s, a man called Michael Barry was made Head of Drama, overseeing all the plays and serials produced by the Drama Department. Amongst other things, he helped to develop the style of programme that's now more commonly known as the drama-documentary, mixing factual evidence with re-creations of the events surrounding it. At that time, they drew heavily on the wealth of material left over from World War II.

In 1953, Barry took a dangerous gamble by allocating his entire budget for scripts that year on one single six-part serial. This was understandable for an elaborate adaption of a Charles Dickens novel or one of the works of the Brontë sisters, but this was science fiction! That particular genre had not been presented to an adult audience with anything more than a single play at that time. Nigel Kneale's *The Quatermass Experiment* had to hold viewers for over a month, and everybody knew that it could so easily fail if they didn't take it seriously.

It proved to be more successful than Barry could ever have anticipated, and this was in no small part due to the high quality of Kneale's storytelling and the unique style of Rudolph Cartier's direction. Although it's now a standard plot device to have astronauts returning to earth having been infected by an alien spore, and thereafter mutate into multi-tendrilled creatures intent on causing mayhem, it was then something that the audience had never seen before – especially in the comfort of their own front room. The series enthralled the nation.

Kneale and Cartier joined forces again the following year with George Orwell's *1984*, starring a young, pre-Hammer Peter Cushing as Winston Smith. The adaption caused outcry over its torture scenes involving hungry sewer rats trying to attack Smith's head through a tube linking their cage to the glass helmet over his head. Demands were made for the second performance, due on the Thursday night following the first one the previous Sunday, to be stopped, but Barry held firm and even introduced it himself.

At the end of January 1955, the same team made *The Creature*, again with Cushing as Doctor Rollason leading the expedition to the Himalayas to find conclusive proof that the Yeti really does exist. Shortly after this, Kneale was approached by Barry with a view to writing a second story about Quatermass, with Cartier once again directing. *Quatermass II* was scheduled for screening in the winter, just as ITV was trying to establish a regular audience. As predicted, the sequel won the majority share of the ratings.

The importance of the Quatermass serials can never be underestimated; they laid the foundations, making it acceptable to watch stories from a genre that was normally relegated to cheap paperbacks or children's programmes. Without them, it's certainly debatable as to whether anything as fantasy orientated as *Doctor Who* would ever have seen the light of day, and certainly by the time the third serial, *Quatermass And The Pit,* was made towards the end of 1958, the Professor's name (picked at random from the London telephone directory when Kneale couldn't come up with a surname for his character) had become part of the English language, just like the word Dalek would a few years later.

Undoubted successes though these programmes were, they didn't help to remove the reputation the BBC had for its mundane, 'safe' style of programming. ITV programme makers had been heavily influenced by American television's attitude and approach towards light entertainment and drama productions, and the difference between the BBC and its rival was all too clear. Former *Doctor Who* producer, the late Innes Lloyd, recalled,"It was certainly a joke at the time to say that if you worked for the BBC, you had to smoke a pipe and own a particularly nice cardigan..."

Doctor Who director Morris Barry confirms that there was certainly a high level of bureaucracy in operation at the time; something that ITV seemed to be relatively free from.

"A vast majority of the producers and directors, much like myself, had come from a military background and had been involved in the War. The precise, ordered way of doing things that had been instilled in you in the army had been carried over. There was paperwork that had to be signed in triplicate twice, that sort of thing..."

Peter Cushing in **The Creature.**

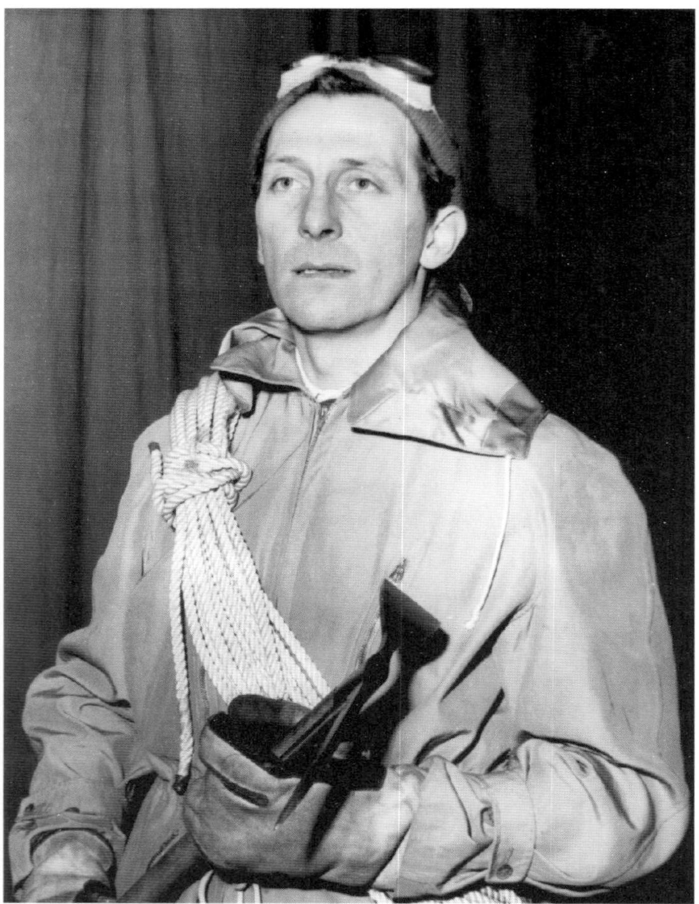

"There was a big, big difference between the approach the BBC had and what America was doing," Lloyd explained. "We seemed to be plodding along quite happily with *Dixon Of Dock Green,* while they had *Dragnet* and *Highway Patrol,* but don't get me wrong on this point. *Dixon* was right for that time, right for that era..."

By the beginning of 1956, the regional sectors into which the ITV network was divided, were beginning to come to life, with such now-familiar names as Granada in Manchester and Anglia Television in the east leading the way. With an insufficient number of programmes being made to fill the regions' different schedules, a number of variety and drama shows were made by independent TV contractors, such as Associated-Rediffusion, ITC and ABC Television.

ABC was a company formed as an offshoot from a large chain of theatres, which in turn provided a substantial amount of funding for their filming. The territory their output covered was the Midlands and the North of England during the weekends. A programme had to be of exceptional quality to warrant a network screening across all of the ITV channels. If not, it was just seen in the region covered by the channel that commissioned it.

Competition was stiff. ATV had already cornered the prime Saturday and Sunday night viewing slots with its popular mix of light entertainment shows and film serials, including *Sunday Night At The London Palladium* and *The Adventures Of Robin Hood.* ABC was determined to fight back...

In 1956, they launched their groundbreaking series of plays that went out under the title of *Armchair Theatre,* but it was not an instant success. The problem was that the only material available for them to adapt were set-texts, already established as long-running theatre productions. Though the finished product was generally of a high standard, there was nothing 'new' to grab the viewers' attention, or more importantly, to warrant a network screening. A producer was needed who would inject his own vision into the series and revitalise the concept of presenting theatre on the small screen. As it turned out, the man who would eventually take the job had a reputation for doing just that.

During 1957, tele-recordings of several plays made by the Canadian Broadcasting Company were shipped over and broadcast by the BBC, with titles such as *Flight Into Danger,* written by Arthur Hailey. This simple 60-minute play would become the template for all future air-disaster movies and inspired Hailey's own best-selling book and hit film, *Airport.*

One name linked all these plays, which were getting a more favourable reaction than most of the output from the two UK channels combined. Their producer, Sydney Newman, was quickly targeted by Michael Barry as someone to bring over to England under contract to the BBC.

"Sydney Newman certainly had a flair for the dramatic. He liked things to be crystal clear for the viewer, things were always done in broad swoops." The late Dennis Spooner, scriptwriter and one-time script editor on *Doctor Who,* also remembered seeing *Flight Into Danger.* "I don't think anyone else could have made it look as though there was a Boeing in a studio the size of a garage. Though, knowing Sydney as I later did, I wouldn't have put it past him to have the TV company build the studio around the Boeing!"

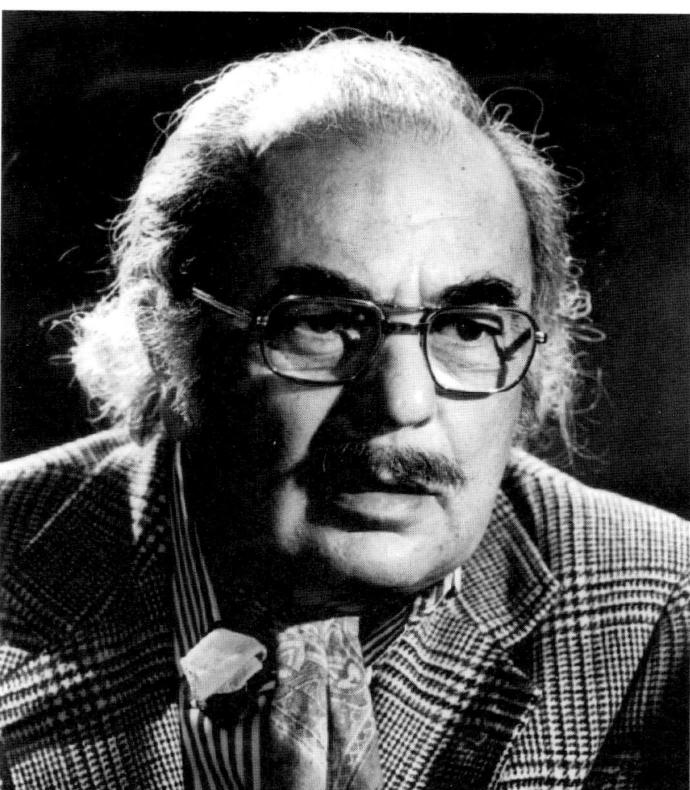

Sydney Newman in 1979.

Newman came to England, and while he was negotiating with Barry, ABC made what was possibly the shrewdest move in their history by offering Newman the chance to take over as *Armchair Theatre's* producer. He accepted the job, moved over from Canada with his family, and that's when a revolution in television began.

The first thing he did was change the policy about the content of the plays, insisting they become contemporary stories about contemporary issues, and used writers from Canada to achieve this effect until he'd found the kind of British talent he thought would be suitable for the task, including such names as Alun Owen and Harold Pinter.

Armchair Theatre changed beyond recognition, and within a short period of time, Newman had made television the most exciting theatre around. The key element behind its success was realism; there were no punches pulled, life was seen as it really was and the term 'Kitchen Sink Drama' evolved because of the series gritty storytelling. One critic even went so far as to rename it 'Armpit Theatre' because of this. Hugh David, who worked as a director on *Doctor Who* during Patrick Troughton's era, was working as an actor in the late 1950s, when all this took place.

"It was suddenly acceptable to have an accent that wasn't refined or Etonian. drama schools broke their backs mass-producing students and teaching them to drop their natural accents. Suddenly, casting calls were going out for TV plays asking for native Leeds accents, Sheffield, Manchester, places like that, and people just couldn't do it. That's when Albert Finney and Richard Burton really hit the big time, as that sort of thing was no problem for them. It was the era for angry young actors – Alan Bates, Robert Stephens, Peter O'Toole – they're all from that time, that generation..."

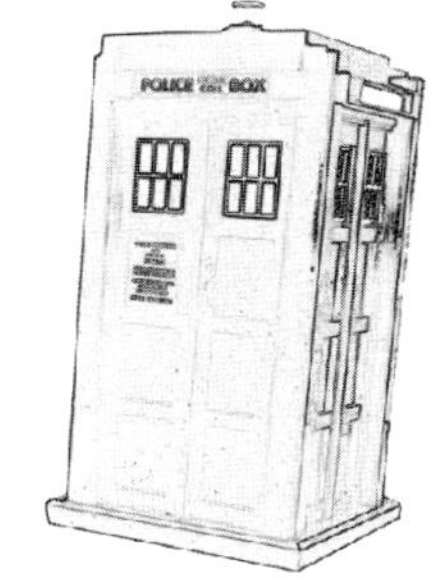

When compared with the size and scale of the BBC, it has to be said that ABC was actually a very small set up, but they compensated for that with sheer skill and enthusiasm. Newman injected his own particular style into everything they made, and if something wasn't working, it was quickly killed off. In some instances, this was only done so that certain elements could be revived a few weeks later, as with *Police Surgeon*.

The dramatised casebook of Doctor Geoffrey Brent, a pathologist working in the Bayswater area of London, seemed to work fine on paper but it quickly became clear after a few weeks of broadcast that the series was not popular. Newman could see that his lead actor, Ian Hendry, had a certain charismatic quality that was ideal for a crime-cum-thriller series, so he killed off *Police Surgeon* after only twelve episodes and held Hendry to his contract with ABC with the promise of a rethink.

A new character was created for Hendry with a similar penchant for solving crimes, but Doctor David Keel was far more idealistic, and when teamed with a sinister secret agent called John Steed (Played by Patrick MacNee, who had been a TV producer in Canada during the 1950's and knew Newman from that time), a legend was born in the shape of *The Avengers*. Hendry left after the first batch of twenty six episodes, making way for Honor Blackman as Mrs Cathy Gale for the second series, and after she arrived, the series went from strength to strength.

Children's programmes were also being made by the ITV companies, but the shadow of the BBC's reputation in that area always loomed over them; *The Silver Sword, Five Children And It, Huntingtower, The Secret Garden*: all of them classics, all expertly done, but the area where the BBC fell down in was science fiction for the younger viewers.

There were serials such as *Stranger From Space, The Lost Planet* and it's sequel, *Return To The Lost Planet* in the early 1950s, but the BBC had only done science fiction for adults up to that point, and then only twice with *R.U.R.* in 1938, a 25-minute play by Czech author Karel Capek, and the previously mentioned *The Time Machine*. By 1956 they were presenting *Space School* where Mum went along on the ensuing adventure with her kids. They were definitely off the mark with an audience that was into *Dan Dare*.

The *Eagle* comic had hit the stands at the beginning of the 1950s, and the lead picture strip of Dan Dare's battle against the evil alien warlord, the Mekon, and his army of towering green reptile soldiers, the Treens, entranced a whole generation. Back in Canada, Newman had experimented with making a science fiction adventure series, based around *20,000 Leagues Under The Sea*, using the cliff-hanger format, which he decided to try and adapt for a Sunday afternoon 'tea time' viewing slot. Malcolm Hulke was hired to write the serial, along with Eric Paice, who told the press at the time:"The idea is to try and bring a style of storytelling to life akin to the *Boys Own* adventure strips. You can't present today's child (by now 1960) with a man whose face is painted silver, and tell him it's a robot. They can see through that as clearly as you and I. Their minds need stimulating with a series of science facts that will then naturally lead to science fiction. And what better way to achieve this than by sending a child up in a rocket?"

And that's exactly what they did with *Target Luna*. Accidentally blasted into space inside his father's rocket ship from a base on a small island off Scotland, little Jimmy Wedgewood spends the rest of the serial being guided back to Earth by a team of scientists. The story was a success, and a follow-up quickly went before the cameras as the first part of a trilogy that Hulke and Paice penned between them.

The first story was *Pathfinders In Space*, where the Wedgewood children, led by the *Dan Dare*-esque figure of Conway Henderson, played by Gerald Flood, went to the moon and found evidence of an ancient alien race in the form of their children's toys. Arriving on the red planet for *Pathfinders To Mars*, they encountered deadly lichen based life-forms, and in *Pathfinders To Venus*, they finally found humanoid life in the shape of savage primitive ape-men.

When people started to query how it was possible for the Wedgewood's pet hamster, Hamlet, to survive such journeys, any child would quickly reply that Hamlet had his own space suit, which indeed he did. Flood told the press prior to the transmission of *Pathfinders To Venus:*"It's truly fantastic! A totally alien world has been created. It's strange, being able to walk through it and touch such strange architecture...(For *Venus*, Newman brought one of his colleagues over from CBC who had been involved with the *20,000 Leagues* project. Designer Tom Spaulding created a world that was entirely based around triangular shapes.)...This is going to be our greatest adventure yet. We even find that there are dinosaurs on Venus!"

It's clear that as work on the stories progressed, the confidence of the production team increased. The saga had gone from the basic rocket-bound setting of *Target Luna* to building jungles and caverns, stretching right across the studio at Teddington, for *Venus*. The sheer cost of trying to mount such 'miniature epics', as one critic dubbed them, was a severe problem, but the important lesson being learnt was that if the drama was kept claustrophobic and the number of sets to the minimum, small wonders could indeed be achieved.

A memo from the ABC vaults gives evidence to suggest that the cost of the sets on *Venus* made the programme go way over budget, and that Newman cancelled a proposed fourth *Pathfinders* serial due to this fact. Instead, he used the same trick he'd done on *Police Surgeon*, and kept Flood and Steward Guidotti under contract from the cast, and gave them new characters for a new trilogy of adventures.

As Mark Bannerman and Peter Blake, they moved across the *Plateau Of Fear*, and down to the *City Under The Sea*, with a direct sequel to that story coming next, *Secret Beneath The Sea*. Their *Pathfinders* Director, Guy Verney, was now acting as the producer for this trilogy because by the time that the final story was broadcast in the Spring of 1963, Sydney Newman was long since gone...

Towards the end of 1961, Kenneth Adams, the Managing Director of the BBC, was trying to find a suitable replacement for Michael Barry, who had decided to move on from his post as Head of Drama. Newman had refused an initial offer to go to the BBC as a producer, clearly wanting to move forward in the industry rather than hold back, so when Adams came back giving him the chance to take over from Barry, Newman was all too happy to accept. He arrived at Threshold and Union House, the BBC's Shepherd's Bush offices, on 15 December 1962, and as Dennis Spooner recalls:"I wasn't at the BBC at the time, but I heard from friends who were, and from what I understand, there was a certain degree of resentment towards Sydney's appointment. One or two of the in-house producers were grumbling about how it should

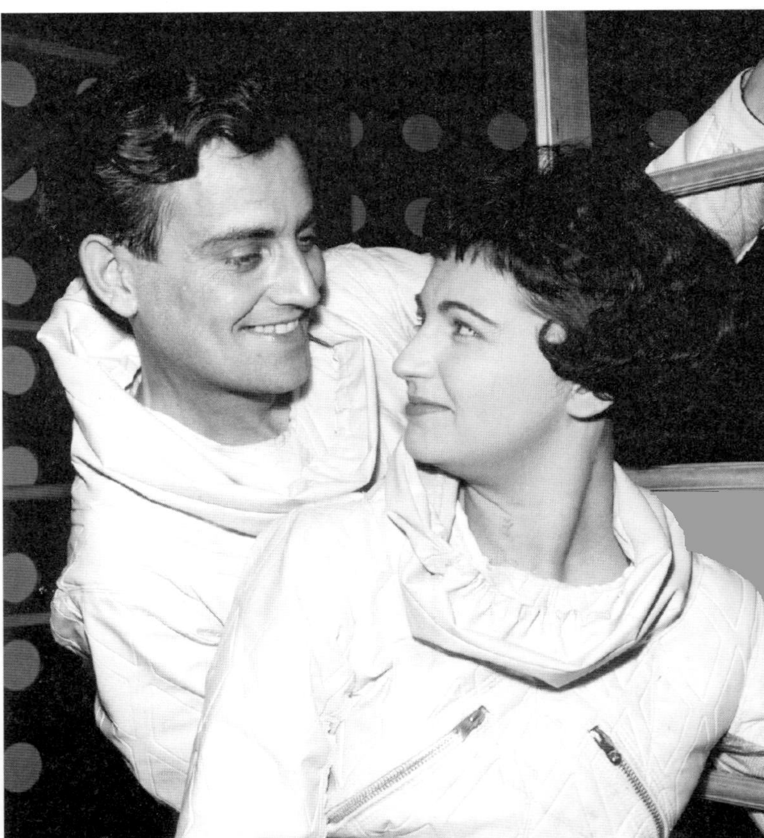

ABOVE: Gerald Flood and Pamela Barney in **Pathfinders to Mars**.
LEFT: **Target Luna** (L-R) Michael Craze, Sylvia Davies, Michael Hammond. Craze later played Doctor Who companion Ben Jackson (1966-67).

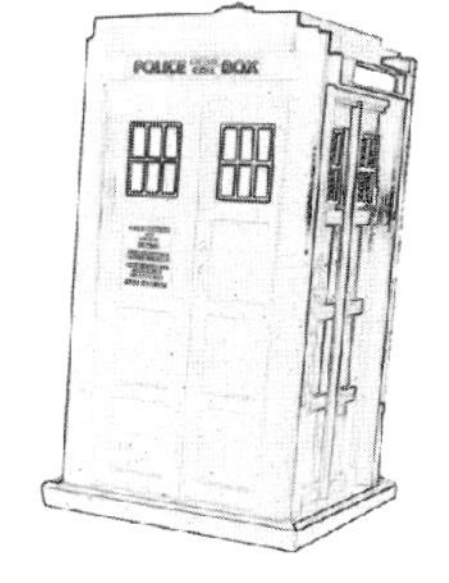

have been their job. He was just like Ceasar walking into the senate, and I'm sure that he must have been aware of how some of them felt...it's just that they all underestimated how bulletproof he was. This Ceasar had a daggerproof toga!"

The plan he instigated made it easier to run the department as a whole. Under Barry, everyone had been answerable to him in the drama area, no matter what kind of programme they were making. Newman divided everyone up into three sub-departments: Drama Series, Drama Serials and Plays. Each sub had its own departmental head, who in turn answered to and worked directly with Newman. To achieve this, several other smaller departments had to be closed down or merged with others. It is no understatement to say that chaos ensued while this was taking place.

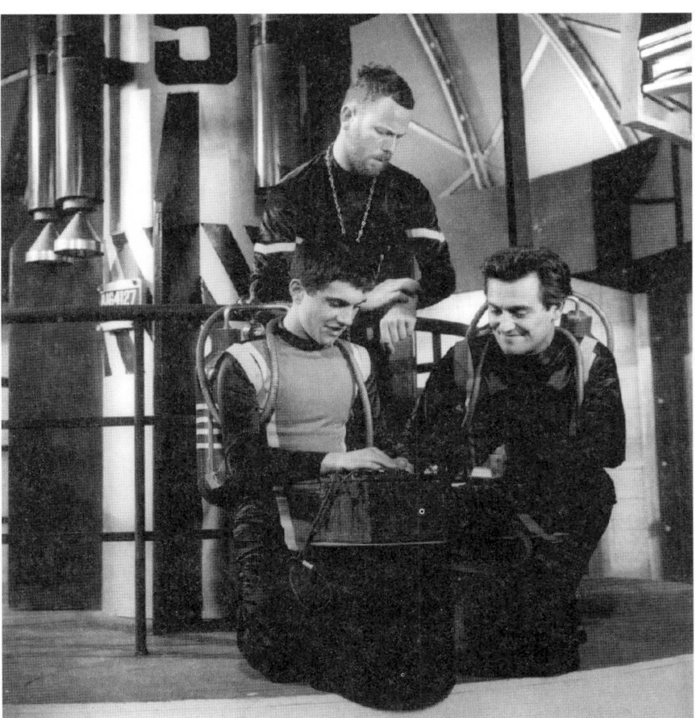

Towards the end of February 1963, while Newman was orchestrating the division of the Plays Department in order to have three separate series running (by the end of 1964, they were the relatively inexpensive *The Wednesday Plays*, the more costly *Play For Todays*, and the expensive epics, *Play Of The Month*), Donald Baverstock, who was the Controller of Programmes for the BBC, decided that something special was needed to fill a gap in the Saturday schedules. The area that was in need of bridging was the half-hour period that linked the afternoon and evening viewing.

Baverstock had a reputation for being the 'Whizzkid' of the BBC, having broken new ground in his early thirties by creating the popular current affairs magazine programme, *Tonight.* He worked on it as a producer with Alisdair Milne, and it had a healthy run from 1957 to 1965.

"It was clear that science fiction had become acceptable to mass-audiences," Baverstock recalls. "Nothing too outlandish; adventure serials were more palatable, as Fred Hoyle's shows had proved."

A Professor of Astronomy and Philosophy at Cambridge, Hoyle had a theory that the first true contact that man could ever have with an alien intelligence would be through radioastronomy, and

LEFT: Gerald Flood, far right, in **City Beneath the Sea.**
BELOW: Donald Baverstock, second from left.

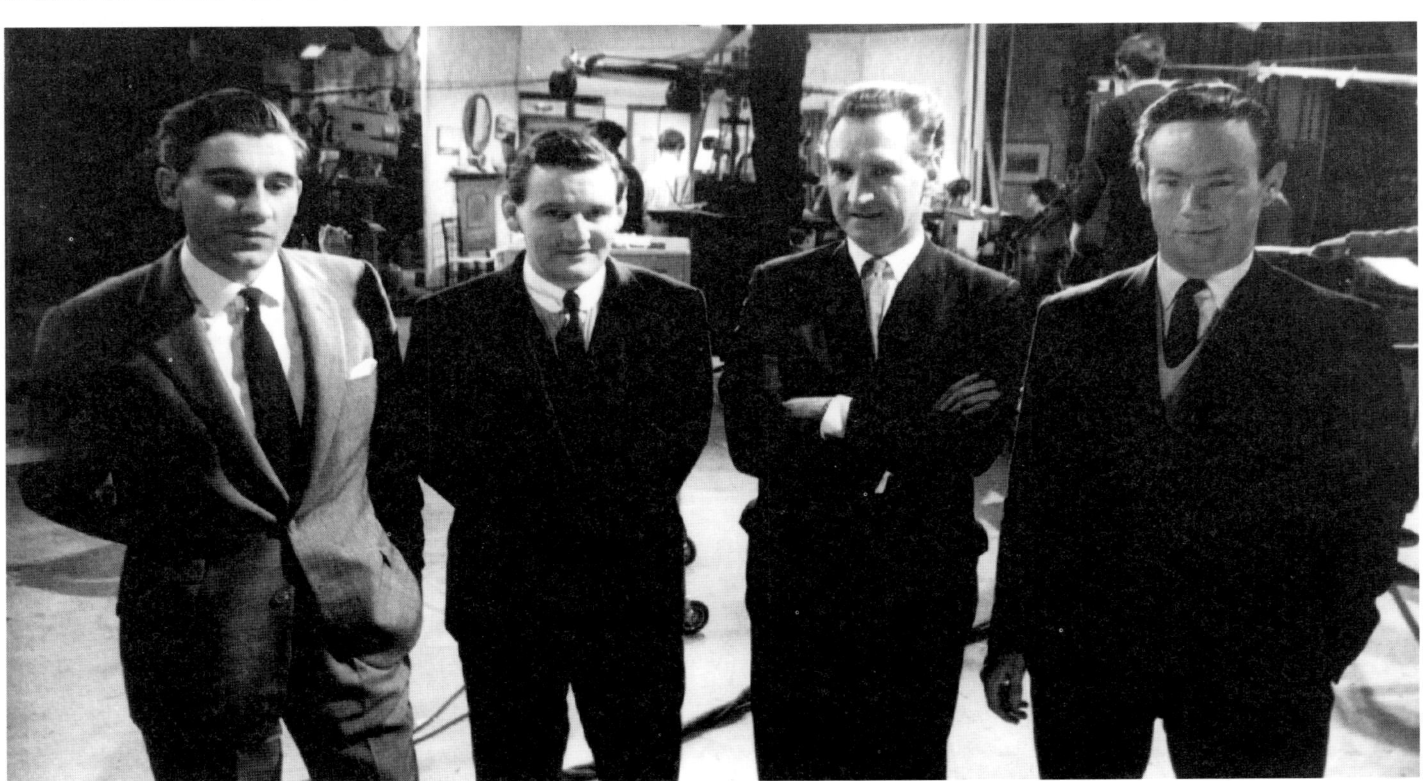

that formed the basic idea behind *A For Andromeda*. Co-written with John Elliott, the story revolved around a brilliant young scientist called Doctor John Flemming, who constructed a computer based on instructions received as signals from outer space, deep within the constellation of Andromeda. Scientists worked with the computer, experimenting in genetics, and created a human being, a beautiful girl with incredibly fast learning abilities whom they named Andromeda. The girl was played by Julie Christie, who would quickly find international fame in such films as *Darling* and *Far From The Madding Crowd.*

The series was a huge hit and the demand for a sequel, revealing what happened to Fleming and Andromeda in the aftermath of the computer's destruction at the first story's climax, was intense. Within a year, *The Andromeda Breakthrough* was broadcast, to even greater acclaim.

During that year (1962), a careful study was carried out into modern science fiction literature, under the supervision of the Head of the BBC's Script Department, Donald Wilson, who would later go on to produce the most addictive viewing of the late 60s with the sprawling epic, *The Forsythe Saga*. With a team of writers, he researched the inherent elements that made the more successful books in the genre work, and in turn ascertain whether they would translate to television.

Wilson was undoubtedly toying with the idea of starting a new project, with a time machine as a central plot device. Whether it was as a result of Wilson's findings or not, Baverstock recalls that an adaption of the *Foundation* trilogy by Isaac Asimov was certainly suggested, but ruled out due to the extreme costs that would be involved.

Although nothing came to fruition immediately, the research would prove invaluable later on. Science fiction was the 'in thing', there was a buzz about it in the air and the BBC did not want to miss out on it. *The Twilight Zone*, with Rod Serling hosting many self-written tales of the strange and even stranger, had just arrived from America on ITV, and following their alien invasion undercover thriller called *The Big Pull* at the beginning of the year, the BBC put out *The Monsters* during the Autumn, a four-part serial dealing with the mystery of the Loch Ness Monster.

Actor Hugh David recalls being sounded out about a science fiction project for children at the start of 1963.

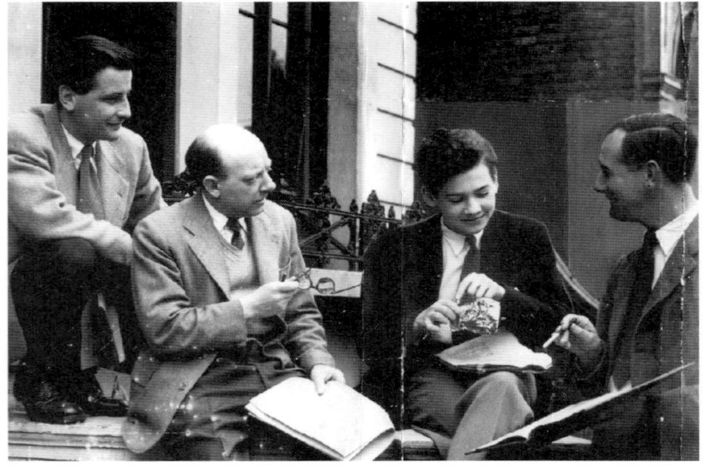

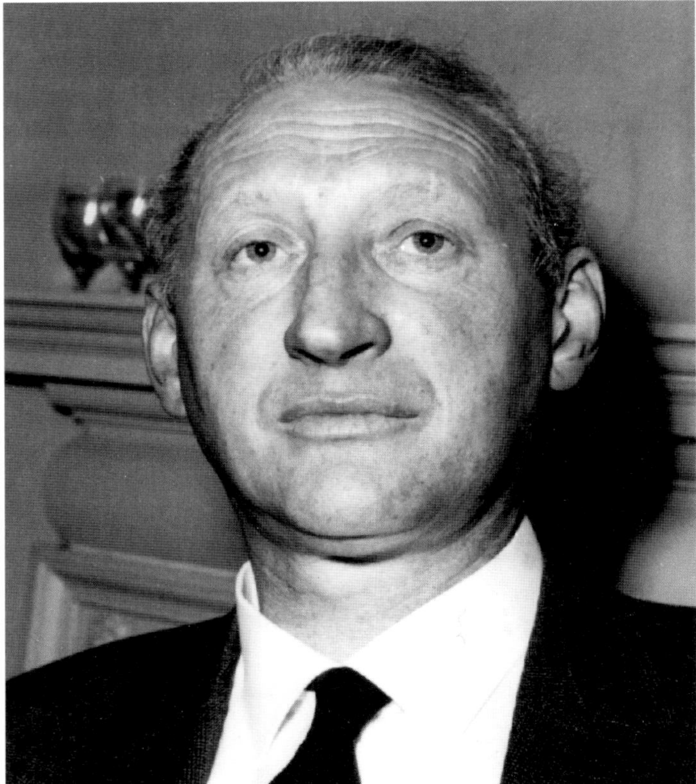

Donald Wilson in November 1963.

"I was asked to play the lead in an adaption of *War of The Worlds*, for something like *Children's Hour*...It was obvious they couldn't do the full whack, with the war machines marching across Surrey and Big Ben getting blown to bits, so they had to get round that, and I think it must have been Rex Tucker who cracked it."

Tucker was both a producer and director of children's programmes during the 1950s, a job that existed as one in those days. Newman's regime had split the job into two, so that the producer looked after the finances and the director looked after the creativity. Tucker's reputation for making quality programmes was renowned, and *War Of The Worlds* would most likely have been planned as a Sunday afternoon 'tea time' serial, aimed at the same kind of audiences that the *Pathfinders* serials were attracting, but very little is known about it as it never saw the light of day, as David explains:

"There were only going to be a few survivors, just a handful of people trapped in an underground station, and they were reminiscing about what had happened. You never saw the Martian machines, you heard them moving across the surface as they went past, but that's all. There might have been a metal tentacle that came in and probed around the rubble a bit, but I'm not sure. I remember it clearly because Rex was a good friend, and shortly after it was pulled, he tried to get me in on *Doctor Who*..."

Tucker was in a position to do this because by the end of March 1963, Baverstock's request for a filler was quickly becoming a reality. He had made it clear to Newman that he wanted something ready for broadcast in September, and as Head of

Rex Tucker (right) directing **The Old Grad** in July 1954.

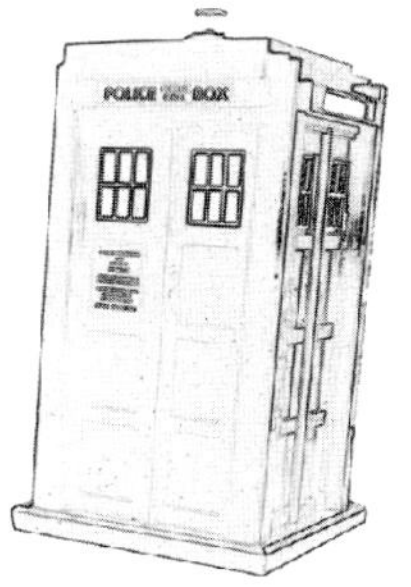

Drama it was his job to get the production up and running. Rex Tucker had been brought in to act as the project's producer.

Baverstock's recollection of why *Doctor Who* was brought to life makes the whole process sound alarmingly simple.

"A typical Saturday afternoon's viewing was non-stop sport for a few hours with *Grandstand*, then there was David Jacobs' pop show (*Juke Box Jury*), but there was never anything in between that made any impact. It would have been too easy to put on a Laurel and Hardy film, or a handful of old cartoons, but that was avoiding the issue... some form of drama, an ongoing series to hold audiences from week to week, was needed.

"There may well have been talk of reviving the old *Flash Gordon* serials again (which, even by the primitive standards of the 1960s, were beginning to look dated, having been made during the 1930s.) but it simply became a case of 'Why not make our own?', and that's how *Doctor Who* came about. The way it worked was that I'd given Sydney a brief on what was wanted, and he would have gone to the script people to see if there was anything they had that could be developed."

Anything that could be termed as an idea or concept was handed to the Script Department to be nurtured, and it was Donald Wilson who took on the main responsibility for handling what would eventually evolve into *Doctor Who*. The notes from his research into science fiction literature were dusted down, and several brainstorming sessions with his staff writers took place, the main one to be drafted in being C.E. Webber. Morris Barry worked with Webber on the long-running soap opera, *Compact*, during the mid-1960s.

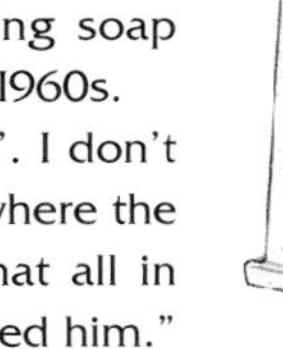

"Everyone called him 'Bunny'. I don't have the foggiest as to why, or where the name came from, but that's what all in Threshold and Union (House) called him."

While Tucker looked into basic production areas, Wilson started to develop the format and Webber spent time drafting up the main characters. The plan was for the series to run for fifty-two weeks, with an underlying plot that would last throughout its run.

It was also decided that there would be a cliffhanger ending to each episode, with the last moments being replayed before the beginning of the next installment, much in the same way that the *Pathfinders* serials had done.

Webber plotted out four main characters, with a male lead (a schoolteacher), a female lead (another schoolteacher, and possible romantic interest for the male lead), a young girl (a teenage pupil of theirs) and a mysterious, ancient old man (a traveller from another world). The 'machine' that he owned was a miraculous contraption able to blend in with its surroundings. At one point it was suggested that this phenomenon be explained by having the time traveller claim that he painted his machine with a substance that would reflect the immediate area, thereby rendering it invisible. The machine could also travel through time and space and

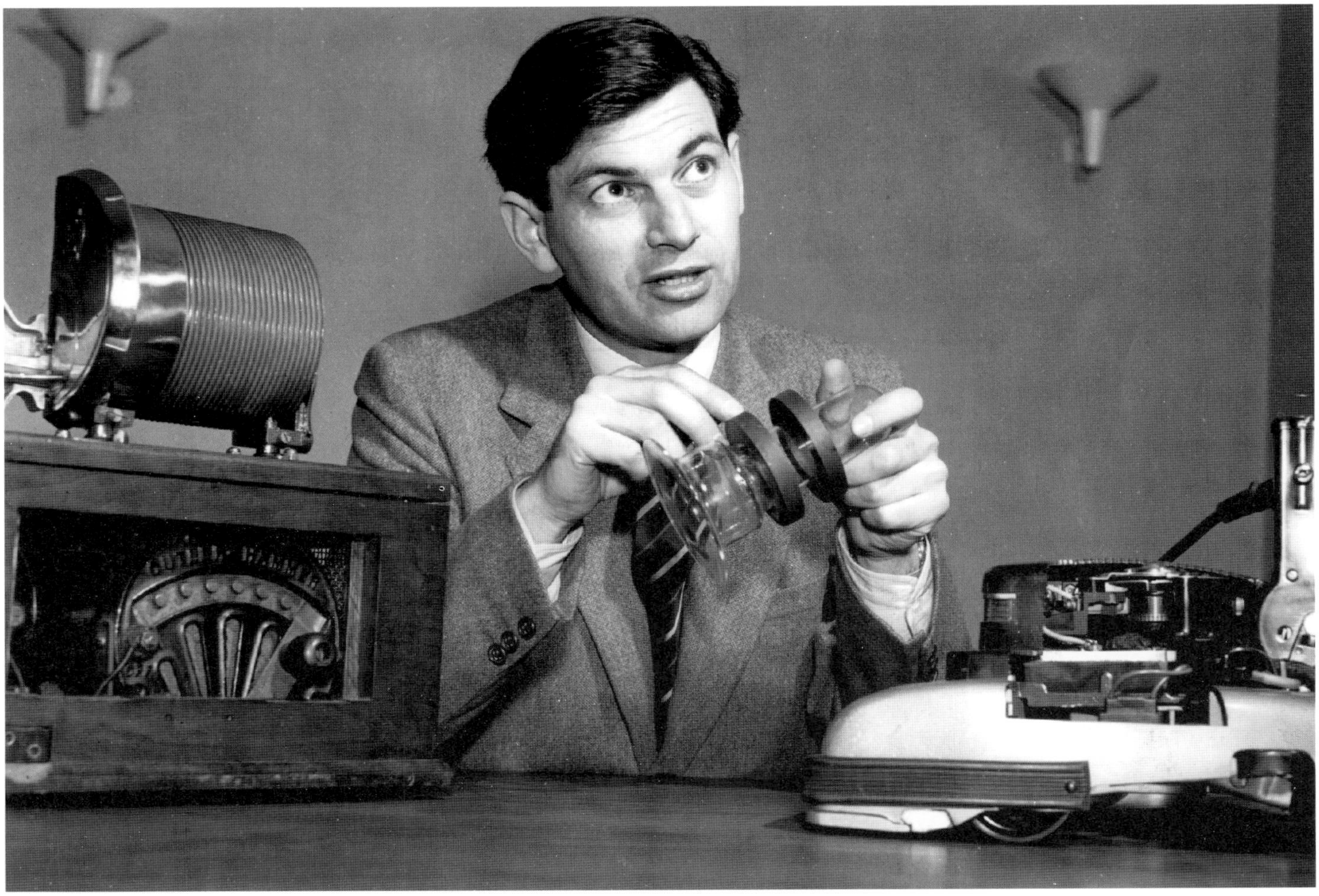

Hugh David as Mr. Marvel in **Meet Mr Marvel** *– August 1956.*

had come to rest on modern-day earth, according to Wilson's plan.

The catch was that the old man had no idea how to pilot the machine properly, as it had a vast control room of amazing and confusing equipment, and this created the running thread of him trying to get the other characters back to their own era after the machine takes off in the first episode.

Newman was adamant that no matter how elaborate the adventure the characters encountered, there always had to be a factual reality behind the resulting story. If, for example, they travelled through time and arrived back at the battle of Waterloo, the characters they encountered would have to be historically accurate, from the way they spoke (with emphasis on avoiding modern slang) down to the clothes that they wore, with costumes being made of material that wasn't obviously from the modern era, and if they travelled to the moon or Mars, the environment they encountered would have to be based on the data that was currently available, with no elements of fantasy added. In other words, he wanted it to be more of a case of fact than fiction.

Mr. Marvel in one of his historical disguises.

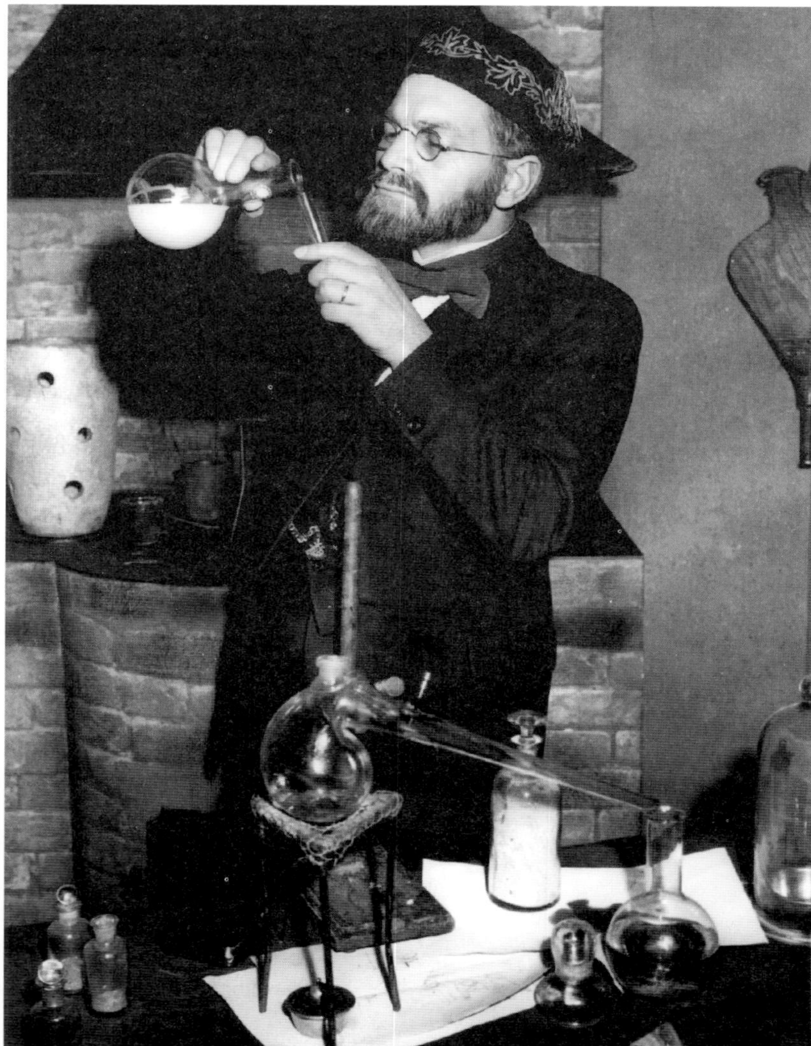

Although the exact origins of the title for the show will probably never be known for sure, Baverstock offers a possible answer.

"I remember there was a dinner at Easter, where Rex and his writers were scribbling down all sorts of names on a napkin. One of the names was *Doctor Who.* It was circled in pencil. I'm sure that napkin would be worth a fortune now!"

By the middle of May, all the plot ideas and character concepts that were flying around had been distilled into a brief guide to *Doctor Who*, which was no more than a few pages long. All the vital elements were present. The machine was now a time machine that could travel across the dimensions of space and time. The four main characters travelled in it (it was not until the scripts for the first story were written that their writer, Anthony Coburn, created its more familiar name, Tardis), and the proposed plot for the first story had been drafted.

Called *The Giants*, it was centred around one of the 'Travellers-Against-Science-Fact' scenarios that Newman favoured, with the time machine, now established as having the exterior of a modern Police Box with the internal control room larger than the outside shell could physically allow, shrinking to a minute size and landing in a teacher's school laboratory. A matter of a few steps across the room is a frightening and lengthy journey for the travellers at the size they're reduced to, compared to a normal human. Webber's story was exactly the kind of adventure the show needed. It was at this point that Tucker got in contact with Hugh David.

"Rex asked me to play this old man who could travel through time. Sort of 'The Nutty Professor', but with a darker side to him. I really didn't want to know, to be honest, having just done my time on *Knight Errant* (a series about an adventurer for hire, in which David played one of the leads for a couple of series), and pretty much decided to quit the acting game and move into production by taking the BBC director's course.

"The only reason I can think of for him having asked me was because of my days as Mr Marvel. Rex used to write for that and do the odd bit here and there, and I suppose there are similarities with *Doctor Who* in a way."

Meet Mr Marvel was made by Associated-Rediffusion in 1956, when David was 28 years old, a Bachelor of Science and a medal winning Drama student. The premise was simple enough: modern technology was creeping in on suburbia at a rate of knots – Vacuum cleaners, washing machines and television sets were beginning to be found in every home. As a result, there was a certain amount of what could be called 'Techno-Fear'. Housewives were unsure of these things, and it was Mr Marvel's job to reassure them.

The series was presented by a fictional scientist who was based in what the script called 'his fantastic laboratory.' The translation of this was a wooden bench facing the camera, with a few diagrams and a blackboard on the wall behind him. To the left was a door, and that played the most important role of all in the programme. While explaining how a telephone worked, Mr Marvel would look up and suddenly tell viewers that his lab had travelled back through time to the moment it was invented, and by going through the door he would step into Alexander Graham Bell's workroom and become part of the ensuing action. Although there was no sign of the laboratory, the door would be on the wall as though it had always been there.

Halfway through its run, Mr Marvel was joined by Sylvia Young as a 'curious housewife', who travelled with Mr Marvel as he explained all. So, he effectively had a time machine that blended into its surroundings unnoticed, and he also had a companion with him. Each episode ended with a mystery that would have to be solved the following week. Sounds familiar? It was not uncommon for educational series of that period to have the presenter become part of a historical re-enactment, it was just that *Meet Mr Marvel* seems to have been more inventive that most.

After David turned *Doctor Who* down, Tucker asked John Slater to consider the role, as he was a popular character in *Z-Cars* and was familiar to younger viewers for having done time as a straight man to *Pinky And Perky.*

The hard task of getting the plot points that had been decided down on paper, in order to form the script for a pilot episode, was handled by C.E. Webber. Morris Barry recalls Webber's script work as always having a strange lyrical quality to the dialogue, showing that he was a sensitive writer of considerable skill, and it's perhaps because of this that his initial draft was not favoured by anyone. Innes Lloyd remembered Webber as being, "A hugely articulate man, incredibly well read with a passion for great literature. You always felt like some form of murderer when you cut into his lines, it was so obvious he'd gone to great lengths to get them just right ... but he was always so affable about it."

The basic draft was handed over to Anthony Coburn, who was one of Donald Wilson's staff writers. Webber had come up with a plot, which was set in part during the stone age, with the miniaturisation plot having been put to one side. Coburn worked from this structure when he began planning the first four part adventure's scripts.

It would be wrong to imply that Webber's contribution to the programme had been made redundant – nothing could be further from the truth. Without his contribution, the first episode would not have made the impact that it did. Coburn merely redrafted the script to bring it down to a more commercial level of storytelling.

Wilson needed someone to take over the everyday editing work on the scripts as they were coming in, and brought in another of his staff writers, David Whitaker, who had won a position in the department in the first place through his work in rep theatres as both a writer and director. Having survived the rigours of last minute rewrites on plays that were changing every week in the theatre, he had gained an acute sense of structuring that made him the ideal choice for a series that had such a variable format. Baverstock was at this point given a breakdown on the kind of series he would be presenting for broadcast.

"The initial plot I was told was underway sounded too good to be true. One moment there would be some sort of adventure in the past, the next it was in the future, then there would be some wild flight of fantasy into one that was pure science. I was certainly happy with the way things were going.

"One of the things I insisted on was the ages of the people on board the space ship. I knew that *Doctor Who* was meant to be as old as the hills, but there had to be a normal couple and a young girl... The varying ages made it easier for viewers to relate to them. Nobody was alienated by feeling that they wouldn't share the same reactions to the fantastic sights they were seeing."

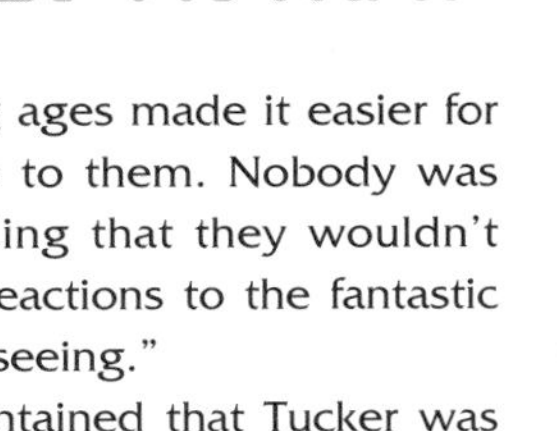

It's been maintained that Tucker was always seen as the temporary producer, just in office to get the programme underway.This can hardly be true in light of the fact that he was actively seeking out cast members and approaching other key personnel, including Tristram Cary to handle the musical scoring – not the kind of moves a temporary producer would have been making. Secondly, his artistic involvement was extreme, working on the background to the characters with Wilson and Webber. This is again, hardly the kind of effort a temporary producer would make. What is clear is that, after all this initial hard work, Tucker went on holiday, and when he returned he was offered the job of directing one of the early stories, with another producer in office.

Newman had brought in Verity Lambert, who had worked with him at ABC as a Production Assistant, and had gained a lot of experience from a brief period of time when she worked for American television. She had gained a sense of commercialism there that the BBC teams seemed to lack, and she was not afraid to argue over points with Newman, who was full of admiration that somebody actually had the guts to do this. Lambert was 28, and when she moved to *Doctor Who*, she became one of the youngest producers the BBC had ever employed.

Wilson was extremely worried about the scale of the demands that the job would put on her. It was not as though *Doctor Who* would be a typical run-of-the-mill production, so he persuaded Newman to make one of the more experienced staff producers the executive producer. Mervyn Pinfield, who was close to retirement at that time, came to the series with an invaluable knowledge of the technicalities of filming and of the kind of administration that was involved. Spooner remembers him well.

"Mervyn was not a young man, but he was like some form of walking encyclopedia. When I took over as script editor (during the second season from 1964 to 1965), I didn't know the ropes of the BBC that well, so everybody kept saying if I wasn't sure I was to ask Mervyn because he'd know. Invariably, he did.

"Hartnell had a hell of a lot of respect for him. I think he was actually one of the few people on the team who was older than him, and Bill (Hartnell) liked that. He was someone he could talk to without the 'I've-been-in-the-business-so-long' attitude, which he certainly tended to use with the younger directors. Mervyn just got on with his job and smoked his pipe."

The first of the directors due to work on the show had also been selected, by Donald Wilson, and the 25-year-old Anglo-Indian Waris Hussein was waiting in the wings. He had several plays to his credit, with the main bulk of his c.v. at that point consisting of directing episodes of the soap, *Compact.* He arrived at the same time as Lambert, when the characters had finally settled with the names that would become so familiar.

The male teacher, previously called Cliff, was now 27-year-old Ian Chesterton. His fellow tutor, Miss McGovern, was now Barbara Wright, while the most radical changes had taken place with the teenage girl. Originally Sue, she was now Susan Foreman, the old man's granddaughter. This was done because there was a certain degree of concern over having a decrepit old man travelling round with such a young woman, but these implications were ironed out by having them related. The Doctor's character had remained enigmatic and mysterious throughout the stages of script development, and the problem ahead was how to cast him.

The immediate solution was to go for a classical actor, with Leslie French and Cyril Cusack both being names that were seriously considered, but it was Lambert who hit upon the idea of asking William Hartnell. Hartnell was a stalwart character actor, who had been in films since the 1930s and was a familiar face on television, having spent the past few years playing the permanently angry army sergeant in *The Army Game*, a sitcom revolving around the most incompetent platoon in the service. He'd most impressed her, however, in *This Sporting Life*, a movie that was shot at the beginning of 1962, with Hartnell playing a grumpy rugby talent scout. That performance showed the qualities that Lambert was looking for and, after some initial reluctance, Hussein and Lambert persuaded Hartnell that playing the Doctor would free him from the type-casting of playing crooks and military figures. In 1967, Hartnell recalled: "I didn't know how to do it. He was a barmy old man, and I'd spent years shouting at soldiers. It was a complete contrast, but I quickly realised that children would love it. Just as I thought I'd done everything, I was going to be a hero, someone that every child would know was their friend."

William Russell, who had proved he could carry a series as the lead with *The Adventures Of Sir Lancelot* in the 1950s, was cast as Chesterton, as it was clear from the actor's work that he had already experienced the rigours of the kind of work schedule he'd face on *Doctor Who*. Jacqueline Hill was offered the role of Barbara Wright. She was someone Lambert knew she could trust and had first met through Hill's husband, Alvin Rakoff, who had directed several *Armchair Theatre* plays when Lambert was at ABC.

The role of Susan Foreman was offered to Carole Ann Ford, whom Hussein had seen working in television centre, the BBC's relatively new main base of productions, and was known for her work on drama productions such as *Man On A Bicycle*. Baverstock recalls the first reaction to his choice: "Everybody wanted Julie Christie. She was the first name that sprang to mind, having done the first *Andromeda* series, but I think she was in Yorkshire doing *Billy Liar* (directed by John Schlesinger in 1962), or something like that. She was a star by the time *Doctor Who* was shown."

By the middle of July, other scripts were being formally commissioned. John Lucarotti was working on *Doctor Who And A*

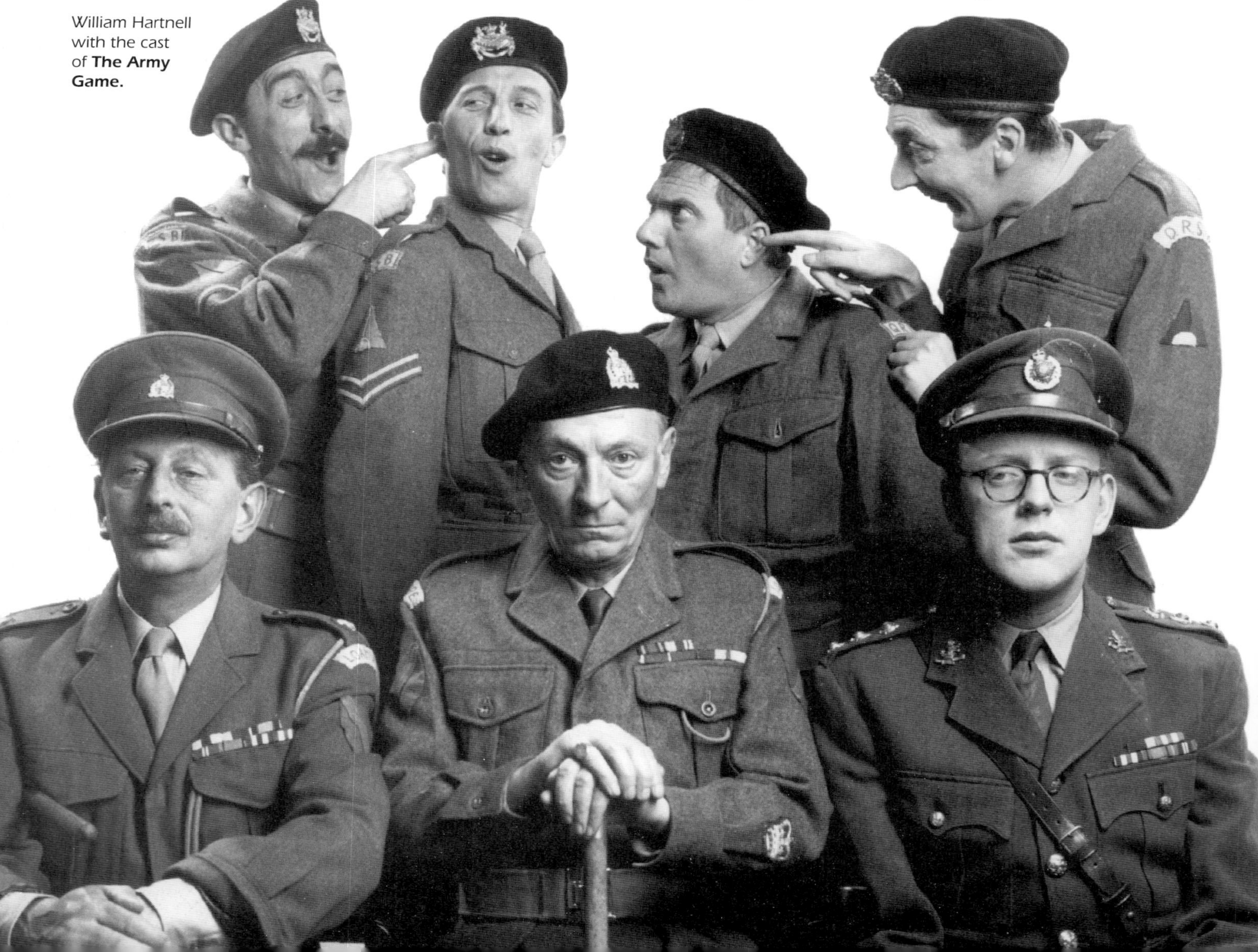

William Hartnell with the cast of **The Army Game.**

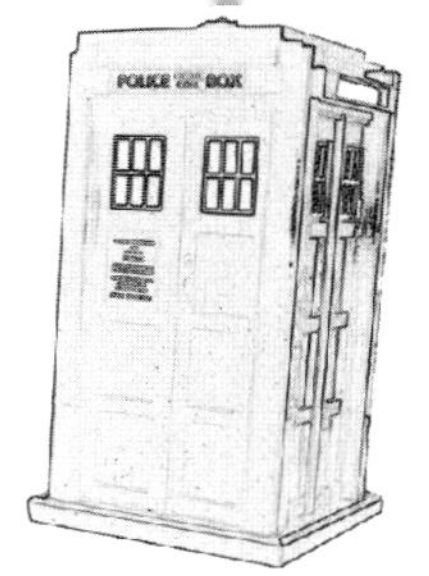

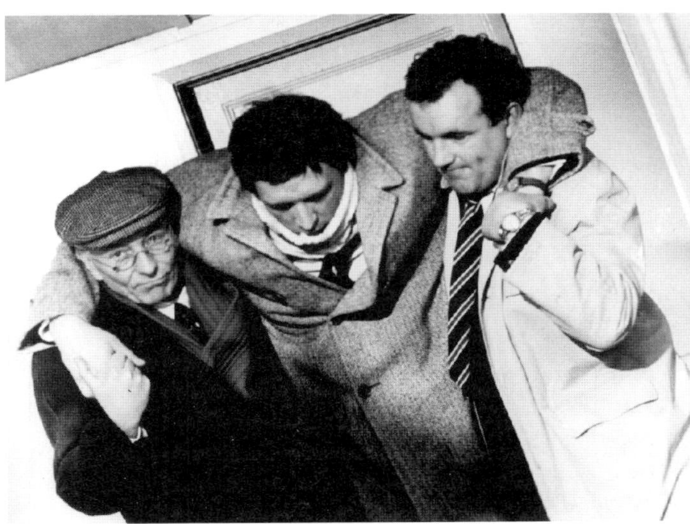

William Hartnell, far left, in **This Sporting Life** (1962).

Journey To Cathay, where the four travellers encounter Marco Polo. The writer had done a fifteen part radio series on the subject for CBC and his work was known to Newman, so when he was asked to write a historical romp, it was the most obvious era for him to choose and central character for him to work with.

David Whitaker was seeking out ideas that fell into the three distinctive story categories, working under Newman's insistence that there be heavy fact behind the fiction, with serials based in the past (*Like Tribe Of Gum*, Anthony Coburn's opening serial), some would use journeys through space, and others would have futuristic elements, such as *The Survivors*, which Whitaker formally contracted Terry Nation to write, having remembered his work on *Out Of This World*.

Nation had spent the best part of that year touring the country with Tony Hancock. Hancock's career was in decline. He had split from his writing team of ten years or so, Ray Galton and Alan Simpson, who had effectively made him a star with their work on *Hancock's Half Hour* on both radio and television. Without their material, the spark of genius was still there, but it just wouldn't light, as had been proved by his first series away from them with ATV. The initial excitement and high viewing figures, due to his return on television, soon waned as viewers quickly realised that this wasn't the same Hancock they knew and loved. That series was where Hancock had struck up a rapport with Nation, who wrote several of the episodes and was subsequently asked to rework Hancock's cabaret act for a national tour he was planning.

What sounded like a brilliant offer, with the potential to gain Nation the reputation as the man who saved Hancock's career, started to go horribly wrong. Nation's new material was never used, for as soon as Hancock got on stage he reverted to his old routines that he'd been using since the early 1950s, and Nation was being paid £100 a week to do little more than act as a minder, making sure that Hancock got from venue to venue.

When the offer from Whitaker came through, Hancock dismissed it as being utter nonsense, deriding the thought of Nation lowering himself to work for a 'kids' programme', but shortly after that, the two of them fell out and Nation found himself out of work once again. Both he and Hancock had shared a room on the tour, and after a show Hancock would often stay up half the night debating with him on the fate of mankind. The comedian was certain that mankind would be wiped out, and had a fascination with contemplating what form of life, if any, would survive.

That line of thought led Nation to write *The Survivors*, with its story of a race devastated by eons of warfare, who had mutated to the point where they could only move around in armoured machines. They were called the Daleks. Towards the end of July, the cast were issued with their contracts and everything was ready for filming. Newman was happy with the way things were going, having watched the programme's progress like a hawk. Innes Lloyd recalled: "I remember Sydney summing up the characters very lyrically. 'They're like curious souls, lost in the universe, trying to understand, on a never ending journey.' He really cared about *Doctor Who*, and if it wasn't for him pushing it continuously, I doubt whether it would ever have been made.

"You have to understand that the BBC didn't like to take risks on that scale. Sydney was a showman, if he said it would run for 52 weeks, it would do exactly that. People were nervous, they just couldn't see how it could possibly last more than thirteen weeks. Little did they know..."

But there was still a long way to go before take-off.

William Hartnell with his grand-daughter Judith Anne Carney.

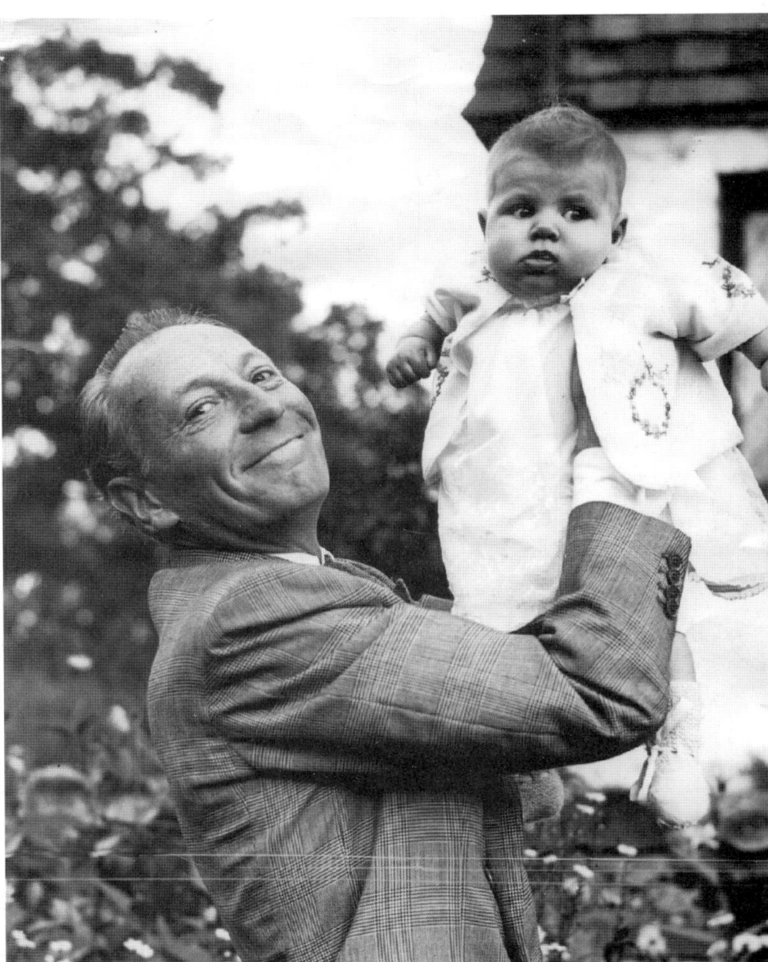

CHAPTER 2

THE GHOSTS OF SATURDAY NIGHT

"It wasn't as though I was taking over from a failure – it was the opposite....William Hartnell was Doctor Who in everybody's minds. I was the enemy, the intruder... I was the one who got blamed for taking 'their' Doctor away..."

PATRICK TROUGHTON interviewed – September 1985

'This church is closed at present, but for those who are working with the BBC, the vicar has left the key under the mat.'

So read the hand-written sign taped to the window by the main doors of Saint Mary's Church Hall, down the far end of Latimer Road in London, and there it stayed for many years while the respective casts of programmes varying from *Z-Cars* to *Till Death Us Do Part* went through their paces, bringing their scripts to life in rehearsal.

It may not have the same ring of authority as today's 'BBC Rehearsal Room Facility', or 'The Acton Hilton' as it's affectionately known, but for a large part of the 1950s and 1960s it was one of many such buildings that the BBC used in the absence of any formal facility.

That particular church hall is where William Russell remembers the first formal readthrough of *An Unearthly Child*, episode one of *100,000 BC*. It took place during the third week of September 1963. Talking about his career when he eventually left the programme in 1965, Russell said:

"Jackie (Jacqueline Hill), Carole Anne (Ford), myself and Bill Hartnell first met in a church hall round the back of White City (the BBC's main London base, and very near Latimer Road). I remember because I asked where Bill was when I arrived, and somebody pointed to the pulpit where he was standing looking down on everyone like some Edwardian headmaster. He was very cordial, very much the host – It was his show."

Doctor Who rehearsals spent a large majority of their early days, certainly up until Patrick Troughton left in 1969, being moved around from empty drill halls to back rooms at the BBC Training Centre, as everything was carefully planned out before any recording took place.

Movements were orchestrated using white tape marks on the floor to represent where walls were positioned, where doors were and where stairways began, as the actors would have to wait until they got into the studio before they had proper sets to work around. A simple chair could represent anything from a computer to an elaborate control panel on a spaceship.

As Patrick Troughton later said:

"You had to suspend belief or you'd crack up and get told off. The villain could be holding you hostage with a gun in your back, when you knew damn well that it was really a coathanger. You had to be children again. It was cowboys and indians time, and you got paid for it!"

Timothy Combe, who would later go on to direct two stories with Jon Pertwee's Doctor, worked as a production assistant on the Hartnell story, *The Reign Of Terror*.

"Being in the Training Centre was good, because we were always near the canteen, so there were plenty of refreshments, although I have to admit that the food was pretty dreadful. Anyway, if we were rehearsing in Latimer Road, Hartnell used to get very tetchy if there was no 'Camp Coffee' there for him. I don't think I can actually recall ever seeing him drink anything else. So, it was nearly always up to the PA to check if there was any there, and dive across to the corner shop and get some if there wasn't, before Hartnell had a chance to notice."

There was a huge amount of secrecy surrounding what was going on in the rehearsals for *100,000 BC*. Part of this may have been due to the fact that there was a certain amount of resentment with the children's drama producers, as they felt that *Doctor Who* should have fallen under their auspices, and not the drama series department's. The cast, and for the first episode this only involved the four main leads, were told to regard the content of the scripts as confidential, and only a select few had seen the designs for the interior of the 'Machine' – The elaborate Tardis Control Room set, which was the creation of Polish-born BBC staff designer Peter Brachaki.

A large percentage of the overall budget that had been allocated for the first block of thirteen episodes of *Doctor Who* went on constructing the set. It was vast, and when it was erected in Lime Grove's Studio D it took up nearly half of the studio space. There were many problems with its layout over the next 52 weeks, with Brachaki's design being so complex that successive directors started to remove bits of it, as Barry Newbery did, who would go on to take over as Designer from Brachaki on *100,000 BC*. He recalls: "Peter had things like ornate pieces of antique furniture decorating the set, things that I suppose the Doctor had collected travelling through time – but they were impractical as directors had to work around them, and as a consequence they'd get annoyed because their camera movements became restricted.

"As the stories progressed, the pieces were quietly removed and returned to the hire company, which actually saved money as it was quite costly to keep them long-term. I'm sure that if you compare the first story to one of the later ones, it's clear that the Tardis is smaller and less cluttered."

The set had three walls positioned around a central control console – a free standing hexagonal prop, with a central glass column that could be manipulated off-camera to rise and fall. It was

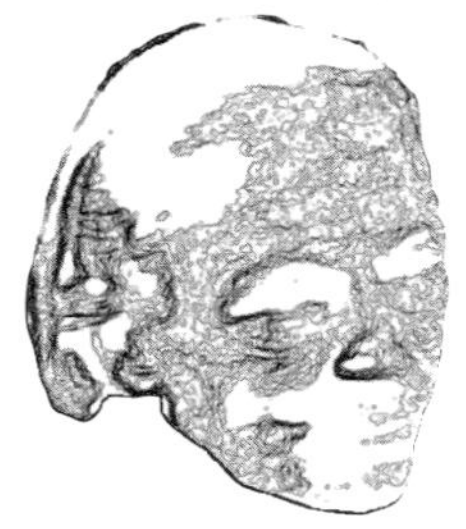

built outside the BBC by a freelance prop company called Shawcraft Ltd. The reasoning behind all the controls for the ship being positioned around one unit came from 'Bunny' Webber's original idea, as Anthony Coburn remembers:

"One thing I remember being impressed with on the original scripts (Webber's) was that there was an incredible sense of ordered logic about some things. I think it was pointed out that if an elderly man was piloting the Tardis, he'd have to have everything in one place, so he wouldn't have to go wandering all over the place to just throw one switch. I'd never have thought about that kind of thing."

The wall to the left of the console held the thick double doors that opened inwards, moved off-camera on cue as the appropriate switch was thrown. The second wall, behind the console, basically acted as a backdrop, and like the left one, it was covered with a symmetrical pattern of roundels which glowed with the aid of some back-lighting. These were among the first casualties to suffer in storage between stories, as Newbery explains:

"The roundels were opaque and made from a very delicate pressed plastic, and quite frankly they shattered very easily. We ended up using a much cheaper material called Cobex to replace them, and when you back-lit them like the others, you couldn't tell the difference on screen.

"The third wall was a problem; it took more time than we had anticipated to put it together properly, so it was quietly phased out. When they reached a point where the characters had to cross

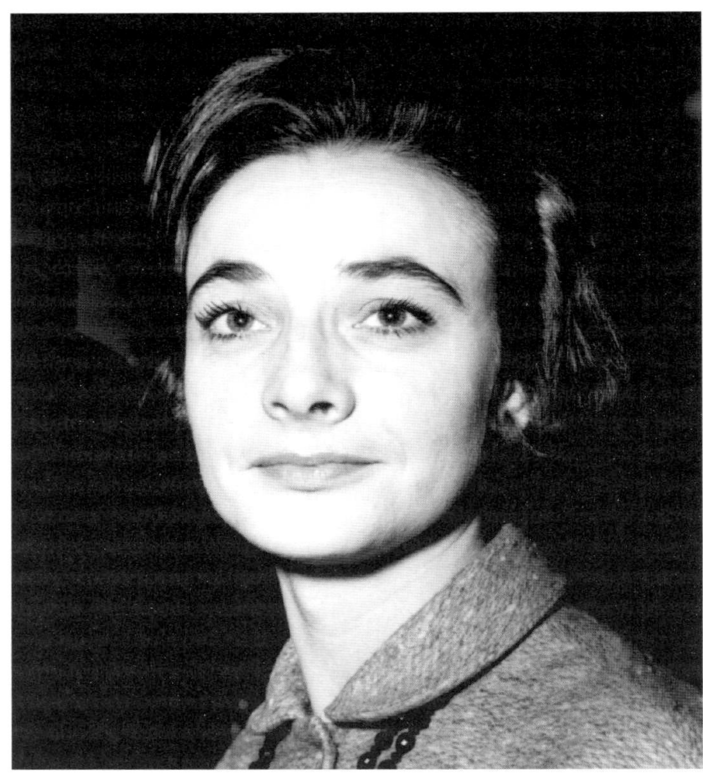

ABOVE: Jacqueline Hill
BELOW: Hartnell, Russell and Ford in studio rehearsal for the remount of **An Unearthly Child**.

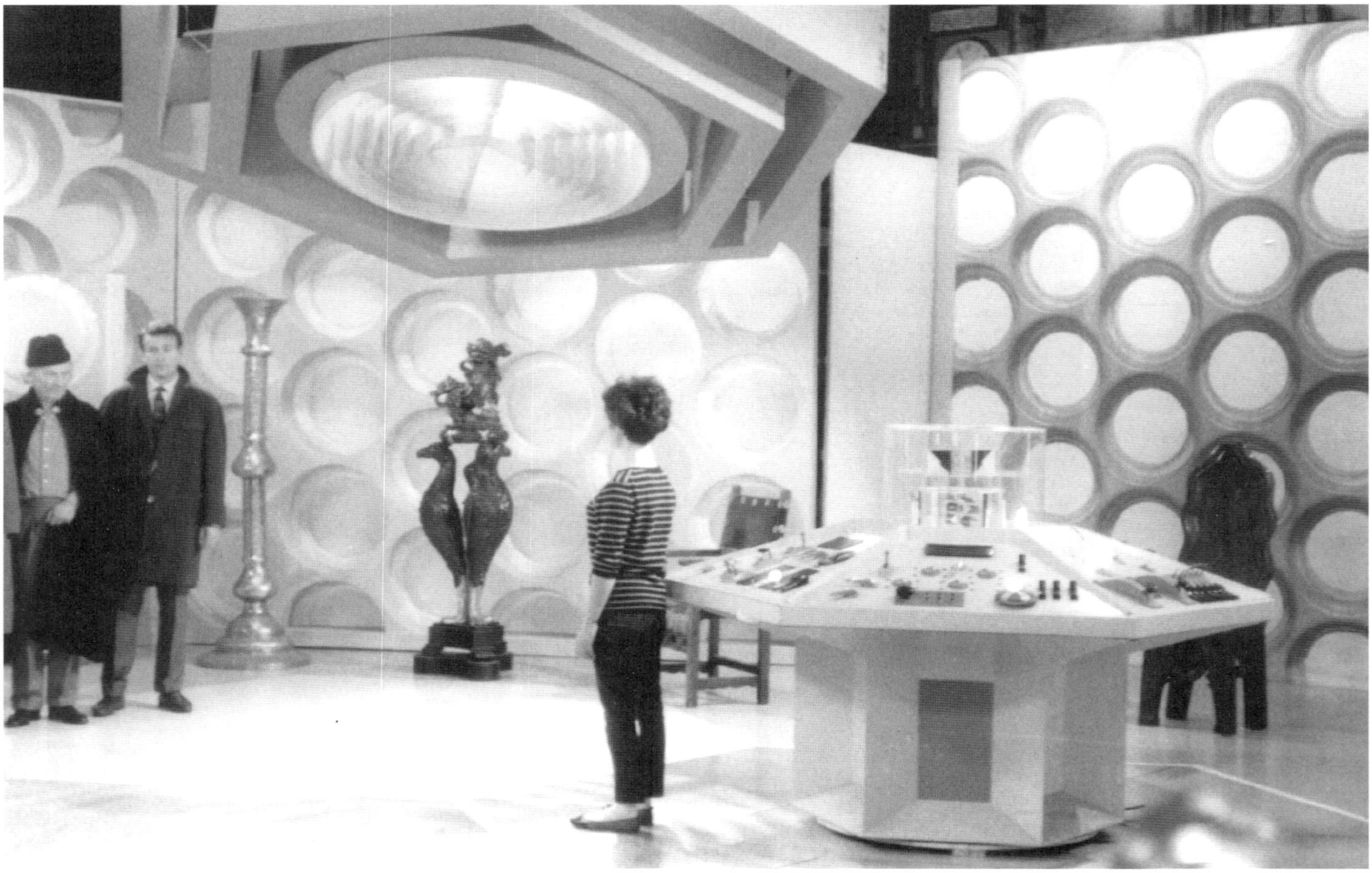

the room so you would see it, a much simpler surface with a small recess was constructed. It saved time, money and blended in more effectively with the rest of the set with the shared pattern of roundels."

Hartnell thought the design of the set was brilliant, particularly the console, with which he insisted he be allowed to practise, carrying out a set routine of switching levers and dials in order for the Doctor to control the Tardis. He even stretched this point to the rehearsals, as Dennis Spooner recalled:

"Bill had his favourite table, which was roughly the same size as the Tardis console, and he'd insist it was there in rehearsals so he could go through the motions of turning all the switches. If it wasn't there, there was hell to pay for the P's, and he always took new Directors to one side and showed them his routine."

Shaun Sutton confirms the story:

"He was always worried that he might get careless and hit a wrong switch and that a letter would arrive from some child asking why he didn't hit the normal buttons. He knew that children were observant, and he was very respectful about that fact and didn't want to get caught out. He knew that something that small could break their belief in him, and that would never do."

Present with the cast at rehearsals were Lambert, Waris Hussein, Pinfield and Douglas Camfield, the PA for the first story. Camfield had joined the BBC in the mid 1950s, and was working his way up the ladder through the BBC with a view to becoming a director, which he would eventually achieve and go on to direct more episodes of *Doctor Who* than anyone else. It was actually Camfield who carried out the first filming session on *An Unearthly Child*, in the week prior to the rehearsal.

Before any of the cast were needed, the climax of the episode had to be shot, with the Tardis landing on a rocky, barren landscape in the stone age, with the credits rolling over the resulting cliffhanger as the ominous shadow of a caveman looms over the police box. All of the main sequences for the episode were due to be shot at Lime Grove, but this brief sequence was staged at the Ealing film studios, and was completed in an afternoon.

As it turned out, the six days of rehearsal did not guarantee that the actual filming would go smoothly. The problematical first full day in the studio took place on 27 September, with the episode completed after one and a quarter hours filming. As the

Behind the cast is the part of the set later removed to improve camera access.

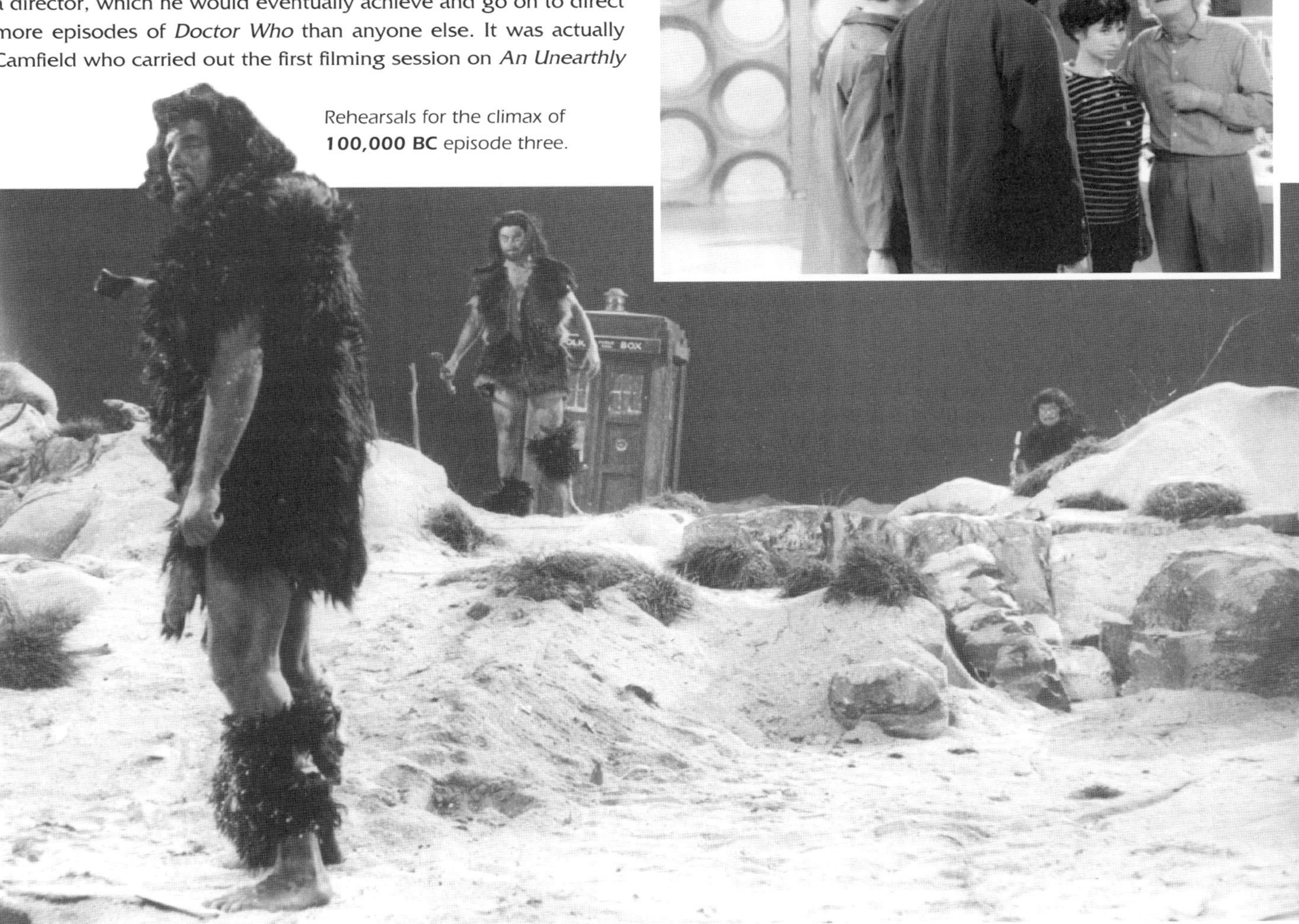
Rehearsals for the climax of **100,000 BC** episode three.

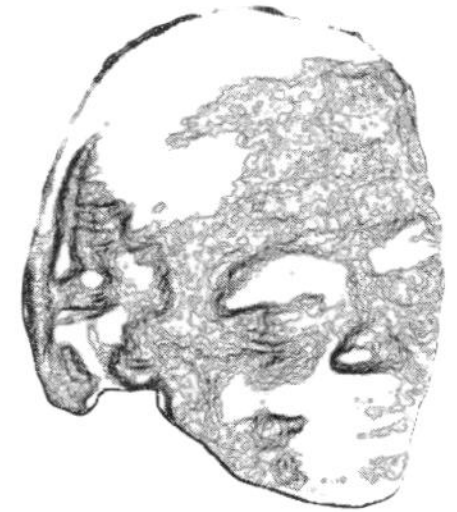

late Douglas Camfield remembered: "It just didn't work out. Hartnell played it far too aggressively, the Tardis doors wouldn't close... we had to do it again and again. In retrospect, I think everybody marched in full of confidence and didn't realise what they were trying to do until it started to go wrong."

Ideally, the material that was 'in the can' would have been used as the first broadcast programme, giving the production team a bit of breathing space as Donald Baverstock's new deadline of 16 November was looming fast, but it was quickly decided by Newman that this was an impossibility. It just wasn't good enough.

Newman had pushed the project forward, he had guided Wilson and Webber through the latter stages of development, he had put so much into it that there was no way he could allow the episode to go out as it was. He felt that it had totally failed to realise its potential. The cast were obviously floundering, and there was little of the edge of mystery and suspense that he knew the series could achieve.

Hussein and Lambert were told what Newman thought was wrong with it, and that he didn't want to give up. Normally the production would have been closed down, but it was just the pilot episode that was abandoned in this case – the production team were told to try again.

By the beginning of October, David Whitaker was revising the script, getting rid of such plot points as Susan mentioning that both she and her grandfather are from the 43rd century, and some of the costumes were redesigned, with Hartnell's changing to the more 'Eccentric Victorian' look that would become so familiar, while Carole Anne Ford lost the futuristic top she had worn in the pilot, simply wearing more modern clothing. A remount of the first part of *100,000 BC* was approved for the third week of the month, with the same production crew on board, apart from Peter Brachaki.

Barry Newbery took over as Designer due to Brachaki being taken ill, and being unable to fulfil his workload. Newbery reworked the junkyard set that was needed, and the school classroom sets, for the sequences where Chesterton and Barbara Wright are seen at work, but left the main set of the episode alone. He takes up the story:

"I didn't touch anything that Peter had done with the Tardis control room set, because to tell the truth, there just wasn't the time and it had already cost over two and a half thousand pounds. So if I'd have gone to Verity and asked for a larger allowance to redesign the set, it wouldn't exactly have gone down that well.

"As each story progressed, there was a tendency to tinker with the Tardis set, with designers trying to simplify it as much as they could, but for that first one, to be honest, I had more things to worry about with the stone age set."

A broadcastable version of *An Unearthly Child* was completed on 18 October, with the revised version now winning the complete approval of Newman. Hartnell had changed his performance and was now presenting a mysterious, enigmatic figure with a mischievous glint in his eye, and all attempts to suggest the strange 'alien' quality of Susan Foreman had also been toned down. The character now came across as a hyper-intelligent schoolgirl.

With Baverstock's approval, work now began on the full series. Due to the decision to abandon the pilot episode, a week had been lost which caused a shift of seven days for the initial broadcast date – *Doctor Who* would now make its debut on 23 November.

It was a matter of necessity to have at least four to five weeks between the recording and broadcast of any *Doctor Who* episode, to allow for the time needed to edit in filmed inserts, and other technical details. A tight 'weekly turnaround' schedule was brought into operation to combat this.

As far as the actors were concerned, it worked as follows: midway through working on one episode, the script for the following installment would arrive. There was very little time for learning lines (basically, that was done on Sunday, their day off), and the week would start with a general read through on the Monday morning, with the afternoon spent editing sections of dialogue if the text ran over 25 minutes.

Tuesday and Wednesday were spent blocking out the moves, planning out which set was where and what scenes were to be done there, while Thursday was spent finalising this and allowing the Costume Department to solve any problems the actors had with their characters' clothing. Friday was 'D-Day', with the actors rehearsing in the completed sets, and after dinner in the evening, the episode went before the cameras. By 10pm, the entire episode had to be 'in the can'.

Seven days after *An Unearthly Child* was completed, *The Cave Of Skulls*, the second part of *100,000 BC*, was recorded successfully. The filmed inserts for this and the next two parts, where scenes or effects had to be staged at Ealing had been carried out two weeks earlier, once again under the supervision of Douglas Camfield.

While the actors started work on the third episode, Terry Nation was back, working with David Whitaker on a second story for the series. Nation's *The Red Fort* saw the crew of the Tardis landing on the outskirts of Delhi in 1857, where they were split up and held by the rival factions involved in the infamous civil uprising that took place in that year. Work on *The Mutants* was now completed as far as the scripts were concerned, and the story was well into pre-production, with Lambert having decided to assign two directors to the project.

The story was seven episodes long, and by giving it to two people, the workload would not be as intense. So Christopher Barry, who had been with the BBC as a staff director for some time, and Richard Martin, who was then a relative novice, were put under contract. Barry was given episodes one, two, four and five to helm, while Martin took on numbers three, six and seven.

The original designer proposed for the story was one Ridley Scott, now internationally famous as the Director of such cinema blockbusters as *Alien*, *Blade Runner* and *Thelma and Louise*. Years later, when it was pointed out to him in an interview that he was nearly the man who designed the Daleks, and he was asked what he would have done with them, Scott cryptically replied: "Look what I did with a B-Movie monster in *Alien*..."

On the first day of November, *The Forest Of Fear* was in studio, with Newbery's complex cave sets being used to great effect. Newbery remembers that the actual substance used to create the cave walls was highly flammable, and that he went into the studio to supervise their construction only to find one of the scenic crew

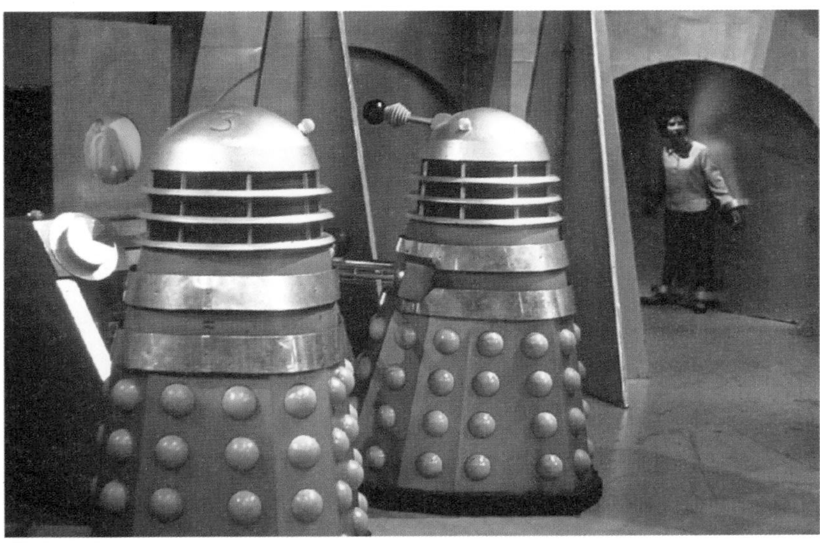

Daleks in rehearsal. Note the number on the back of the Dalek on the left.

trying to heighten the smooth look of the rock surface by melting it with a blow torch!

The cost of the episodes was beginning to push the limits of their budget, and Lambert did not want any money to be carved off the allocated amount for *The Mutants*, which would be the next tale to be shot. To compensate for this and save money, she asked Whitaker to come up with a cheap 'filler' story which could use sets that already existed. The obvious answer was to use the Tardis control room. David Whitaker refered to the event in some correspondence towards the end of the 1970s:

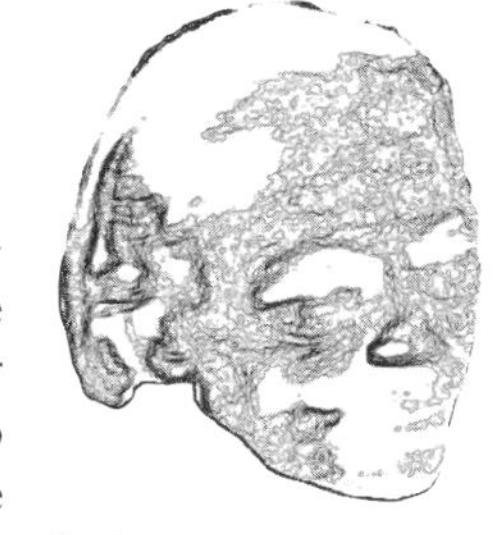

"Verity had an idea about setting a story in the Tardis, which cost so much money that she wanted to show it off a bit. I saw it as a chance to solidify the four main characters by putting them in a situation that would tell the viewers a bit more about them but the question was how to do this.

"I remembered that there was a film that Alfred Hitchcock made about a group of people trapped on a lifeboat, and how they were forced to reveal their innermost secrets to each other (LIFEBOAT, made in 1944). That's where the idea of putting the Tardis crew in a similar situation for a couple of weeks came from."

Whitaker started drafting out *Inside the Spaceship*, and in doing so brought the episode count for the first three stories up to 13, which evened out the budget as Lambert had planned. By

The regular cast meet Marco Polo.

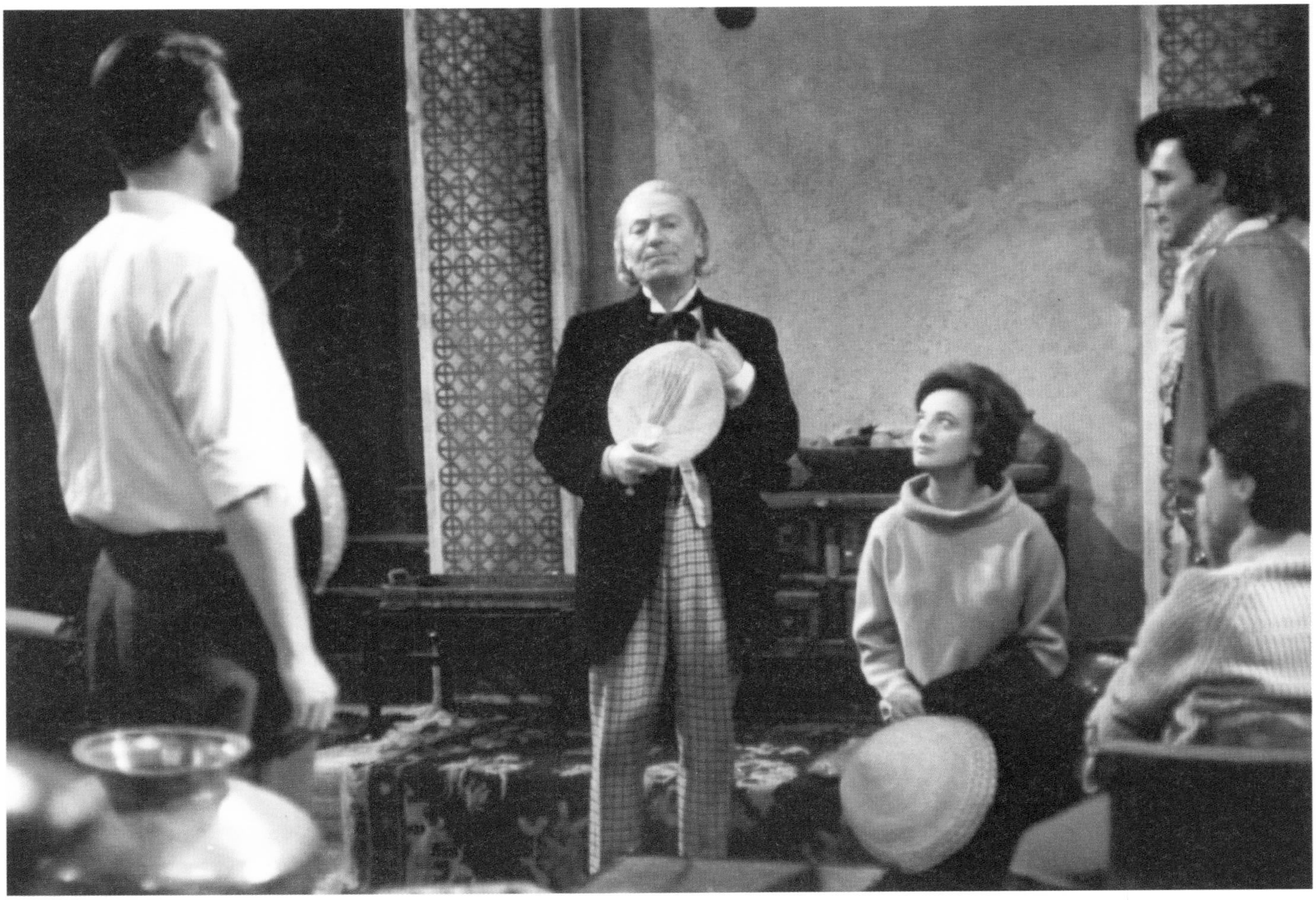

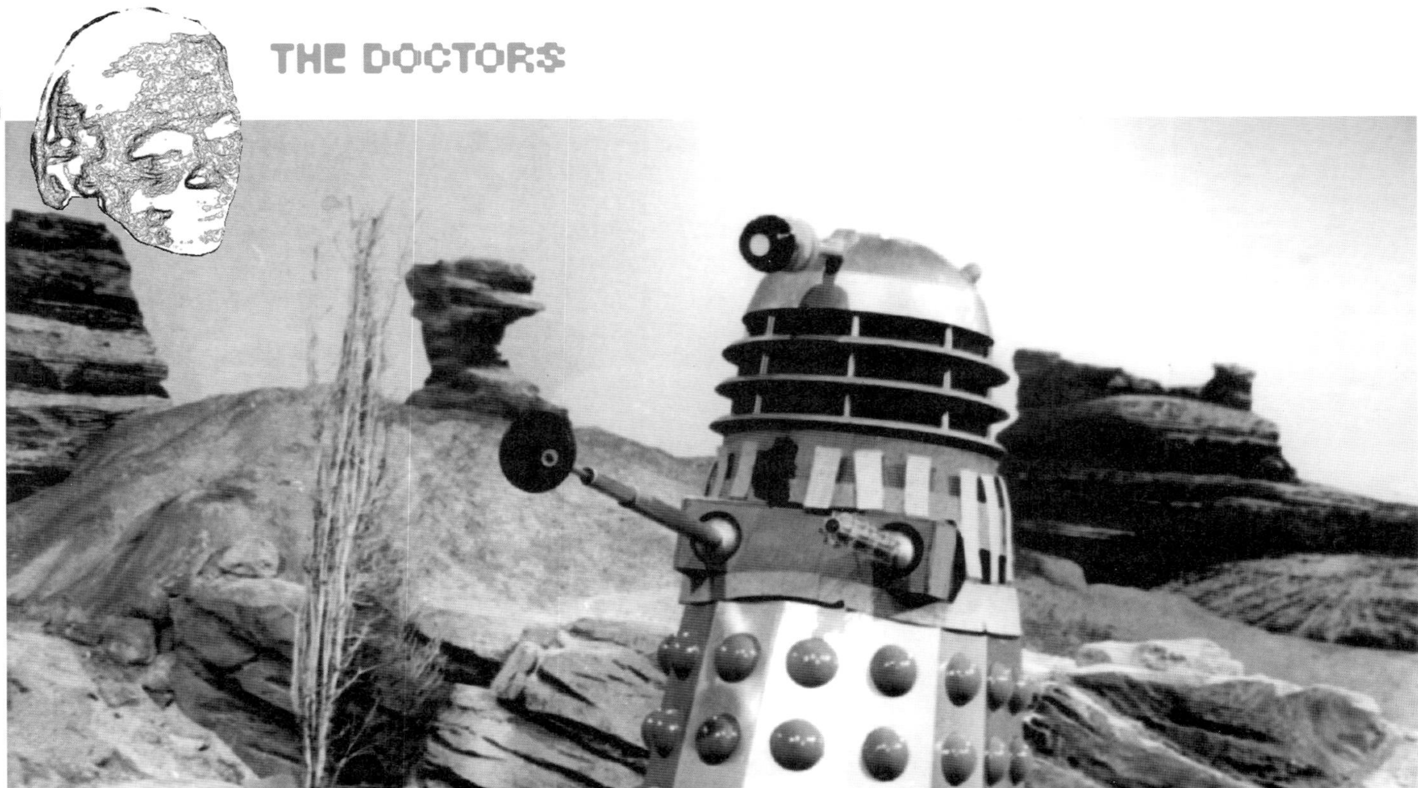

This well-worn Dalek was about to be blown up. Note the hole in its casing where the explosives were inserted.

mid-November, the second batch of 13 episodes was planned to include the seven-part Marco Polo epic, followed by a more science fact-based story, Robert Gould's *The Minascules* (which seems to have also been known as *The Enemy Inside*). The plot was based around the miniaturisation scenario that 'Bunny' Webber had first mooted with *The Giants* earlier in the year. Anthony Coburn's *The Robots* was due to follow that.

One plotline submitted at the time, although not directly attributed to Gould, suggests that the Tardis should materialise inside a human body, having shrunk to the size of a pinhead. The Doctor wants to observe the ship's passage through the blood stream on the monitor and gives Susan strict instructions not to open the doors, which, being an impetuous youngster (as the plotline describes her!), is exactly what she does. She is caught in an air bubble and dragged outside and the Doctor has to try to guide the Tardis after her, with Chesterton ready in a diving suit to rescue her, hopefully before the air bubble reaches the brain of their host and induce an embolism. The climax of the first episode revolved around Chesterton finding Susan, and their struggle to get back to the Tardis sharing an oxygen mask between them. As they find the time machine, it's being attacked by a group of gigantic white blood corpuscles.

Apart from being a production designer's nightmare, the story seems to have been finally dropped because of a similar story which was being turned into a film, as Dennis Spooner explained:

"I remember working on *The Daleks' Master Plan* (made during the third year of *Doctor Who*), and John Wiles (the producer at that point) had a story that he desperately wanted to do about the Tardis landing inside a human body. It had been kicking round since I first started working on the show, and I had to tactfully point out that he'd probably end up facing a vast legal case, as *Fantastic Voyage* was being shot at the same time. I think it was dropped there and then."

By November 8th, Hussein completed work on *100,000 BC* with the final episode, *The Firemaker*, recorded on that evening. Donald Wilson spoke about one thing in particular that bothered him about the first story:

"I don't think we should have had Doctor Who smoking. I remember that William Hartnell was quite worried about this, not wanting to be seen as a character who drinks, or anything like that, but the script called for him to be quite clearly seen lighting a pipe. I accept that it was a necessary plot point that someone had a box of matches, but I would rather have had one of the other characters own them."

It seems that nobody was entirely happy with the first story. In fact, for a short period, Coburn's scripts were dropped while another story, called *Living World* by Alan Wakeman was seriously considered as a replacement. There are no formal records of what the story was about, but one clue can be found in some notes made by Spooner. When he took over from David Whitaker, he went through all the old material left by his predecessor to see if there was anything worth recommissioning. He dismissed it, jotting down in his notes:

'*Living World* – Idea about rocks, trees, etc being dominant species. Control humans and DW & Crew with silent sound. Difficult to pull off without laughter at moving rocks...'

In retrospect, he's quite right in saying that the resulting special effects would have been ludicrous, and it was *100,000 BC* that was made, even though Lambert, Hussein and Wilson felt it was not right for an opening story. Speaking in 1965, William Hartnell clearly had reservations as well:

"I have the greatest respect for Verity Lambert, but I do think that the caveman story was a mistake. I asked her whether she actually believed that children would accept that these primatives could speak English. I certainly didn't, and I was certain that the children would feel the same."

Work was steadily progressing on *The Mutants*, with Christopher Barry joining the production office in mid-October and carrying out some insert filming for the first two episodes at the end of that month.

Staff Designer Raymond P. Cusick was brought in, and alongside Newbery, he shared most of the workload of visualising the first year of *Doctor Who* serials.

Newbery comments:

"I did all the historical stories, which varied from the stone age to the French Revolution (*The Reign Of Terror*), while Ray handled the more fantastic ones, where monsters and spaceships were needed, which suited me fine..."

The first appearance on screen of a Dalek was not due to take place till the second episode of *The Mutants* serial, *The Survivors*. The climax to part one, *The Dead Planet*, following the time travellers discovery of the apparently empty Dalek city, had Barbara being confronted by one of the creatures for the first time but all that was seen heading towards her was one of its armatures.

Like *100,000 BC*, the first episode of *The Mutants* only featured the four main leads, with the rest of the 'human' cast not appearing till episode three. In 1967, William Hartnell spoke about this:

"The beginning of the early adventures always had a wonderful air of isolation about them. We were on our own, and the people at home knew that the mystery would begin and a monster would appear at any moment. It took time for the story to unfold, people just don't have that patience any more."

It's interesting that he liked the scenes where he was working only with the companions. Innes Lloyd recalled that he was never comfortable with guest casts:

"He had an incredible sense of loyalty to the regulars and found it difficult to get on with the main visiting actors. They were strangers, and the show was his territory. Just as he was getting used to them, the next story would come up and a new cast would arrive, and it made him increasingly edgy."

Hartnell made his feelings known in an interview conducted when Patrick Troughton was halfway through his time in the role.

"I don't like the modern approach to *Doctor Who*, with him simply arriving in the middle of some event where there is a crisis going on that he solves in an instant. I don't like it at all. He seems to deliberately find trouble, whereas I merely chanced upon it."

As well as having strong views about storylines, Hartnell was very clear about the form his main adversaries, the Daleks, should take. He made it quite clear that he saw the Daleks as being anything but humanoid. He wanted to avoid the cliche of which Sydney Newman was all too aware, the 'Men In Strange Costumes' brand of monster, although this was very nearly the way the Daleks appeared, as Ray Cusick recalls:

"I was talking to Mervyn Pinfield because, quite frankly, making science fiction was an entirely new area for me, and I wasn't sure of how to approach the Daleks. He said, 'Get some cardboard tubes, use one for an arm, one for a leg, a larger one round the body. It will make a suit, if you paint it silver that could be your Dalek.' He was missing the point, as this was exactly the kind of thing we were trying to avoid."

Cusick wanted to disguise the human figure totally, leaving enough flexibility for the actor inside the costume to be able to move it around.

Cusick continues:

"I hit upon the idea of making the Daleks so that the actor was totally unseen, and I wanted a shape that would make the viewers think twice about whether anybody was in it. The way to do that was to make them just a bit shorter than the average human, and make them squat and quite fast."

Nation wanted to have the creatures with a flat base, mechanised arms and the only indication of anything at face height was to be a metal eye-stalk. The idea of giving the Daleks smooth, flowing movement came from the writer watching a performance on television by the Georgian state dancers. David Whitaker offered this memory of the event:

"Terry phoned me at the office. He was terribly excited because he'd seen these strange dancers where the women wore these vast, hooped skirts which hid their feet and made them seem as though they were floating.

"I knew what he meant, but I couldn't see how this could apply to the Daleks until I saw what Ray Cusick did with them. His designs were breathtaking, and I'm quite sure that without them, we would not have got beyond the first handful of stories.

"The Daleks actually caused quite a stir when the first ones arrived at Lime Grove. One man nearly walked into a wall when he saw them being pushed into the studio. People would either look

William Hartnell at the height of his popularity as Dr Who appearing on **Junior Points of View**.

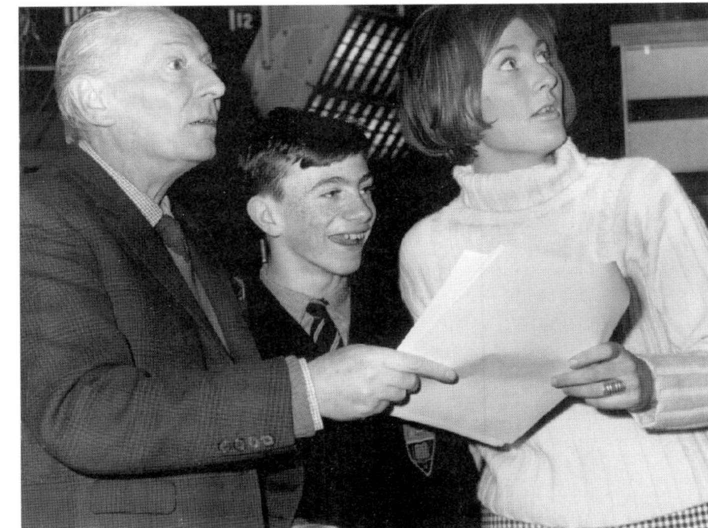

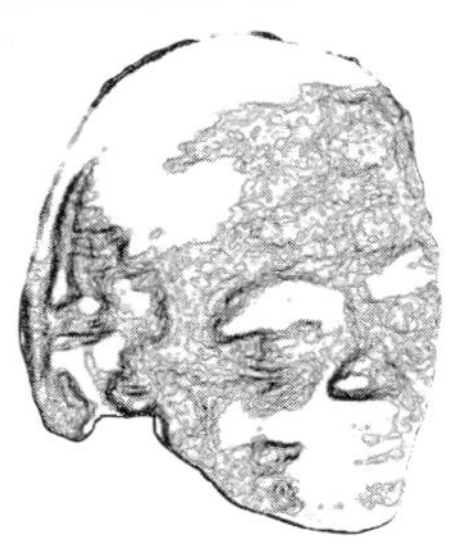

on in awe or laugh nervously. I think it unnerved certain quarters, making them think twice – perhaps we weren't the joke that they thought we were after all.

"I remember that one of the actors brought his son to the studio on the second one we did *The Dalek Invasion Of Earth*, and I saw him standing a few feet in front of where the costumes had been left for the lunch break. He was just staring at them, so I asked if anything was wrong, and he said that he didn't like to see the Daleks looking sad. I laughed and asked him how on earth he could tell, and with the most truthful look I've ever seen, he said that it was obvious as their eye-stalks were drooping!"

Four Daleks were built by Shawcraft Models, who were becoming familiar faces on the *Doctor Who* set with their regular work making special props repairing the Tardis console, which they'd built.

The designers handled all visual aspects of the series that were seen on screen, with one exception being the costumes. Any special effects had to be supervised by them as well, with the BBC effects unit not becoming formally involved with *Doctor Who* until the end of the fourth series. The pressure was intense, as Cusick testifies:

"It was highly pressurise, the sheer amount of things that had to be done nearly always led to seven day working weeks. That's why other designers were brought in for the second year, to take the workload off Barry and myself. It was genuinely too much for us alone to cope with."

The Dead Planet went before the cameras on 15 November, with an apparently smooth run-through. It was only afterwards that Christopher Barry discovered that all the footage that had been recorded was unusable. Electrical interference had caused damage that was beyond repair.

There was no alternative other than to keep the story in production, and go into the studio on the following Friday with *The Survivors*. Like *An Unearthly Child, The Dead Planet* would have to be remounted, but there was not the kind of spare time that was around before. There was now just under six weeks until transmission, so a day would have to be found at least a week before transmission to allow Christopher Barry the editing time he needed.

Fortunately, *The Survivors* experienced no problems, other than general confusion as to which Dalek housed which actor in the technical rehearsals on the set. This problem was solved by taping numbers to each casing so that Barry could call the movements by referring to 'Dalek 1', 'Dalek 2', and so on. In the euphoria of success that the programme experienced once the creatures had made their debut, one anonymous production crew member spoke to the press, commenting that, "William Hartnell was not amused by the Daleks having numbers taped to them. He came up alongside me, waved his walking stick at them and said, 'The most terrifying race of beings in the universe, and they look like ballroom dancers!'"

The second episode was finished on the evening of 22 November, as news was beginning to filter across from America of the assassination of President John F. Kennedy. The following day, both ITV and the BBC were swamped with coverage of the tragedy, and as news items began to come over and normal programmes were cancelled to make way for them.

Almost unnoticed, at 5.16 pm, the schedules began to return to normal, and *An Unearthly Child* was broadcast. There was little in the way of pre-publicity, and only a few newspapers carried the odd comment from Hartnell and Lambert about how they saw this new series. If anything, the press seemed more concerned with the fact that an untried show was getting such a long run. Lambert said, in a comment that seemed to try and reassure fans of the more classical science fiction literature:

"Our aim is to present a drama series in the best tradition of classic adventure stories, like *The Time Machine* by H.G. Wells, or the works of Jules Verne.

"*Doctor Who* is for the whole family. The stories will be more factual and there will be no monsters as such, that are normally associated with science fiction."

This seems an extraordinary statement, as Lambert was certainly aware of what would follow *100,000 BC*. Perhaps it was a case of just keeping quiet; Donald Wilson had made his feelings quite clear on how intensely he disliked the scripts for *The Mutants*, questioning the morality behind the storyline, and Sydney Newman was totally unaware of what was going on.

Newman had distanced himself from the programme once production was underway on the first story, satisfied that it was running smoothly and that he could leave Lambert to get on with it. The Daleks represented exactly the kind of 'Bug eyed monsters' that he had forbidden the production team to use. Lambert must have known that there would be hell to pay when *The Survivors* went out.

The Escape went into Studio D on 29 November, with Richard Martin now directing, and the following day saw Baverstock sanction an extraordinary move. *An Unearthly Child* was repeated immediately prior to *The Cave Of Skulls* being broadcast.

Baverstock explains:

"The shock of the Kennedy assassination and the news coverage that followed caused chaos. There was a lot of money riding on *Doctor Who*, so the repeat was cleared to try and pick up any viewers that may have missed the first showing."

Towards the end of *IOO,OOO BC*, an average of between six and a half to nearly seven million viewers were hooked. But, this was nothing compared to what was to come.

With just over two weeks to go, Christopher Barry took *The Dead Planet* in front of the cameras again on 6 December, to meet the 28 December broadcast date. This time everything went smoothly, and the actors who were due to feature in *The Ambush*, the episode which should have been shot that day, had the luxury of having an extra week to learn their lines.

Shaun Sutton visited the rehearsals midway through the story, and recalls Hartnell getting angry with some of the extras:

"He was in the middle of a scene where he had some important words to say to his companions, and there was this line of Dalek actors behind him without their shells. One whispered in another's ear and made some joke, and all three of them started to giggle.

"Old Hartnell spun round like one of those army sergeants he was always playing, and bellowed at them, 'You, Sir! Third Dalek from the left, Sir! I will not have laughter in my rehearsal time!' And, you know, they didn't say another word after that!"

By the end of December, episode five and six, *The Expedition* and *The Ordeal* were finished, and it was only after *The Dead*

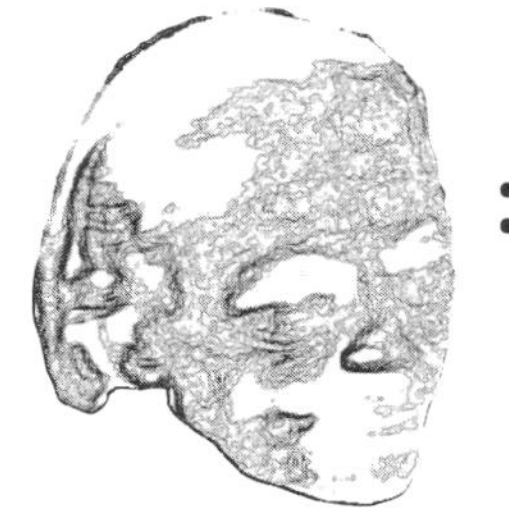

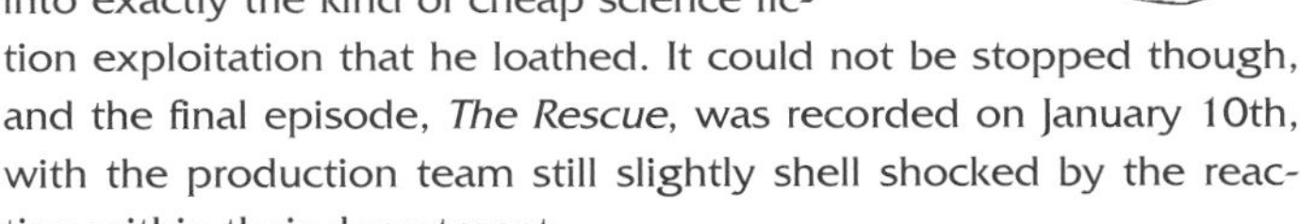

Planet had been screened that speculation began to mount as to what was to come.

David Whitaker:

"I certainly remember phone calls coming in with people in the building wanting to know what was going on, and asking what on earth it was heading towards Barbara at the end of the episode. After the first two or three calls, I was just saying watch next week, but by the twentieth, I was beginning to think that we might be on to something..."

The second Doctor, Patrick Troughton, even saw *The Dead Planet* .

"I remember the kids making a hell of a fuss about *Doctor Who*, and I remember watching the first Dalek episode and thinking, 'Wait a minute, what the hell's that?', when this damn great sucker-stick started heading towards one of the girls. Let me tell you, I was there on the floor with them the following week, just as eager to see what it was!"

The reaction to the broadcast of *The Survivors* was twofold. Firstly, Sydney Newman went through the roof. As soon as the episode had finished, he was on the phone to Lambert, telling her to come to his office first thing Monday morning. Donald Wilson was shocked as well.

"I remember talking to Mervyn (Pinfield) about the programme the day after the Daleks appeared. We had both seen them in the studio, and I had certainly given my nod of approval to the designs, but it came across like a horror film. We both agreed that any child who watched it must have been terrified."

They were both very wrong.

Newman told Lambert in no uncertain terms that he felt she had betrayed the concept of *Doctor Who*, and turned it into exactly the kind of cheap science fiction exploitation that he loathed. It could not be stopped though, and the final episode, *The Rescue*, was recorded on January 10th, with the production team still slightly shell shocked by the reaction within their department.

Lambert approached Paddy Russell to direct *Inside The Spaceship*, but she proved unavailable (though she would go on to direct several stories later on). The immediate solution was to offer the job to Richard Martin, who was under contract already with the Dalek story, but he was only free to handle the first of the two episodes, *The Edge Of Destruction.*

Whitaker was rumoured to have written the story in two days, which was not unusual as Nation freely admitted that he had drafted out *The Daleks* at the rate of one episode a day.

Whitaker elaborates:

"I certainly hammered out the bare bones of the script over a weekend, but it was a matter of having to. There was too much work to do on Terry's scripts to be able to take time off to write it properly. As far as I can recall, I basically tinkered with them while the Dalek story was being made until they were needed, by which time I'd finished them."

At this point, the viewing figures for *The Escape* came in. They had jumped dramatically, rising by two and a half million viewers.

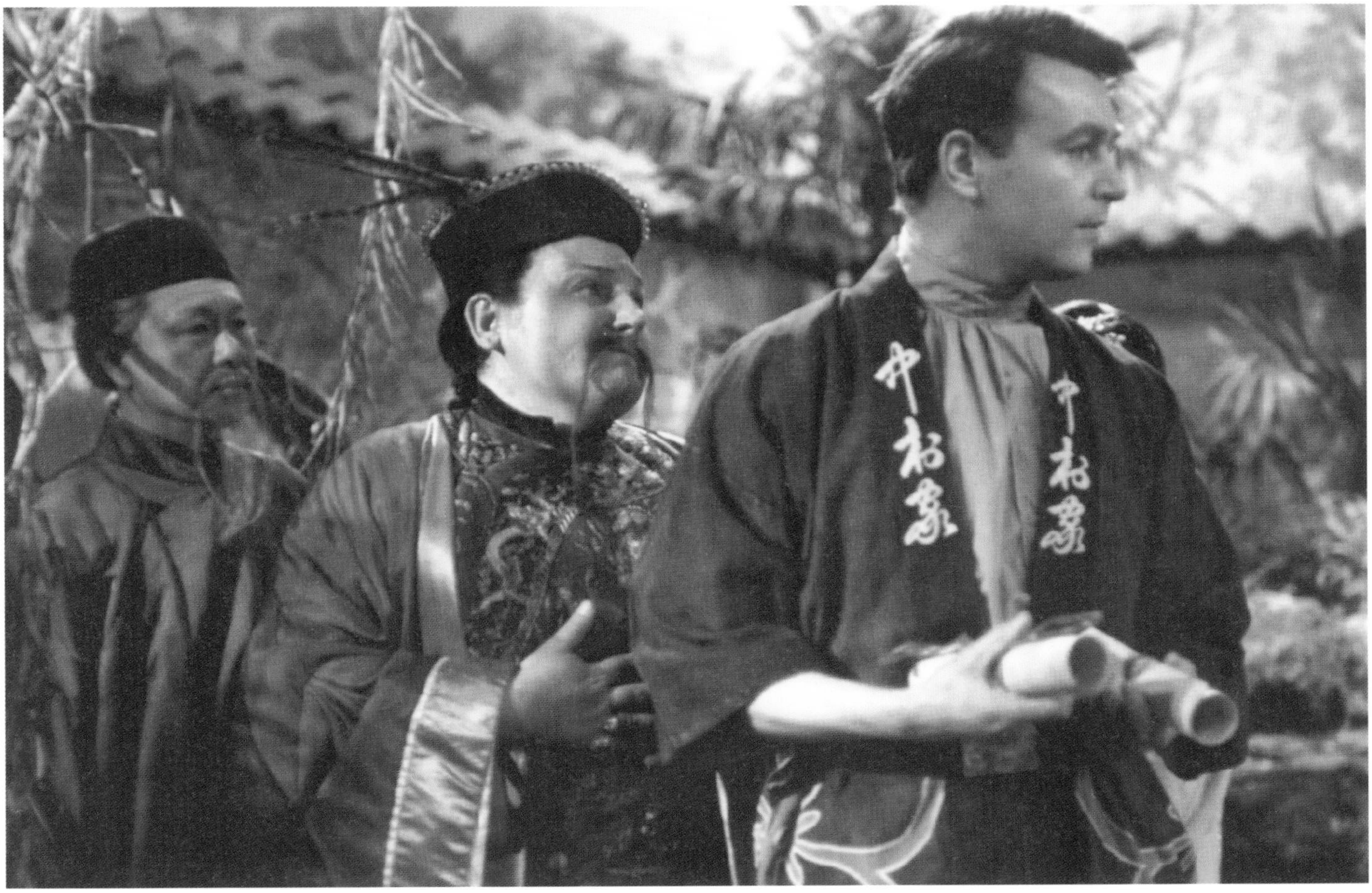

William Russell in **Marco Polo**.

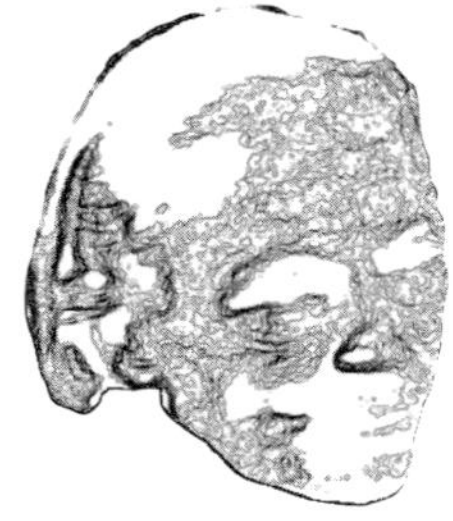

The second phase of the reaction to the Daleks was beginning to kick in. Episode four gained another million, and letters started to flood in – not by the handful, as had been the case after the first episode of *100,000 BC*, but by the sackload. There were literally thousands.

Ray Cusick:

"Verity called me into her office, saying, 'Look, Ray. Look at these.' She was sifting through piles of letters. The mail started to flood in as soon as the Daleks were seen, all from children who were desperate to know more about them."

The ratings continued to climb, and by the end of the story (which was now referred to as *The Daleks* as a more general title, rather than *The Mutants*), it was drawing over ten million viewers. It was a huge hit.

Lambert had been vindicated, and the combination of Nation's writing and Cusick's skillful realisation of his monsters had ensured that the show would certainly run for its planned first year, and perhaps even longer. The kind of reaction it was getting could not be ignored.

William Hartnell, in 1965:

"I had confidence in what we were doing. I felt certain that we would be a success, although there were very few who agreed or shared that opinion with me. It was only after Mr Nation's Daleks appeared that they started to see my point."

The final seal of approval came from Huw Wheldon, the BBC's Director of Programmes, who ultimately had the power to stop a programme being made if there was an adverse reaction to it. Anybody who raised the fact that they felt *Doctor Who* was too frightening for children was promptly cut-down to size, with Wheldon happily saying they were talking 'utter nonsense', and that his own children were imitating the Daleks at home, running round with baskets on their heads shouting 'Exterminate!'

Wheldon commented in 1964:

"*Doctor Who* is a prime example of the BBC at its best – accommodating for what the audience wants and fulfiling their expectations to the last letter. I certainly watch it; in our house Saturdays always grind to a halt the minute the police box appears."

Lambert's search for a director brought her to Frank Cox, who had just completed his BBC director's course and was hired to handle *The Brink Of Disaster*, the second half of *Inside The Spaceship*. Cox trailed Martin, observing him to learn the ropes, as he took *The Edge Of Destruction* into rehearsal on 13 January.

The production schedule *Doctor Who* directors had to cope with was now tighter than ever. With the reshoot for *The Dead Planet*, a week had been lost and there were now only three weeks between recording and transmission dates. One advantage was that the cast were now working well as a team, with a rapport having been quickly established between them.

Kubla Khan's elaborate palace set.

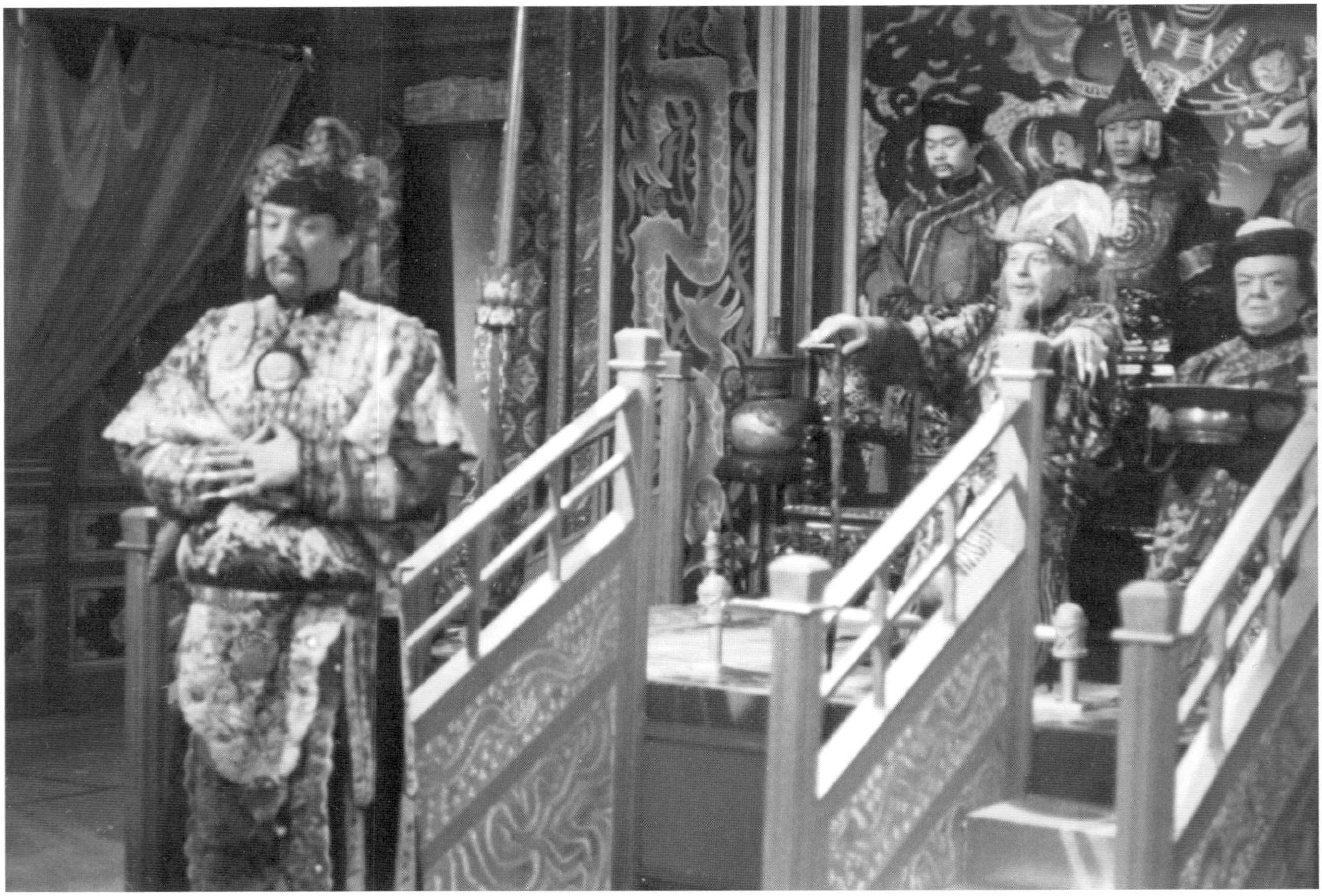

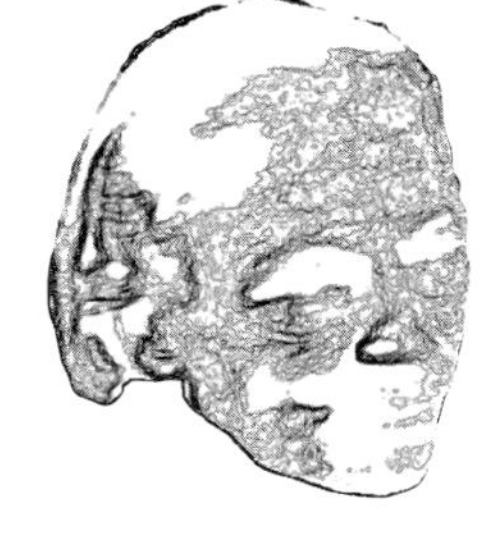

Jacqueline Hill comments:

"I was told that Bill used to tell people he thought of us as his second family. He used to bring in little presents, sweets and cakes that Heather (his wife) had made. I remember he used to get very protective towards us when directors started to get annoyed in rehearsals.

"There was one, a Hungarian I think (probably Henric Hirsch, who Directed *The Reign Of Terror*), who was not actually a well man. He was getting quite angry over something that Carole Anne Ford was doing, and Bill lost his temper and threatened to stage a walk-out if he didn't stop picking on her. He really cared about us."

Waris Hussein was now back with the production team to start work on *Marco Polo*, the final overall title that was given to Lucarotti's scripts which were based on Polo's diaries, *Description Of The World*.

Hartnell claimed credit for the story idea:

"I liked the idea of meeting famous figures in history, because it would show that there was no equal for *Doctor Who* – he could match any of them. I wanted Aristotle, Nostrodamus, Freud, Henry VIII or any of the kings. The closest we ever came to my suggestions were when we met Marco Polo and Richard the Lionheart (*The Crusades*). I liked to think of him travelling through time, sampling fine foods and wine and banqueting with kings!"

Lucarotti lived in Majorca, so it took time for the scripts to arrive, leading to the theory that *Inside The Spaceship* was quickly written to allow enough time for his story's elaborate sets to be built.

Two things make this seem unlikely; Whitaker had been working on the idea since October 1963, and, as Barry Newbery observes, the first episodes of Marco *Polo* only needed a few barren landscapes and tent interiors for Polo's encampment.

"The scripts were very clever. As the story progressed, the settings became more and more grandiose as the travellers got closer to the domain of Khubla Khan. At the beginning, they were in the wilderness, by the end they were in palaces and throne rooms. That gradual progression made the journey seem more fantastic."

The cost-cutting explanation is more plausible. What does seem to be the case is that Cusick stayed on as designer for the two-parter, to allow Newbery enough time to research what was needed for the historical adventure, rather than have to lose valuable time on a story where very little work was needed.

Inside The Spaceship needed only a few additions to Brachaki's main Tardis set, with Cusick adding some sleeping quarters for the Tardis crew.

William Hartnell was unhappy with the large amount of dialogue his character was given in the scripts, as Whitaker had crafted several long monologues for him which there was barely enough time to learn in full. It ended up with William Russell and Jacqueline Hill trying to work around him, as Russell explained on leaving the programme:

"We were all trapped inside the Tardis for a couple of weeks. Bill couldn't cope with this at all as they'd given him incredibly long, intricate speeches. He just couldn't get them into his head at all. It ended up with the rest of us trying to ad-lib the points he had to get across and make it sound as though he'd made them. I don't know how we ever got through that one."

One legendary story about the rehearsals details how Hartnell could not remember the phrase 'Fault Locator', with the words coming out continually as 'Fornicator'! As it was, Hartnell did not like scientific dialogue.

"Doctor Who is a man of magical powers and mystery. I would often cut words like 'atomic flow', because they did not have the right mystical quality. I saw him as more of a magician than a scientist – so much more can be achieved with the unexpected."

The Edge Of Destruction was recorded on 17 January, with Cox in attendance to get a feeling of the continuity that would be needed when he went into rehearsal on the 20th. On the 24th, *The Brink Of Disaster* was shot, and the first block of thirteen episodes had been completed. Plans for the next block of 13 episodes had, however, now changed considerably.

Whitaker knew that the arrival of the Daleks would change what was acceptable as science fiction within the programme's format, and that the more 'faction' based stories were no longer appropriate. The first move he made was to stop Terry Nation working on *The Red Fort*, and ask him to write another science fiction adventure story as quickly as possible. He wanted it to fill the six weeks after *Marco Polo*, and complete the second block of thirteen episodes, but there was very little time to come up with a similar, complex story to *The Daleks*. Whitaker came up with a solution.

"Terry had to write his second story in about two or three weeks. I told him that the easiest type of story to write in that space of time was a *Perils Of Pauline* style of adventure, changing the setting each week but keeping the same story running through it. He wanted to do a treasure hunt story, like the *Treasure Of The Sierra Madre* (A classic Humphrey Bogart film, made in 1946), and the amalgamation of the two ideas led to *The Keys Of Marinus*..."

Lucarotti's work on *Marco Polo* had gone down extremely well, with Donald Wilson commenting:

"After the Daleks had been introduced and proved to be a popular hit, I realised that Verity knew what she was doing and that science fiction was not my area after all. I did keep an eye on the historical stories, and was particularly pleased with the Marco Polo adventure and the ones in the Inca city and Culloden (*The Highlanders* – a Patrick Troughton story). They were the kind of thing that Sydney Newman originally wanted for the programme."

Wilson admits that it was at this time that he decided to 'Leave Verity to get on with it', and the Inca story he mentioned was *The Aztecs*, by John Lucarotti. His work on *Marco Polo* had so impressed Whitaker that he quickly asked him to write another historical story, with the plan being to have it follow *The Keys Of Marinus*.

Anthony Coburn's *The Robots* was now abandoned, as was Malcolm Hulke's work on *The Hidden Planet*. In his notes from his time as script editor, Dennis Spooner re-read two submissions that were dated from the first season and had been rejected by (presumably) Whitaker at the beginning of February 1964. To quote from the notes:

'*Doctor Who And The Man In The Ice* (By future *Who* writer Brian Hayles) – Stone age man found in ice in the antarctic (echoing Hayles future story, *The Ice Warriors*), still alive – Business

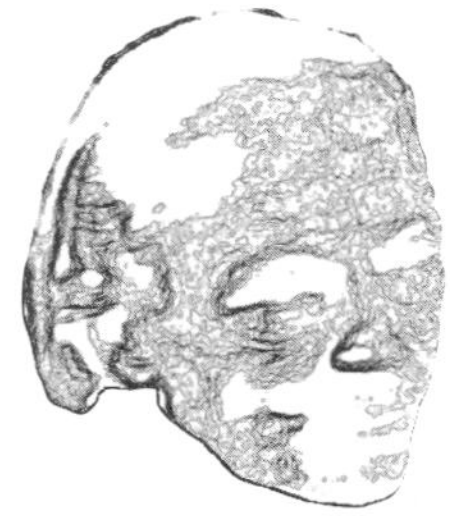

mogul wants to use DNA for strange transplant, as he believes the caveman's genes will give him immortality – Doctor Who rescues cave man to take him back to his own time...'

Spooner noted that this would have been too much like a sci-fi B-movie plot, and was questionable as a story for younger viewers. The second was '*The Great Gamble* (The author is noted as being Oliver Skene, who worked extensively on ITC's series, *The Adventures Of Robin Hood*) – On a Mississippi showboat – Doctor Who has taken his companions there to show them what they were like – The Tardis is taken hostage by a pair of gamblers believing it to be a treasure chest.. Doctor Who has to gamble the lives of his companions in a poker session to win it back...'

Spooner noted that the morality of this story was totally at odds with the ethics of the series, though the idea of using the Mississippi as a location is noted as being sound (though it would never be used). Spooner himself submitted an idea at this time, with *Robin Hood's Last Stand* (or *The Truth Of Sherwood Forest, The Bandits Of The Woods* – it had various titles), in which it's revealed that Robin Hood was not the good guy, and that he terrorised the Sherrif of Nottingham and Prince John, whom the Doctor helps to recover their villainous reputations by plotting to make Robin look like a hero.

Whitaker also had an interesting idea that would have formed another epic historical story. He explained the concept:

"I was always intrigued by the story of Stanley and Livingstone meeting up in the middle of the jungle, and I was toying with the idea of doing a story with Doctor Who trying to ensure that they would meet safely by using the Tardis to move around the continent to direct them. One episode would be helping Stanley, the next Livingstone and then back to Stanley again. As soon as he left them, they'd end up in trouble and he would have to get them out of it the week after the following episode, so there would be a dual series of cliffhangers running.

"It would have ended with the two parties meeting up, with Doctor Who and his companions watching from the side as the famous words, 'Dr. Livingstone, I presume' were said, and then they'd leave, knowing that their work was done. It was never done because the series took a different direction with more and more science fiction stories. Who knows, I might send it in for Tom Baker." (Baker was the Doctor at the time of writing, and Whitaker never did.)

The Roof Of The World went into rehearsal on 27 January, with a large guest cast arriving, including Mark Eden as Marco Polo. In an unusual move, Hussein had been working beforehand on preparing brief animation sequences for the story, which showed a map with a line charting the journey through the course of the episodes that Polo's entourage and the Tardis crew made on their trek to Cathay. Eden would go on to record the narration for these inserts when they were used in each installment. The first episode was recorded on 31 January, and the second, *The Singing Sands* followed the next week, by which time *The Daleks* had finished transmission and a new wave of letters began to arrive.

Demands were being made to bring the Daleks back as soon as they'd been killed off on screen. Lambert spoke to the press saying that if a suitable script was found, it was not an impossibility, but realistically, the truth of the matter was that they would not be seen again until the second season.

The decision had been made to end the first year's run after 42 weeks, though production would keep going for a further 10 weeks, and two more stories would be completed before the production team's summer break. By keeping *Planet Of The Giants* and *The Dalek Invasion Of Earth* back, it reduced the pressure to get material ready by creating a backlog of episodes.

Twelve episodes were still to be filled. Six were committed to *The Sensorites*, by Peter R. Newman, who Whitaker was aware of from his work for the Hammer film studio. This story

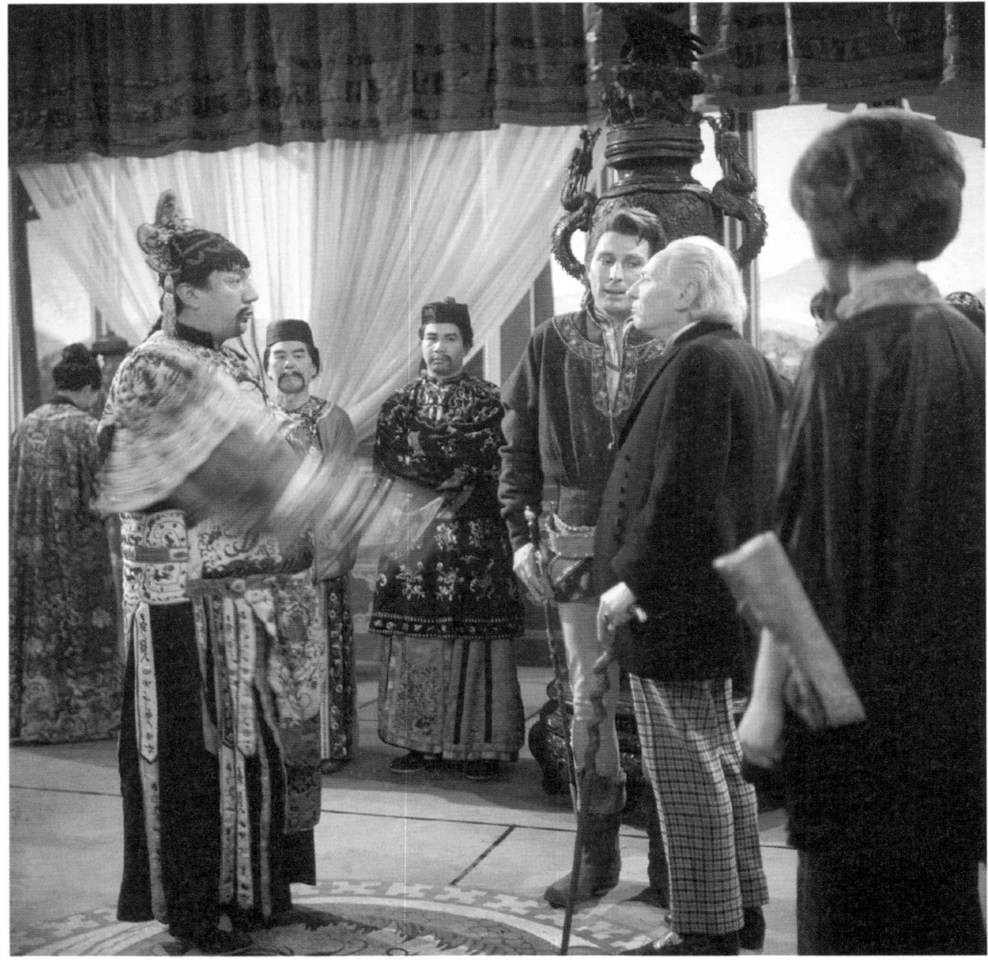

Marco Polo and the Tardis crew arrive in Kubla Khan's palace.

was brought in to replace Whitaker's own, *The New Armada*, which Gerald Blake remembers being approached to direct.

"Verity Lambert actually asked me to work on one of the earliest *Doctor Who* stories, but I never saw a script for it. All I knew was that it had them meeting Sir Francis Drake, and that I'd mentally cast Leonard Sachs. I just don't know what happened. Innes Lloyd also asked me to do some pirate story while Hartnell was still around (probably *The Smugglers*), but I wasn't available for the dates. I finally got to do one when Pat Troughton was in residence (*The Abominable Snowmen*), so I never worked with Bill."

Dennis Spooner's notes indicate that the armada story was certainly reconsidered while he was script editor, but there were far more science fiction stories being written by that point and it remained unused. Spooner takes up the story of how he came to write the final six episodes:

"I'd sent David Whitaker a Robin Hood idea, which he liked but was worried about the amount of comedy in it. He wanted a historical story, and gave me a few options. One was certainly about the invasion of Gaul, a sort of *Doctor Who* meets Asterix, but we agreed to try and do one like *A Tale Of Two Cities*. David was a great literature buff and, *The Reign Of Terror* was the result.

"I think Terry Nation had put a good word about me in his ear, as we'd survived together working for Hancock, so I guess that's why I probably got in there so easily. David always found it hysterical that I'd gone from working with Hancock to *Fireball XL5* and then *Doctor Who*. I can remember him looking at me and saying, 'Comedians, puppets and now this!', before he'd crack up."

The Reign Of Terror was planned as the finale to the series, so eight stories would have been produced in total, out of which only three could be termed as the truly historical stories that Newman had originally wanted.

During the first week of February, Lambert decided to donate two of the Dalek costumes to the orphan village run by the Doctor Barnado's trust in Ilford, on the outskirts of London. The resulting publicity, centering around the fact that children flocked around the Daleks wherever they went, heightened the pressure to bring them back.

To take the pressure off Hussein, Lambert hired John Crockett to come in and direct the fourth episode of *Marco Polo*, *The Wall Of Lies*. This allowed Hussein time between the third and fifth parts, *Five Hundred Eyes* and *Rider From Shang-Tu*, to supervise the increasingly complex studio work that was needed for the final three episodes. William Hartnell always expressed a particular fondness for the story, and in 1967 commented on the sets:

"I always thought it was so tragic that the people watching at home could not see the colours and the patterns of the sets. The

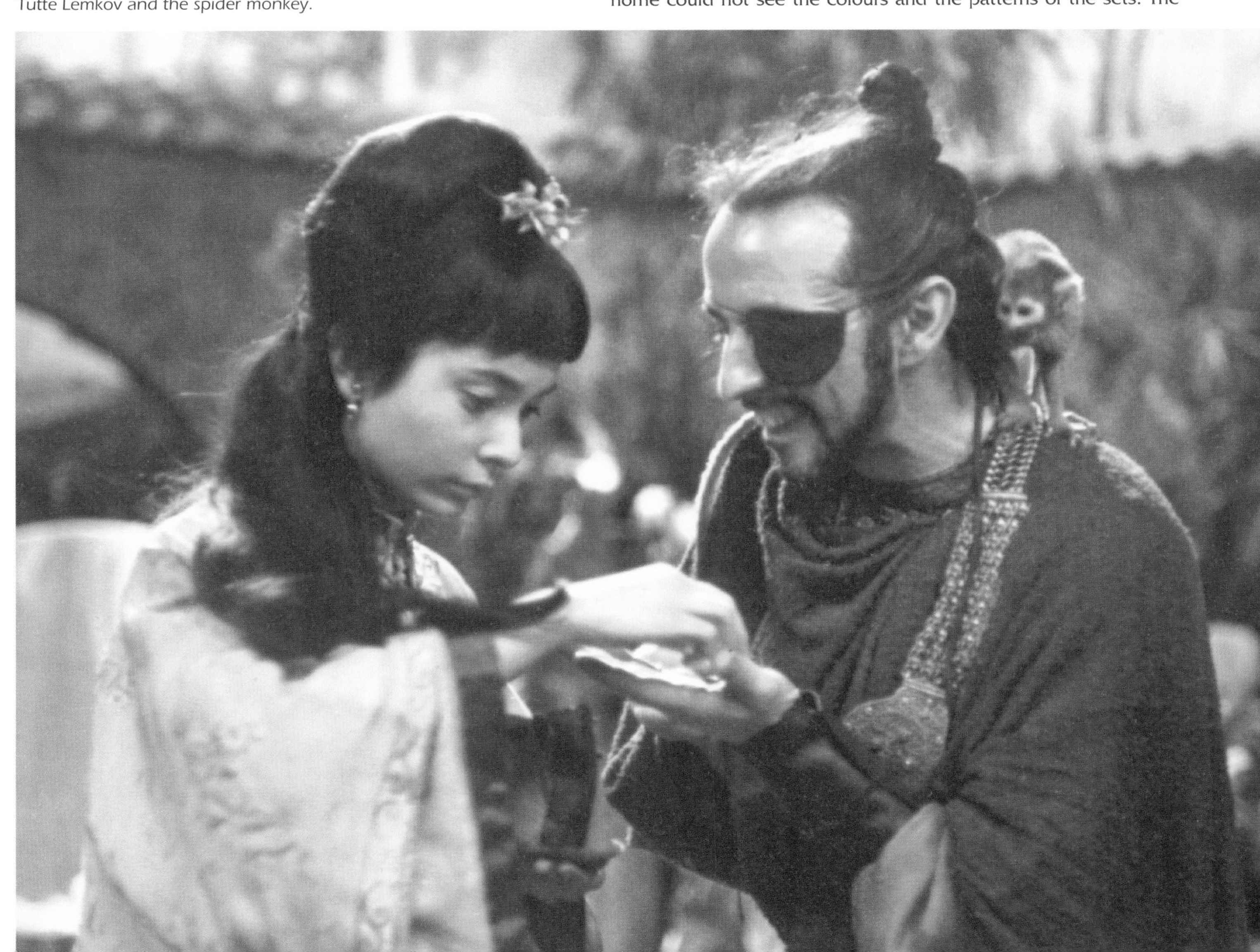

Tutte Lemkov and the spider monkey.

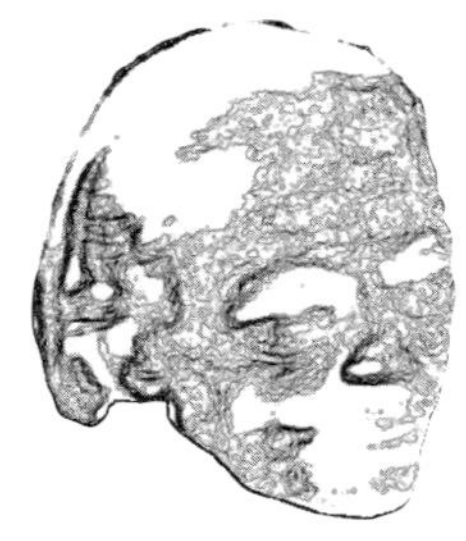

cast would never see them till the end of each week, so when we moved into Lime Grove, and I always felt great anticipation as to what would be awaiting me.

"When Doctor Who met Khubla Khan, there was an air of elegance and grace about the costumes and surroundings that made me proud to be involved with the series. They were breathtaking, and it always saddens me to think that we were the only ones who saw them as they were meant to be seen."

William Russell has a story about Tutte Lemkov, who played Kuiju, and how his scenes involved one of the first instances when live animals were used in the programme.

"Tutte had a spider monkey that was meant to sit on his shoulder and eat grapes during all his scenes, but it just clung round his neck for dear life and stared in terror at the lights. I saw Tutte take it to one side, he talked to it, stroked its head, fed it nuts, and by the time we were recording in the evening, they were the best of friends. I actually think the monkey stole the scenes!"

The final episode, *Assassin At Peking*, went into Lime Grove on 13 March, following *Mighty Kublai Khan* the previous Friday. The fourth episode was transmitted the following day, having been one of the most publicised stories to date, the first ever to feature on the cover of the *Radio Times*, with a photo shot during the recording of the second episode.

Terry Nation had managed to complete the scripts for *The Keys Of Marinus* on schedule, so the first three were ready for the serials director, John Gorrie, to begin work on when he arrived at the end of February. Cusick was back as the designer and faced with an awkward challenge, having to create a new setting for each episode – Nation had created a 'quest' story, as Whitaker had suggested. Five new locations would be needed in total.

Recording for *The Sea Of Death*, the set-up episode of the time travellers' quest to find the Keys of Marinus, took place on 20 March. The story saw the only appearance in the programme's history of Nation's attempt at creating an enduring villain, the Voord.

Skilled assassins, encased in protective armour, their elaborate masks were moulded in vulcanised rubber while their bodies were covered in slightly adapted wet-suits. The overall effect gave them a uniform, shiny black texture that made them difficult to light properly in the studio.

David Whitaker:

"I remember being slightly disappointed by the Voord. You couldn't really tell what they looked like on screen, and that was a shame, because when you saw them in the flesh the effect was rather good."

Mervyn Pinfield, who always tried to reassure the press that any new monsters would not be too frightening, was very fond of the creatures as they reminded him of frogmen from the war.

At the press call on one of the studio days, when press photographers snapped away as Carole Anne Ford grappled with one of the Voord actors (Peter Stenson) who was in full costume, Pinfield commented:

"Our intention has never been to scare children with our monsters. They're there to make the programme exciting. They (the Voord) are not meant to be a successor to the Daleks, whom I'm sure we will see again..."

Dennis Spooner comments:

"Mervyn could never understand why people seemed to prefer the monster stories and it's ironic that when he directed a story (*The Sensorites*), the monsters looked like little old men. One of the costume designers told me that the camera crew called them 'Mervyns', because they thought they looked just like him!"

Although not seen till the climax of *The Velvet Web*, the second episode recorded on 27 March, the Morpho Brain Creatures were the second race of 'monsters' that the story called for. Cusick designed them carefully with air pipes hidden beneath their protective glass chambers so that their skin could be made to pulsate by using air pressure.

In the episode where Barbara Wright discovers the creatures, she tries to smash the jars housing them, and the cost of the containers was such that there could be no rehearsal. There was only one set, and she would have to smash them once, and only once, as the episode was being recorded.

Jacqueline Hill remembers:

"I had to hit them, and there was this resounding thud. Nothing happened. I just couldn't break the glass, and there were the poor things inside wilting on cue, as the supposedly hit them, which it hadn't. We just had to keep going, but it looked as though the shock of someone tapping on their bowls had killed them. It was quite hysterical!"

With the production schedule running for 52 weeks, the strain on the cast was considerable. Lambert had planned for this, with some of the stories being tailored to allow the principal characters

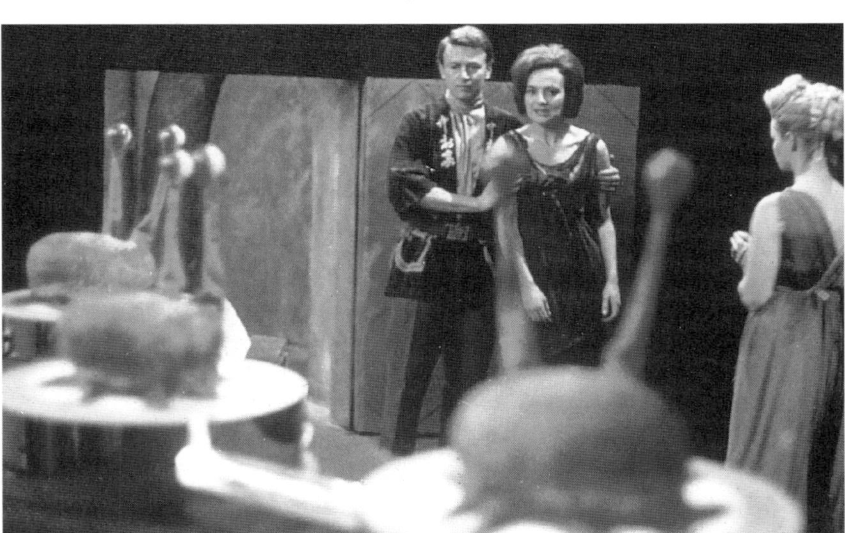

The Morpho brains.

to be absent from the action of the plot for a couple of episodes at a time. *Marinus* saw this brought into effect, with William Hartnell leaving for two weeks as work on *The Velvet Web* was completed, covered by the fact that the next two installments would revolve around his companions' quest to find the 'Keys'.

Dennis Spooner:

"For about four or five weeks after he'd been on holiday, everything was always fine with Bill Hartnell because he'd basically sat fishing and learning his lines so that he was word perfect. It was always the scripts that were handed to him on his return that he started to 'fluff' when we got to them."

The Screaming Jungle was shot on the 3 April and *The Snows Of Terror* on the 10th, with Hartnell back in the rehearsal hall for *Sentence Of Death* on the 13th. Ray Cusick.

"That was the first time the Tardis was seen landing. It was all done as a model shot, and we even had the light on top of it flashing as it appeared. There was also a Buddha-like statue (in *The Screaming Jungle*), which suddenly had to grab Jacqueline Hill.

"The prop was made so that it was hollow, with a large enough cavity for one of the extras to sit inside, with his arms sticking out which were camouflaged to match the rest of the statue. He got terrible cramp because he had to stay in there for ages."

The Voord did not have the same impact as the Daleks at all, although they did go on to appear in the first *Doctor Who* annual, which went on sale at the end of the year. As one viewer observed in a letter to the press:

"Admirably creepy as the current monsters are in *Doctor Who*, they lack the originality of the Daleks, and they don't even have a catchphrase like 'Exterminate! Exterminate!' for children to imitate. Bring back the 'Pepperpots From Space', BBC or at least don't make their successors so sinister."

Crockett went into rehearsal with *The Temple Of Evil*, the first of four episodes that made up *The Aztecs* on 1 May. Hartnell remembered the story with affection.

"The story in the Aztec city allowed me to show a side of the Doctor that I wanted to see more often but the scripts never allowed it. There was a lady in the court he was courteous, civil and charming to (Cameca, played by Margot van de Burgh). He was, after all, a gentleman. I always felt that many of the writers failed to understand that fact."

It took time, but people within the drama department's various divisions began to accept *Doctor Who* and even admire what the production team were achieving.

Gerald Blake:

"*Doctor Who* originally had a bit of a stigma attached to it, it was the skeleton in the closet. One or two producers told me how they'd made formal protests about it to Sydney Newman, and how they were furious that he'd defended it. Six months later the same people were coming up and saying, 'Did you see last night's *Doctor Who*, very clever. Makes you proud to be in the same department'.

'There was an incident around about the time that *Doctor Who* started. *Dixon Of Dock Green* had been going for some time, and there was a reverential attitude towards it, as though you had to ablate in the presence of the blue lamp outside Dixon's police station. Anyway, the police box that they used was kept down at Ealing Studios and it went missing. Someone had written on the floor where it had been, 'Doctor Who Was Here!'. This was the scene shifters' idea of a joke."

Mervyn Pinfield left his duties as Associate Producer mid-way through production on *The Aztecs*, to start preparation on *The Sensorites*, which in the absence of the other regular directors (Hussein, Martin and Chris Barry), he had opted to direct. In a typical one-line comment to the press, he said as the story was launched:

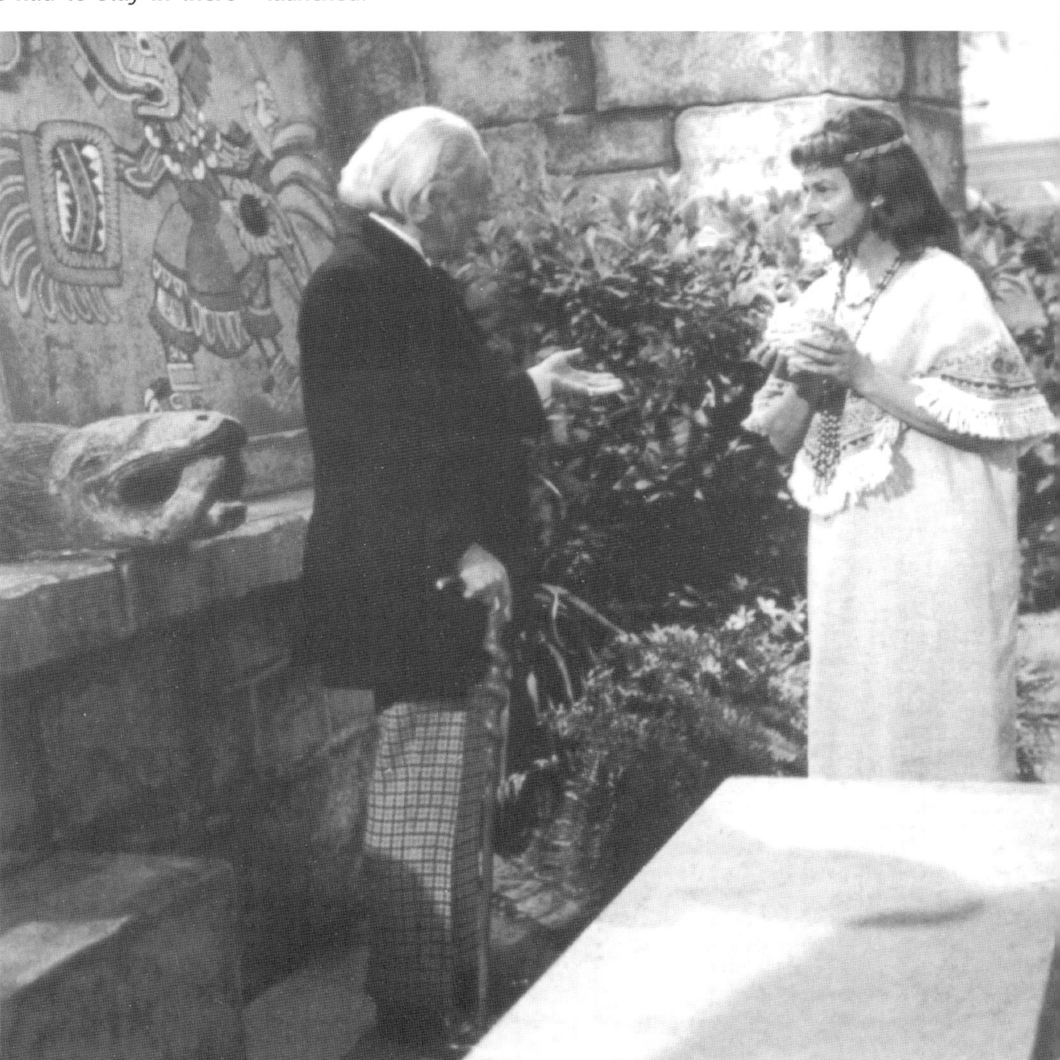

The Doctor with Cameca in the Aztec gardens.

"The Sensorites are by no means meant to scare. They emphasise the point that you must never judge by appearances."

The Sensorites themselves consisted of a simple costume, comprising a body suit with hoops around the feet so that they looked flat and round like plates, while the actor's head was covered with a mask with an enlarged cranium.

The creatures had no mouth or nose, pointed ears and dark eyes, with the sockets on the mask being covered with black

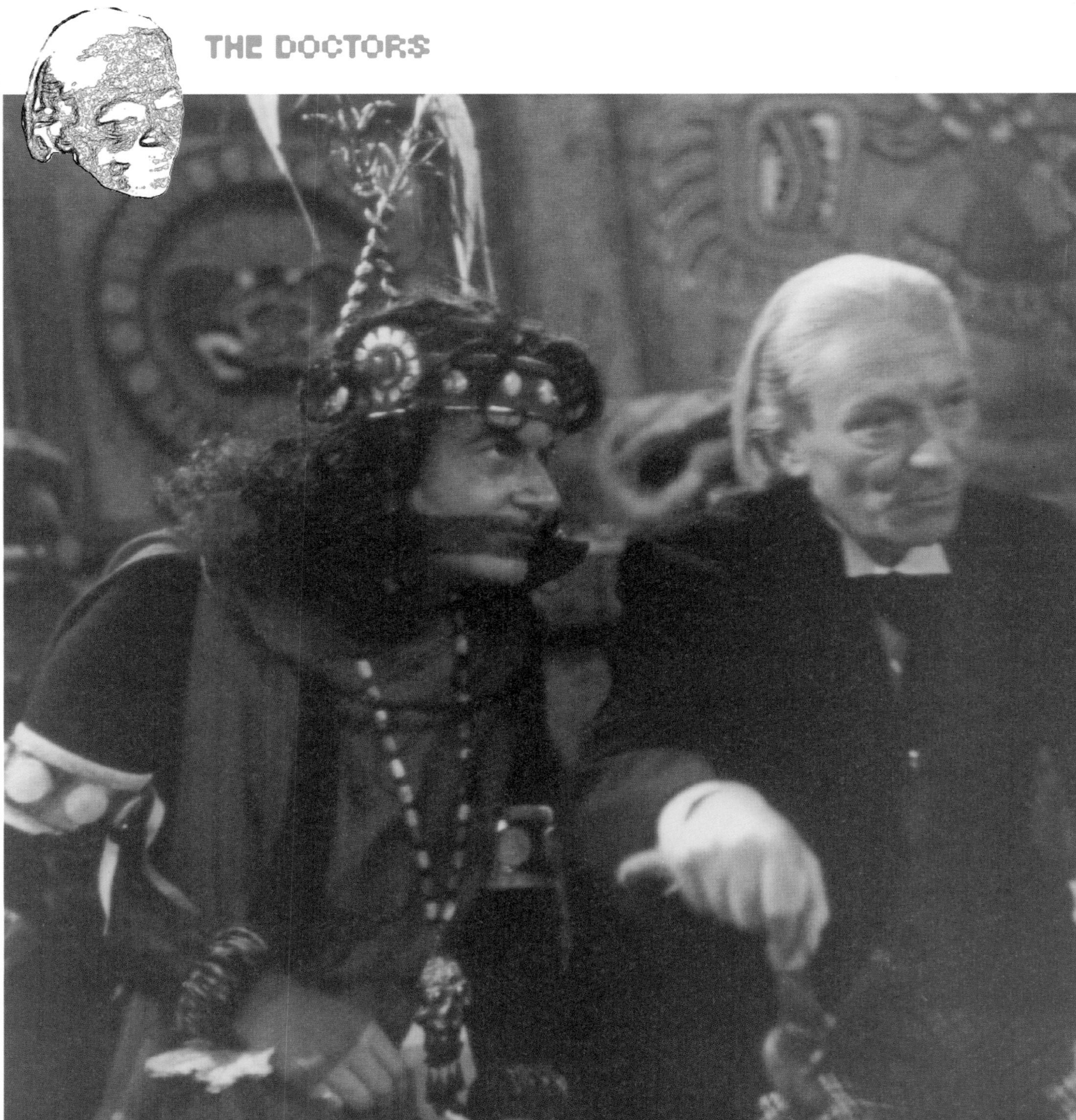

The Doctor and Tlotoxly

gauze on the inside, allowing the actors very limited vision, which frequently resulted in them failing to realise they were standing on each other's enlarged feet.

Ilona Rogers, who played Carol, one of the crew of the spaceship trapped by the Sensorites, remembers:

"William Hartnell thought they were totally silly, but I thought they were rather sweet. He used to call them the 'Pixies', and some of them could barely see at all because they couldn't wear their glasses under the masks."

David Whitaker remembers Pinfield directing the series:

"Mervyn Pinfield was not well for as long as I knew him, he'd been with the BBC for years. There was a joke that he'd held the fuse wire for John Logie Baird when he first invented the TV camera. As far as I can recall, on that first story which he directed there was a decision made to split the workload. Six episodes could take a hell of a toll on a young director, let alone someone as old as Mervyn."

Timothy Combe explains this point further:

"You came in about six weeks before rehearsal to work on the scripts and get the designs done, and then the weekly turnaround of episodes was pretty frantic. The first one I worked on (*The Keys Of Marinus*) was not so bad because John Gorrie (director) was

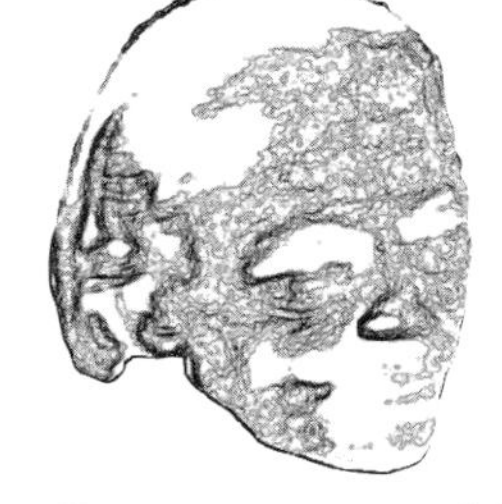

pretty keyed in to what he was doing, but there were horror stories going around of tempers flying with the other directors. The atmosphere could get very tense in the director's gallery and the air could go pretty blue as well!"

Frank Cox returned to take over from Pinfield on the last two episodes of the story. Cusick's work on the sets for the story won praise from the cast.

William Russell:

"The Sensorites story was pretty dull, to be honest, but the sets were superb. There was a wonderful organic feel about them. Someone hit the nail on the head by saying it felt as though you were inside one of the monsters' brains."

The story was completed on Friday nights between 29 May and 3 July. The following day, when the episode *Hidden Danger* was due to be broadcast, an unexpected reprieve in the recording schedule came for the production team. Due to the overrunning of the sports coverage on *Grandstand* that day, *Doctor Who* was postponed for a week. Unexpectedly, the week of lead-in time that had been lost by the remount of *The Dead Planet* had been returned.

The Sensorites.

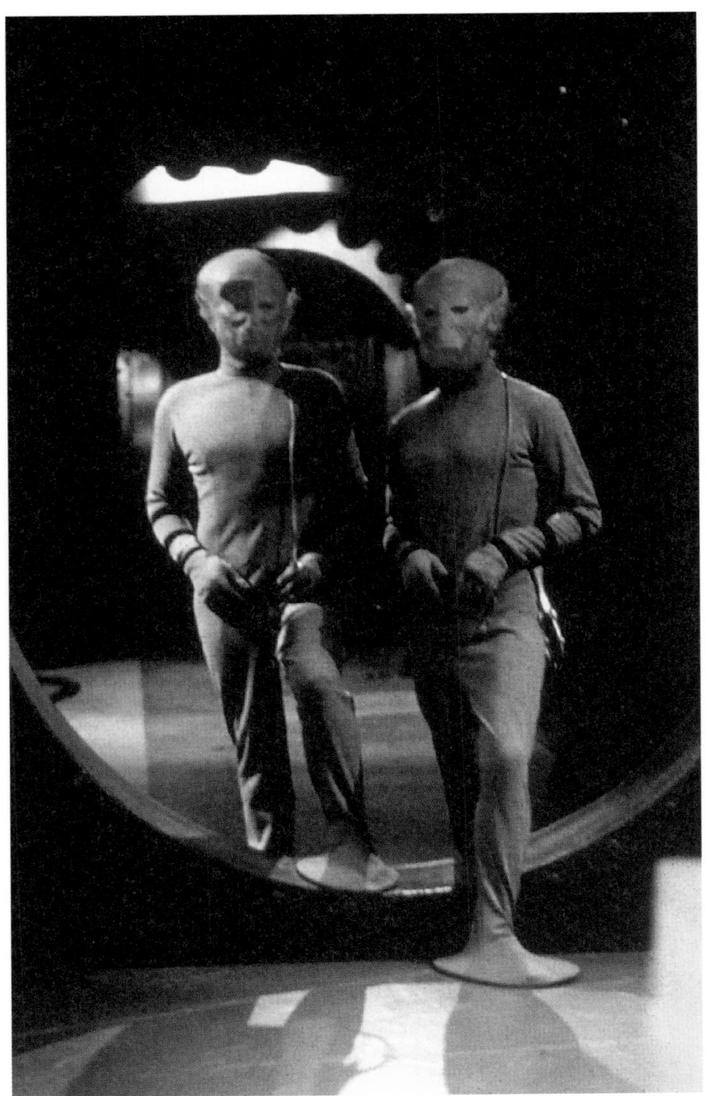

Jacqueline Hill managed to disappear for a couple of episodes on the story for a brief holiday, just as Ford had done in *The Aztecs*, with sequences involving her shot beforehand. William Russell was the final member of the regular cast to do this, filming insert material for episodes two and three of *The Reign Of Terror* when production began.

For the first time, location filming was used in the programme. This was mainly done as a practice run for what was to come with *The Dalek Invasion Of Earth*, as the programme's main film cameraman, Peter Hamilton, explains:

"The French Revolution scenes had about one afternoon's shooting using a double of Doctor Who. It was a dry-run to get a film crew together, because they had the big London shoot coming up with the Daleks (*The Dalek Invasion Of Earth*), and they wanted to iron out any technical problems concerning the equipment before they started."

The double was an extra, Brian Proudfoot, who was used for several brief sequences which were supervised by the Production Assistant, Timothy Combe, on 15 June.

Combe takes up the story:

"Hartnell was rehearsing, so he couldn't do it and they got this poor guy in who he had to train to be Doctor Who. It was hysterical, like watching a great ballet diva training a protege. 'No, no, man! Hold the shoulders straight, walk with dignity! Raise the head. Damn it, Man! Show some pride!' "

A Land Of Fear went before the cameras on 10 July, after a tense week in rehearsal.

Dennis Spooner.

"I certainly went to the run through on the first few episodes, because it was at that time that Verity and David Whitaker asked me to take over as script editor for the second year (David Whitaker was moving to Australia as soon as the first year of production ended).

"I don't know exactly why, but Henric (Hirsch, the director) and Bill Hartnell just didn't get on. I don't know whether he was getting tired because they'd been on the show for a hell of a long time (9 months). The PA was acting like the ref at a boxing match to keep things going."

Combe knew Hartnell well from working on *Marinus*, which was actually completed three months prior to *A Land Of Fear* , and knew how to cope with him when he became irritable.

"Bill and I were actually quite good friends, and I made it my task in life to keep everything happy on that French story. Henric was very charming and suave, but he found *Doctor Who* a hell of a strain. Bill was used to the director's coming in and saying 'Do this, move here, move there', which he could then argue about until they'd agreed on some point. Henric was very much 'Well, what shall we do now?', which annoyed Bill intensely. The situation just got worse and worse..."

Guests Of Madame Guillotine was finished on 17 July, and it was during the week of rehearsals for *A Change Of Identity* when things started to go badly wrong.

Timothy Combe:

"Henric had only done one television play before, which was a James Joyce story, and I don't think he really wanted to do *Doctor Who*. He had no real idea how to plan everything out – I had to

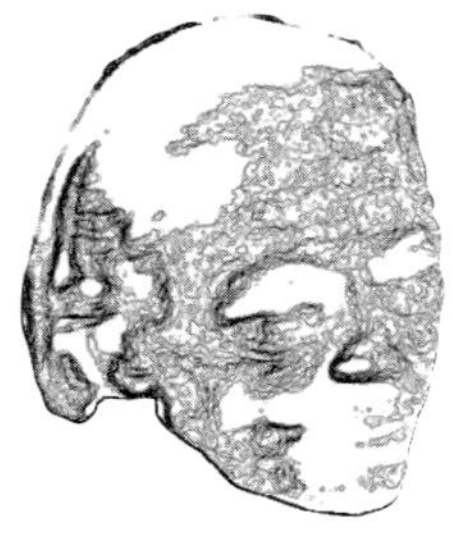

do his camera script for the last few episodes and ended up calling the shots for him. He got very ill through the stress; it was absolutely wrong for him, he should never have said he'd do it."

Hirsch felt unwell during the afternoon runthrough of the episode in studio, and actually collapsed outside the control gallery. Combe took over the rehearsal while Lambert quickly found a director who was free, *Marinus's* John Gorrie, to take over for the recording in the evening.

Dennis Spooner:

"Tim Combe worked minor miracles to keep everything going after Henric had collapsed. It caused quite a shock, and everything was planned much more carefully after that to keep everything calm. I played bridge with Henric nearly every night, and I thought he was a very pleasant character.

"Tim used to go out to dinner with Bill to make sure that there were no problems with him, and it was certainly not as difficult for the last few episodes. Tim wet-nursed him through till the end, calling out the camera shots and blocking everything out in the studio. We got through it, but only just."

Prisoners Of The Concierge marked the end of the first series when it was broadcast on 12 September. The ratings were holding with a steady regular audience of between six and a half and seven million viewers – quite a fall, compared to the height of the season's popularity after the Daleks had made their debut. The success of *Doctor Who*, however, cannot be attributed merely to the arrival of the Daleks or any of the other monsters. Without the central performance of William Hartnell, it's doubtful whether it would have succeeded at all. Hartnell spoke of his first year in the role in 1967:

"The first batch of stories were quite difficult, because as with any play or series, it takes time for you to grow to trust the people around you. I quickly saw that they were people who I could rely on. They became my second family."

Fifty two weeks in a continuous rehearse/record situation would be hard for any actor to cope with, as the casts of *Z-Cars, Compact, The Newcomers*, and other shows that were in the same situation have testified. Learning different scripts from week to week was a nightmare, and the numerous stories that circulate

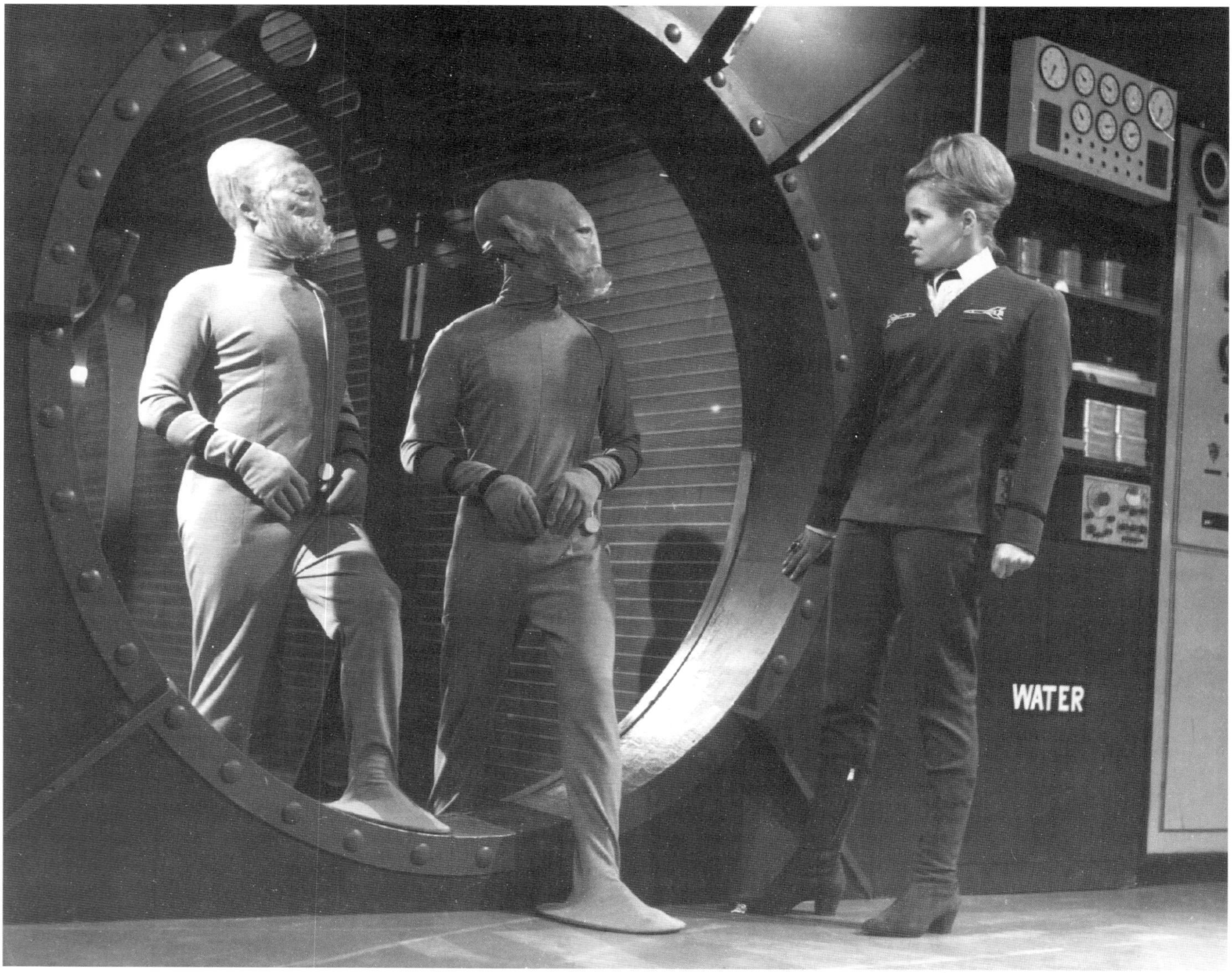

Ilona Rogers confronts the Sensorites.

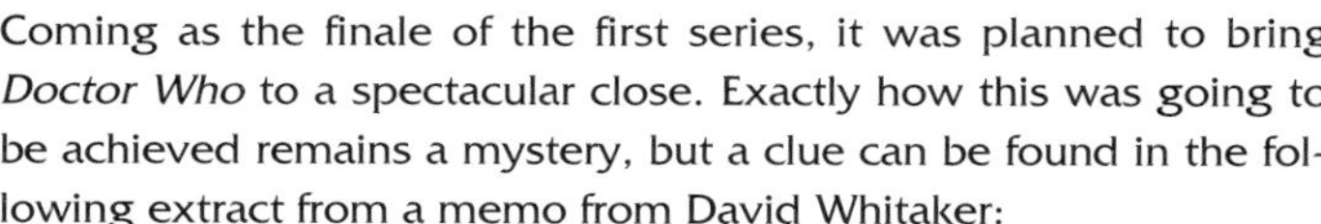

about the cantankerous behaviour of Hartnell on the set are not without foundation.

The strain on him was immense. Apart from carrying the programme as its star, he was suffering the early stages of arteriosclerosis (hardening of the main arteries, resulting in poor blood circulation), which would eventually lead to him retiring from the acting profession towards the end of the 1960s.

Innes Lloyd:

"Bill was not a well man and he tended to keep very quiet about exactly what was wrong with him. He had something wrong with his circulation, and this made it extraordinarily difficult for him to concentrate. He was a perfectionist, and it got more and more of a strain to get the kind of performance he was satisfied with, and more importantly, to get the lines right."

With *The Reign Of Terror* finished, work began on the final realisation of Webber's original idea for the pilot story, with a miniaturisation plot in *Planet Of The Giants*, which was written by the future award-winning drama Producer, Louis Marks. The story would act as the run-up to the return of the Daleks, which the public had been demanding since the beginning of the year.

William Hartnell:

"I began to dread the return of the Daleks, but not for the obvious reason. I admired the design and the skill of the writing, it was just the fact that every time they appeared, I knew I would loose another member of my 'family', so as to speak.

"First there was Carole Ann (in *The Dalek Invasion Of Earth*), then Bill and Jacqui (they left after *The Chase*), and the poor Greek girl (Katarina, played by Adrienne Hill, who was killed in *The Daleks' Master Plan*). I always had this dreadful feeling that one day, the Daleks would come for me!"

Mervyn Pinfield took on the task of directing the story. With his expertise in the technical tricks that could be staged in a television studio, he was ideally suited for such a complex production. He worked closely with Ray Cusick, who was back as designer.

"We had to accommodate the two life-size enlarged sets in the same studio (all episodes for the story were shot in TC4 at TV Centre), so one side had the lab and the garden, and the other had a gigantic sink plughole or giant dead worms in the garden!"

Douglas Camfield was brought in to handle the last of the four episodes that were recorded, between the 21 August and 11 September, and arrived several weeks before to trail Pinfield in pre-production.

Camfield commented:

"It was strange for someone to take over midway through a serial, and I think it was actually unheard of on other shows, but Mervyn was not well, and I think I was brought in as back-up more than anything else."

Although four episodes were actually shot (*Planet Of Giants, Dangerous Journey, Crisis* and *The Urge To Live*), it was cut down to three in post-production.

David Whitaker:

"The *Giant* story was terribly slow moving, because you couldn't have people an inch tall stride across a garden in a matter of minutes – it took them hours, so the plot dragged dreadfully."

Crisis became the episode title for the amalgamation of the two blocks of filming, making the story a three-partner. The press build-up behind the return of the series created a lot of public interest, so when the story was broadcast at the end of October, the ratings averaged out at eight and a half million viewers.

Terry Nation had been commissioned to write a sequel to *The Daleks*, which he initially called *The Return Of The Daleks*. Coming as the finale of the first series, it was planned to bring *Doctor Who* to a spectacular close. Exactly how this was going to be achieved remains a mystery, but a clue can be found in the following extract from a memo from David Whitaker:

"If Doctor Who were to die, I cannot think of a more noble demise than in destroying his ultimate nemesis. If there is one thing that goes against everything he stands for, and brings his anger to the surface, it is the total injustice and tyranny that the Daleks represent.

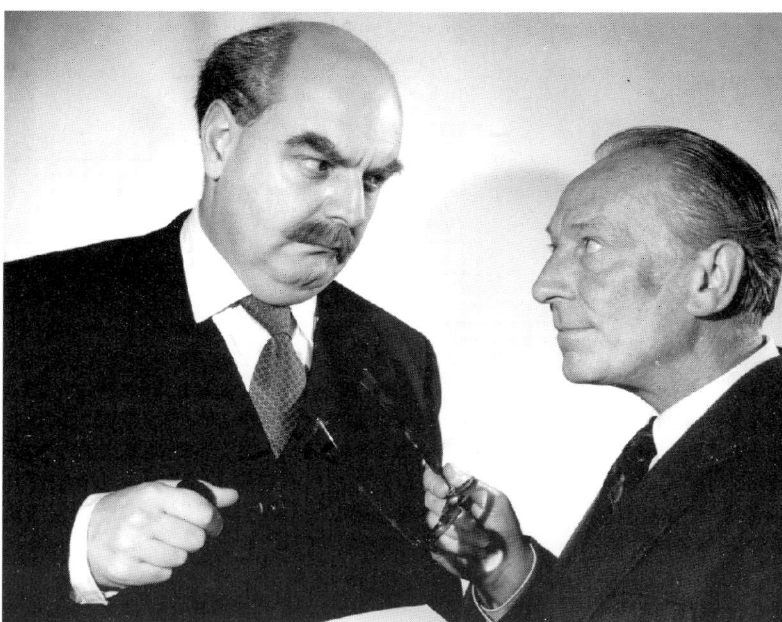

Derek Francis and William Hartnell in **After the Party**, prior to working together again in **The Romans**.

"Doctor Who has regarded the earth as his home for many years, and if there were a threat facing his world that put its very existence at risk, I am sure that he would have very few qualms about making the ultimate sacrifice to preserve its freedom."

With the second season being confirmed by Sydney Newman, the demise of the series was no longer an issue for Whitaker to worry about, and *The Dalek Invasion Of Earth* became the second story of the new series.

Technically speaking, it was to be the most ambitious production that the *Doctor Who* team had ever attempted, with six days of location filming prior to the studio work. Every story, with the exception of *Inside The Spaceship*, required insert filming of some sort – whether it was model work or stunt sequences filmed at Ealing, there was invariably something that had to be shot before studio recording started.

Peter Hamilton:

"It was like being a member of the SAS, getting up in the middle of the night to stage the invasion of London with some BBC props and trying to avoid any straying members of the public. There were always one or two partygoers heading home, who

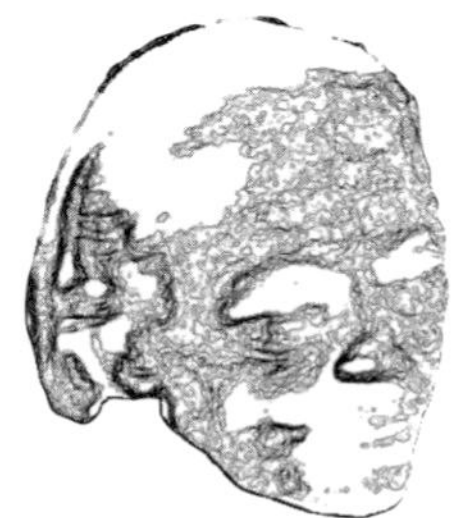

nearly had a heart attacks when they saw the Daleks heading towards them!

"We had a Dalek in the Thames that slowly rose out of the water on a pulley system, with the guy inside in his trunks, and it kept getting stuck. It took ages to get right and when we got back it suddenly struck me, 'What the hell was a Dalek doing in the Thames, anyway?'. I don't think anybody gave me a good explanation."

Richard Martin returned to direct the story, and on 18 September took *World's End* into Studio One at the Riverside Studios, run by the BBC in Hammersmith. With Cusick and Newbery now taking a well-earned rest after close to a year of continuous work on the series, Cusick's former assistant, Spencer Chapman, took on the job of building the interiors of the Daleks' flying saucer and the vast landing bay where it touched down. The whole series was set in and around the deserted streets of London, and as William Russell recalled in 1965:

"I was told by one of the guys inside the Daleks that when it came to the part where they storm across Westminster Bridge, they were waiting for their cue and out of the side of his casing he saw a nun hurry past desperately trying to ignore them. There was nobody else in sight, as the camera team were on the other side of the bridge and the production assistants were out of view. It was about five in the morning, and when they told the others, nobody believed them because they couldn't understand what a nun would be doing there at that time of day. So there was this story going around the set that the Daleks had seen a ghost nun!"

The Daleks made their first speaking appearance in the story in the second episode, *The Daleks*, recorded on 25 September. Four Daleks had been made, based around the casings of the two that the BBC still held from the first story with the chance being taken to slightly upgrade the design to make them more durable, as it was inevitable even then that this would not be their last story and they would certainly have to endure future filming. If they looked the same, their voices certainly didn't carry the same resonance as before.

The Daleks (their first story) used a pre-recorded soundtrack which had been treated by the Radiophonic Workshop, for all their dialogue. The 'ring-modulator', which distorted the human voice into that of a Dalek's, was now housed in the Riverside Studio and the voices were done live, by actor Peter Hawkins.

"I had to use a very precise vocal pattern to get the words out, otherwise they just blurred together and came out as 'babble'. The chaps inside the costumes had to learn the same dialogue as myself, so that they could hit a button inside and make the lights on the Daleks' heads flicker in sync with what they were saying. Thankfully they knew what they're doing and I don't think there was ever a time when they flashed away in silence."

Day Of Reckoning and *The End Of Tomorrow* were shot on 2 and 9 October and on the first of those two there was an unexpected accident involving William Hartnell when he hurt his back during the on-set rehearsal. Whitaker had to quickly rewrite scenes in which Hartnell was involved with a double being used in his place. Although the filming was being closely followed by the press, news of the accident strangely made only one of the evening newspapers, with Lambert stating that, "Mr. Hartnell is fine, and he will only be absent from one of the episodes of the new Dalek story. He expects to be back before the cameras next week."

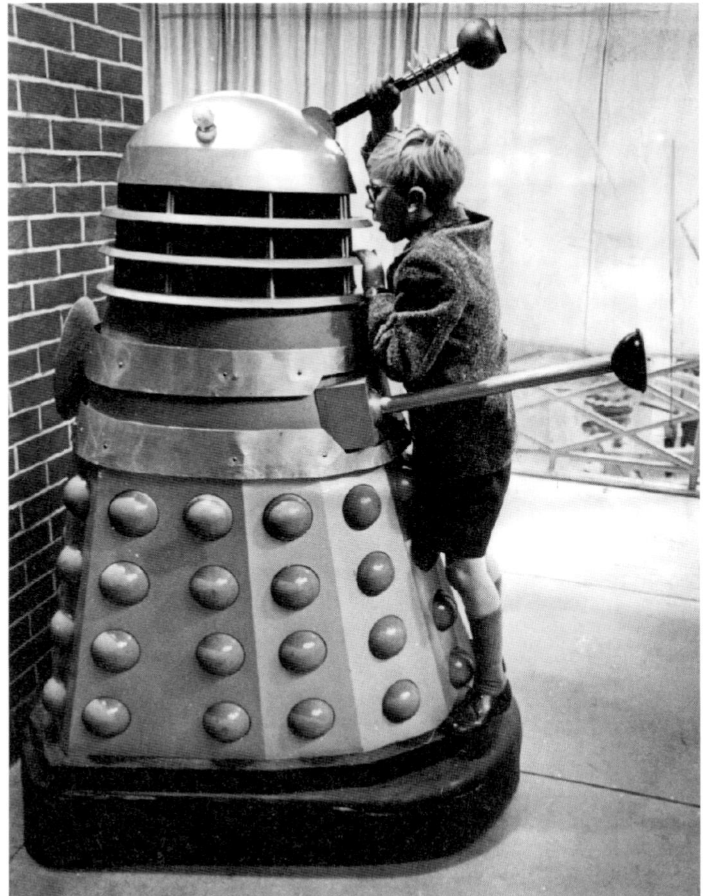

Geoffrey Sawyer, aged 11, examining a Dalek at the Daily Mail Schoolboys and Girls Exhibition in 1965.

The Doctor was knocked out for the duration of that installment, and as Hartnell recalled in 1967:

"There was only one time when I hurt myself, and it was an accident. Towards the end of each year, everyone began to feel the strain and get a bit careless. With all the explosions and chases we had going on, I'm surprised nobody ever got seriously injured."

After *The Waking Ally* (16th October), the final episode saw the first of the significant changes that would take place through the course of the second season. Susan Foreman had left the series, and actress Carole Anne Ford also elected to leave and move on to other projects. She felt unhappy about the way the character had developed and wanted to break free of the series. *Flashpoint* on 24 October was her last time on the Doctor *Who* set.

"Bill was furious," Dennis Spooner recalled. "He was absolutely livid, because the first he knew about it was when he read the script. Carole genuinely wanted to move on and didn't want to be typecast as a schoolgirl for the rest of her life. She was in her twenties then, and wanted to do other things.

"He came storming in to David Whitaker's office, waving his script, saying, 'Why wasn't I asked, why did no one consult me?' And David, who was ever the diplomat, said, 'Surely it's up to Carole to do what she wants.' Well, that floored Bill, and he quietly said, 'But, she was my granddaughter...' Then we both realised

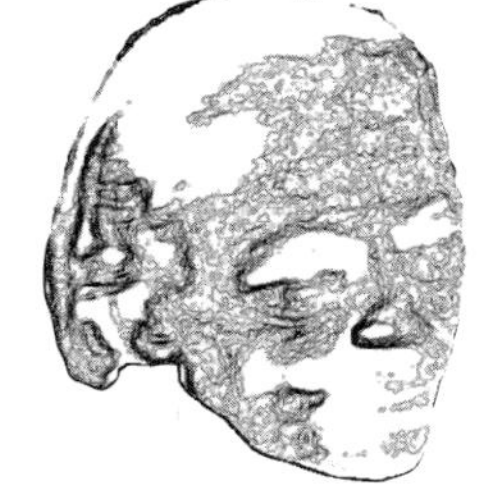

that he was actually quite upset about it, so we took an early lunch and went to the pub with him."

David Whitaker adds to the story:

"Hartnell was very upset when Carole went, but then I pointed out that the series would still keep going without her. He thought about this and came to the conclusion that things weren't so bad, as he still had Bill Russell and Jacqui, and I just didn't have the heart to tell him that they'd already been to Verity and asked if they could leave as well."

Hartnell was, however, getting a lot of feedback from children, which he found highly enjoyable.

"The most charming child comes up to me, a total stranger, and asks if he could shake the hand of Doctor Who. Then I realise that I'm no stranger at all, to him and every other child, I'm their friend. I could not dream of getting a more fulfiling response to my work than this. After years of playing killers and Sergeant Major Bullimore (Hartnell's regular character in *The Army Game*), it's the most refreshing change."

The Dalek Invasion Of Earth was an enormous hit, with a *Radio Times* cover heralding its arrival and a regular audience of over eleven million viewers tuning in. At its peak, the serial was getting just under twelve and a half million. It marked a period when the programme was at its height of popularity, only equalled during Tom Baker's reign.

After the end of season party, the cast and crew went their separate ways, with Lambert taking a brief holiday before returning in the first week of November to start work with Dennis Spooner on the rest of Season Two. The cast were due to return on 31 November to begin rehearsals on *The Rescue*, the last two-part script completed by Whitaker before he left the country.

"Dennis was very accommodating, saying that if ever there was a star I thought the Tardis should visit, or a conqueror Doctor Who should nudge off his throne, to just write and send it in. I was the 'Boss', according to him, and what the 'Boss' wrote got made. I took him up on it. I had time to relax, and *The Crusades* was the result."

Maureen O'Brien was brought before the press just before filming began, revealing how excited she was to be taking on the job of the new companion.'

"It's tremendously exciting. I can't wait to meet the Daleks as I think they're rather cuddly. I'm looking forward to travelling through time as well, as I think the clothing from the past is so wonderful. I hope we go to somewhere like ancient Rome, or meet one of the great kings."

Christopher Barry returned to direct the series, under contract to make six studio bound episodes, as the budget was now tight. Lambert had planned the stories to be relatively confined, to save on money which had been overspent on the location filming of *The Dalek Invasion Of Earth*. She had calculated that this would even out the production costs nicely.

Desperate Measures was completed on 11 December and Jacqueline Hill had fond memories of the story:

"When Maureen came into the show, she had this cute pet monster that followed her around but it got killed, which I thought was a shame. I thought it would have been fun to have it as a pet on board the Tardis, pottering around the control room, but somehow I don't think Bill would have stood for that."

Derek Francis arrived the following week to start work on *The Romans*, as Emperor Nero. Hartnell was delighted to have him join the programme as they'd known each other for years, working on various films and plays together in the past.

In 1976, Francis was interviewed about the time he spent working on *Doctor Who*.

"Billy Hartnell and I had known each other for about twenty years, so it was a bit of a riot for four weeks. Tremendous fun. There was a twinkle in his eye and he'd give me a look that always made me want to laugh, but he didn't get me until the end.

"It came to the bit where Nero goes mad, you know, the Nero fiddles while Rome burns bit, and Billy was standing off camera watching me go rocketing over the top. They called 'Cut', and he just made a quiet 'Tut, tut' sound as he walked away, shaking his head, saying, 'Typical, just typical', and that's when I started to laugh."

The script was by Spooner, and it was the first attempt made in the programme to do an out-and-out comedy adventure – something that Whitaker had advised as being unsuitable for the format when Spooner had submitted his Robin Hood script to him the previous year.

Spooner explains:

"David was always worrying about how Hartnell would react to humour being introduced, but, as I pointed out, he'd just spent years in a sitcom with *The Army Game*, so if anybody knew about dead-pan timing, it was him. He was the master of the disbelieving stare whenever Bootsie and Snudge came up with a scheme (Characters in the sitcom played by Bill Fraser and Alfie Bass).

"I took Bill to one side, and said, 'Do you want to have a go at this?', and he was all for it. So I went to David and told him, and he gave me a helpless look and said, 'Just wait till I've gone, okay?' So I did."

The Slave Traders was completed on 18 December, with *All Roads Lead To Rome, Conspiracy* and *Inferno* following, with allowances being made for time off during the Christmas period.

William Russell:

"The one in Rome was strange, because the week before we were on an alien planet, then we were charging around as though it was a *Carry On* film, and before we knew it, there were giant ants everywhere (*The Web Planet*). I think *Doctor Who* was one of the most unpredictable shows I've ever worked on."

William Hartnell, in 1965:

"The variety of stories never ceases to amaze me. Now, for example, we are in the middle of an attempt by the Daleks to invade the entire universe (he was talking midway through recording *The Daleks' Master Plan*), and as far as I can recall, this time last year we were in ancient Rome."

The Rescue and *The Romans* got ratings as high as thirteen million, but that was peaked by the first new story to go into production in 1965, which was perhaps one of the most costly and innovative ever attempted in the programme's history.

Dennis Spooner explains:

"Bill Strutton had been working on the Zarbi story for ages, certainly well before I arrived. It was one of the stories that Verity set up, because she found him and brought him in to see David Whitaker."

"I didn't have to touch a word when the scripts came in as he'd practically edited them himself, but it was quite clear that it would cost a packet. You had all these ants at war with giant butterflies (the Menoptera), and there wasn't a human in sight. I pointed this out to Verit, and she got quite excited about doing a pure science fiction story, even if it hit the budgets for the next few stories."

Richard Martin arrived at the beginning of December to co-ordinate directing the story, and decided to hire a choreographer to help make the Menoptera more alien, by giving them strange movements and devising an odd, clipped vocalisation for their dialogue. Roslyn de Winter took on the job, and being an actress, she was also hired to play one of the creatures herself.

Filming for all the sequences involving the Menoptera flying (using a kirby-wire system) and the climactic battle between the two races on the planet Vortis was staged at Ealing in the first week of January 1965. None of the main cast were needed for these scenes, so rehearsals for *The Romans* were not affected.

Bill Strutton stated:

"After the Daleks, I thought I had to do something different. I got the idea for the new insect creatures from an encyclopedia, and I'd seen ants fighting in the wilds of Australia, so I put the two together."

The Zarbi costumes were constructed in three main sections – the head, middle and rear, with vinyl leggings held up with braces under the main body shell. Wires enabled the actor inside to manipulate the pincers, and they could see where they were going through a small hole under the head section, obscured from camera-view with black gauze.

The Menoptera costumes were black catsuits lined with rings of yellow fur, which Spooner recalls made them look like 'pacifist bumble bees'. The head was covered with a cowl, and the face painted to match the colouring of the costume. The creatures' vast wings were made from lightweight plastic layered across a frame, which could be spread open to reveal the full wingspan on some of the suits.

William Hartnell:

"The ant monsters, the Zarbi – I was not over-keen on them, but the beautiful Menoptera were different. I thought this showed the potential *Doctor Who* has to present the fact that all is not evil in the universe but I have little interest in finding out for real.

"If I were offered the chance to travel to the stars, I would decline. If man was meant to meet the Daleks, or whatever lives on other planets, he would have been born there."

A venom grub, a Menoptera and a Zarbi.

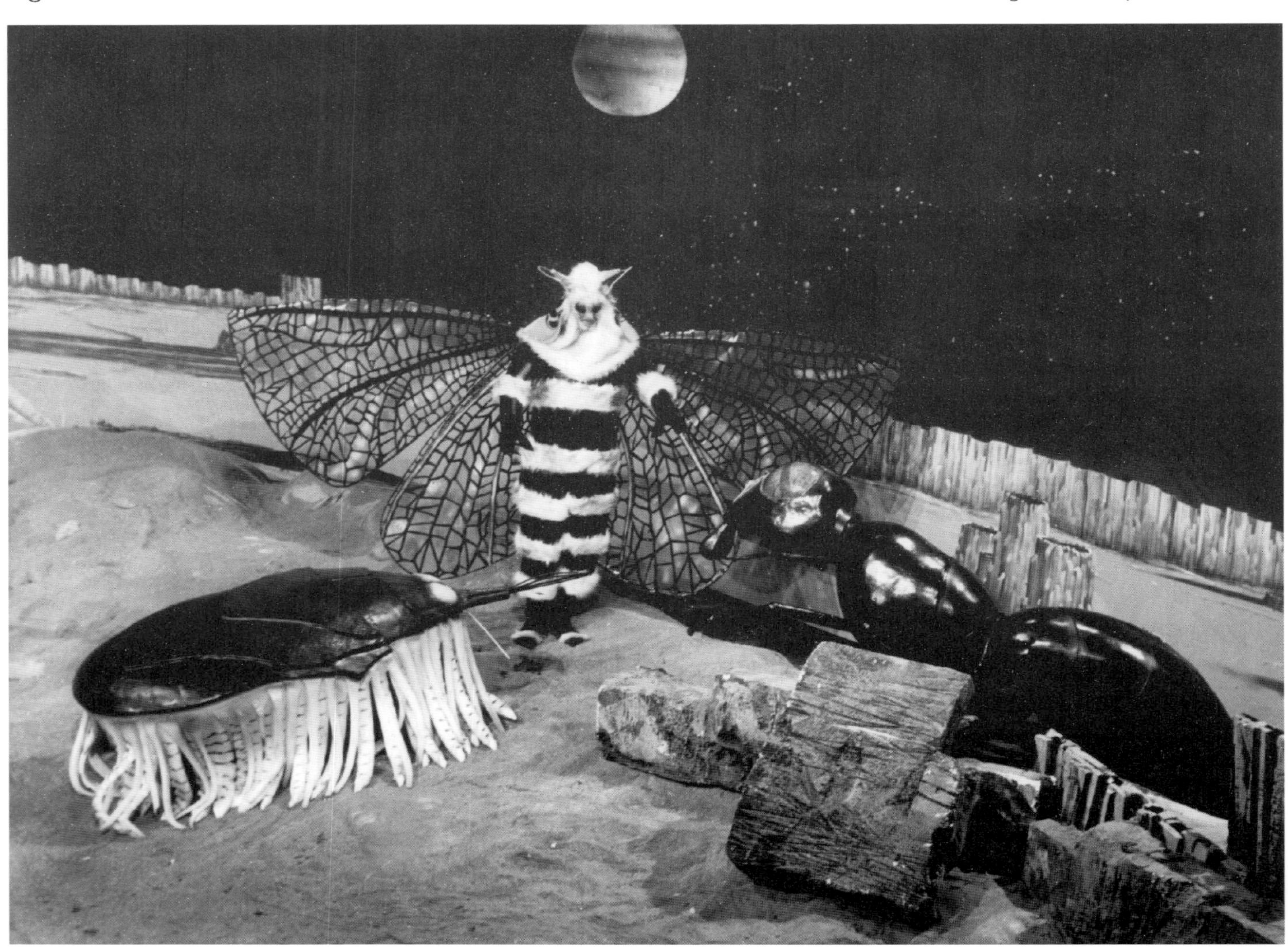

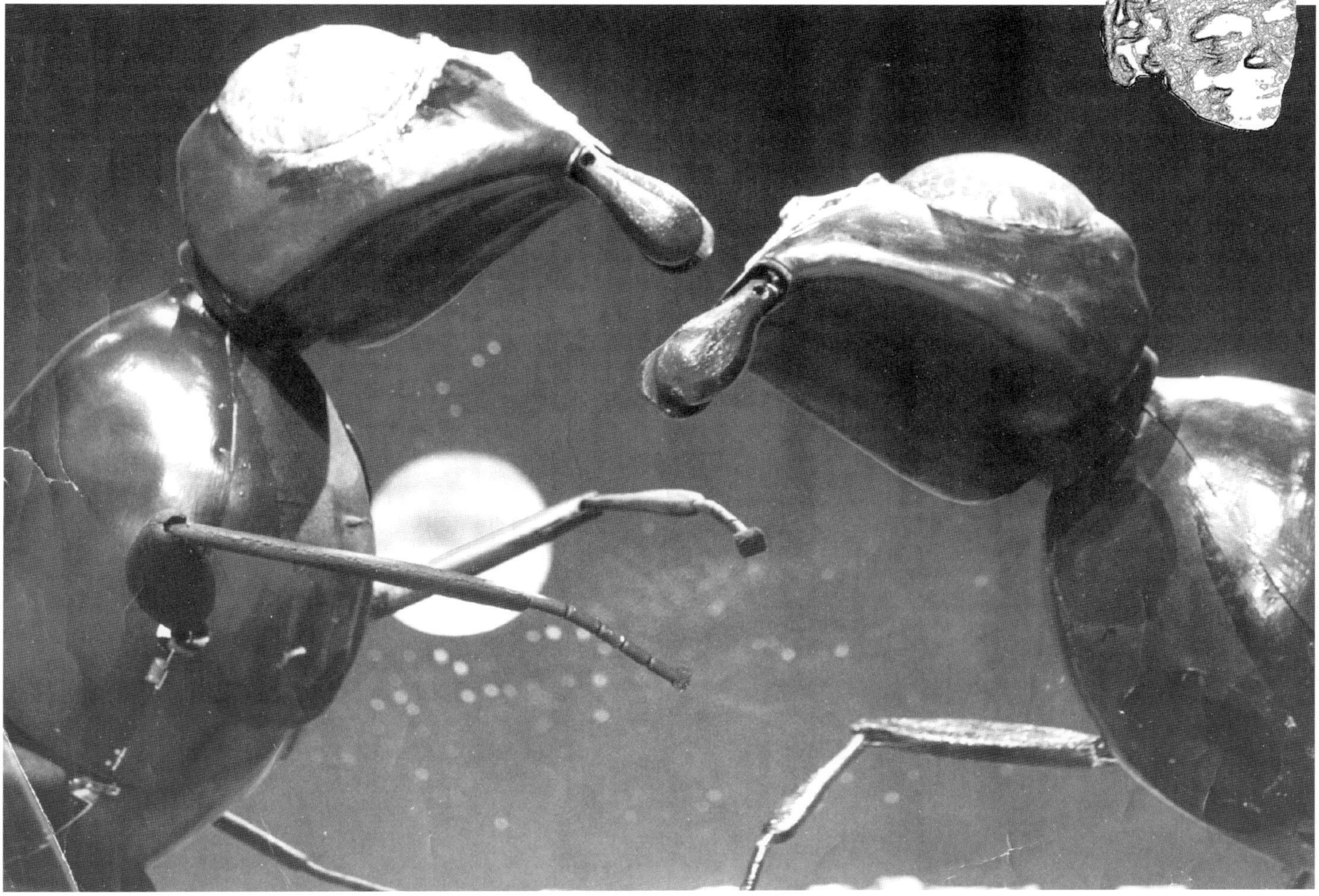

Zarbis in conversation.

Escape To Danger was completed on 5 February, and *Crater Of Needles* on 12 February, with the third race of aliens on the planet being introduced. The Optera were the mutated descendants of the Menoptera, who fled deep within the caverns of the planet when the Carsenome, the parasitical intelligence controlling the Zarbi, first took control of Vortis. The costumes were made of heavy rubber, with the legs held together so that the creatures had to hop to be able to move.

Dennis Spooner:

"Bill Russell though they were hysterical, and they were nicknamed 'The Flowerpot Monsters', because they looked like deranged versions of Bill and Ben."

The final two episodes, *Invasion* and *The Centre*, were shot on 19 and 26 of February, with the resulting costs cutting heavily into the budgets for the next two serials.

Spooner:

"The Zarbi were basically meant to be the next Daleks, I think there were even one or two bits of merchandise that were made, but there was no way we could afford to bring them back, even though the story was a huge hit."

The first episode hit a ratings peak of thirteen and a half million viewers, which would not be beaten until well into Tom Baker's run in the series.

Spooner was right. Toy manufacturers were looking for potential characters to latch on to, particularly monsters, as the demand for Dalek toys during Christmas 1964 was severely underestimated. The market would be flooded with toys, games and books towards the end of 1965, when 'Dalekmania' really took a grip of the country's children.

Terry Nation was already hard at work on a third Dalek serial, which had a working title of *The Pursuers*. Martin was booked to return four weeks after *The Web Planet* had been completed to begin pre-production work on it, although there is a suggestion from Spooner that *The Chase*, as it would finally be called, was not Nation's original idea for the new adventure.

"One of the designers (possibly Cusick or *The Web Planet's* John Wood) wanted to have the Daleks on the moon, reasoning that they were alien and didn't need oxygen, so it could be shown that they could go into any atmosphere and not be affected.

"Terry wanted the Daleks to invade America and have them going to all the famous landmarks, but I can't recall if he ever wrote a draft with them on the moon. Verity wanted a new race of robots that would be as equally dangerous as the Daleks, and the result of all these ideas flying round was *The Chase* which, to be honest, was a bit of a mess."

David Whitaker had spent the past few months completing *The Crusade*, a historical adventure based around the legends of Richard The Lionheart. In many respects, he surpassed all of the other historical stories with what was generally regarded by the production team as some of his finest work on the series.

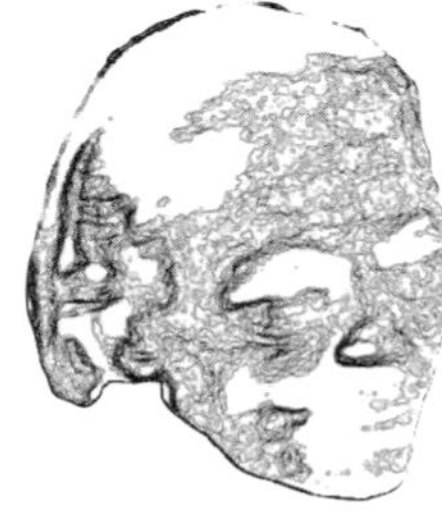

Douglas Camfield:

"*The Crusade* was my first full *Doctor Who* as a director and I couldn't have dreamed of getting a better script. It was beautifully crafted, superbly researched. Whitaker was the 'boss' when it came to *Doctor Who*, and not a word of it was changed.."

Dennis Spooner:

"David had certainly come up with the goods. It was almost Shakespearian in many ways, and I remember that some of the actors came up to me saying they'd never watched the show, and that they hadn't realised the scripts were of such a high quality. I told David, but he didn't see it as a compliment. He was one of the most self-effacing people I've ever met."

The story, which had a working title of *Doctor Who and The Saracen Hordes*, saw the return of Barry Newbery as the designer. Both he and Cusick had requested that other designers come in to work on the show, so the workload was not so intense for them, so John Wood and Spencer Chapman were now regulars of the programme. *The Crusade* was one of the episodes that Newbery oversaw for the second season.

Dalek on location for **The Chase**.

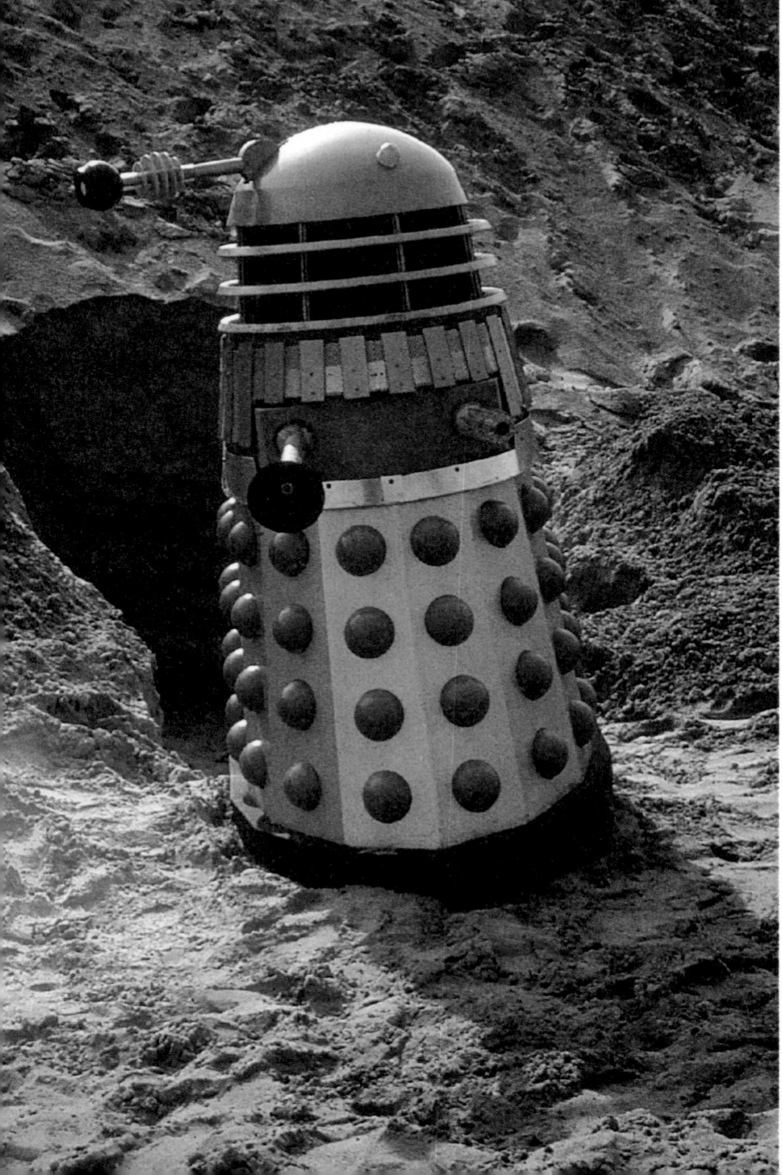

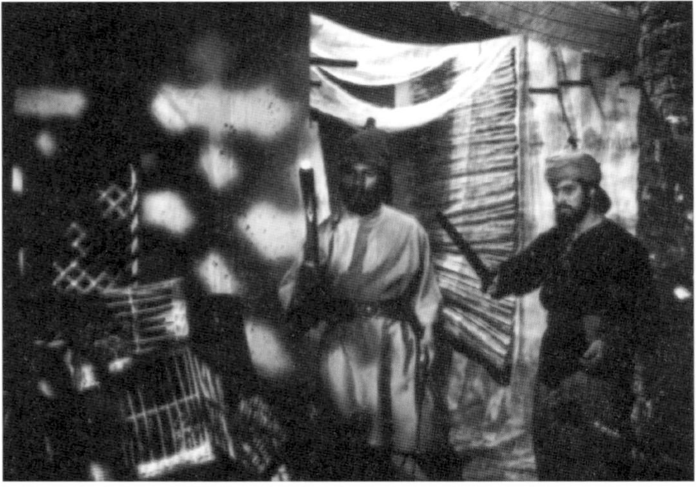

Saracens from **The Crusades**.

Two of the new cast worth noting in this story are Julian Glover and Jean Marsh. Marsh would go on to appear in the third season as a regular companion, while Glover, a respected actor, broke the taboo of appearing in the series.

Douglas Camfield:

"There was a certain reluctance by 'name' actors to work on *Doctor Who*, not wanting to be seen in something as trivial as a 'kid's programme'. I don't have any time for actors who get that precious. Well, Julian didn't have that kind of problem at all. He looked at the quality of the script and considered whether it would offer him any challenges, rather than think about who'd be watching the finished show."

The Warlords finished the story off on 26 March, with Lambert so pleased with the result that she asked if Camfield would be available to come back in May to begin work on another historical adventure which Spooner was writing called *The Time Meddler*.

The money lost on *The Web Planet* severely cut into the money available for the next serial, *The Space Museum*, which Pinfield had returned to direct. Since the completion of *The Dalek Invasion Of Earth*, Pinfield had effectively stepped down as the executive producer, even though he was still getting an on-screen credit every episode.

He had gone to Sydney Newman before the start of the second series, stressing that Lambert now needed no advisors or assistance as she had proved herself to be a more than capable producer through the course of Season One. Spooner recalls that he was offered the job of directing *The Space Museum* for two basic reasons; he would know how to realise the production effectively on the restricted budget, and the complex special effects sequences were ideal for him to handle as few knew the capabilities of a television studio better than Pinfield.

To ensure that the demands from the script could be accommodated, the production team moved back to TV Centre, where the facilities were far more modern.

Spooner:

"*The Space Museum* was a sort of 'Now-Get-Out-Of That' for Mervyn, setting up challenges for him to try and crack on the screen. I remember that there were an awful lot of joke set-pieces in the original version, but the general opinion was that *The Romans* had not worked as a comedy, and that it was best to

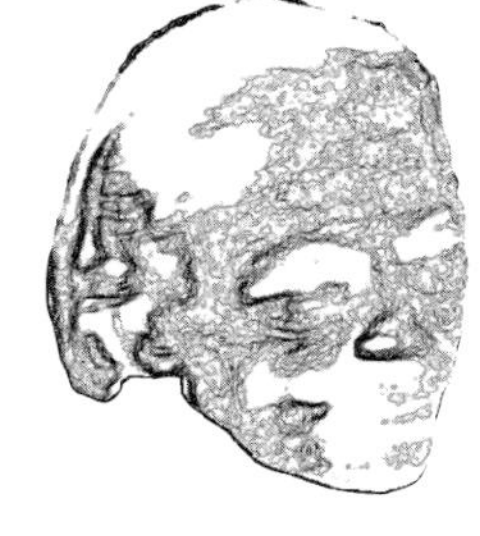

keep the level of humour in the show pretty basic and subtle."

The Space Museum was shot on 2 April in TC4, with *The Dimensions Of Time*, *The Search* and *The Final Phase* following. Pinfield once again made a rare comment to the press as filming began. Nearly every story of that era was greeted with great interest by the newspapers, as it was in the national interest to keep the public informed of when the Daleks would be back.

"Technically, we are attempting tricks that have not been seen in *Doctor Who* before. There are no new monsters, the suspense will come from the situations that Doctor Who will be facing, and how he overcomes them."

Specifying that there were no monsters in *The Space Museum* was a cover-up, to keep hidden the fact that the Daleks appeared at the end of *The Final Phase*.

Spooner:

"*The Chase* was one of the stories that I saw through from beginning to end with Terry, who'd hit a bit of a brick wall over what to do with them. David had given him the idea of doing *The Perils Of Pauline* on a story from the first series (*Marinus*), so we came up with the idea of doing it like a chase-movie.

"He also wanted a rival race for the Daleks to have a big battle with – a set-piece for the end of the serial. That's where the Mechanoids came from, and they cost a hell of a lot of money. We seemed to be doing one expensive serial and that made the next couple suffer. Looking back, it was a haphazard way of doing it. The cheaper ones in between the ones that the money had gone on could easily have lost us some viewers."

Spooner is not altogether wrong on this point. There was certainly a considerable drop in ratings during *The Crusade* and *The Space Museum* compared to *The Web Planet*, and the Daleks' return was seen as an ideal way to boost things again.

During the second week of April, Martin took the Daleks on location shooting for the second time that season. Ray Cusick was sharing the workload of the story's design requirements with John Wood, having already reworked the Dalek casings as he was unhappy with what Spencer Chapman had done with them on *The Dalek Invasion Of Earth*.

Doubles were used for Russell and O'Brien, saving them having to leave rehearsals for *The Space Museum* , and several lightweight Dalek suits were used to show them moving rapidly across the dunes.

Extensive filming sessions were carried out at Ealing for the story, with the most complex set-up involving the battle between Daleks and Mechanoids at the story's climax. The Mechanoids were huge creations, which housed an actor who operated their arms, costing so much that only three suits were built. Lambert stated at a press call during the Ealing shoot:

"Mechanoids are just as dangerous as the Daleks, which is why they fight each other to the death at the end of the adventure. I'm not prepared to say who wins, but I will concede that this is certainly not the last you'll see of the Daleks."

The only other location filming carried out was for the departure scenes of Russell and Hill, who use the Dalek's time machine to get back to modern-day earth at the end of the sixth episode.

Hartnell:

"I tried to persuade my dear friends to stay with me, but they would have none of it. The Daleks had taken part of my 'family' away yet again. Although I enjoyed the company of Peter (Purves, who would take over as a companion in *The Chase*), and all the others, something was always missing for me after that. It never felt quite the same, and it was never as much of a pleasure to go to rehearsal any more."

Hartnell was due to suffer another blow, as Lambert herself was planning to leave by the end of the summer. He was very loyal towards the original set-up, and enjoyed working with Spooner, whom he found to be receptive to his problems with the scripts.

Spooner himself admits:

"I always consulted with Bill and the others, as they played the characters and if there was something they had to say that they weren't happy with, it got changed. They knew the characters better than anybody else."

The production team were now back at Studio One at the Riverside complex, with *The Executioners* being recorded on 30 April. The story was notable for a brief appearance by the Beatles on the screen of the Doctor's 'Time And Space Visualiser', using stock film of the group singing 'Ticket To Ride'.

Spooner:

"There was an idea about asking the Beatles to appear in the show, but their schedules were worse than ours, so it just didn't work out. The gag would have been to have them done up as old men, still singing the same old songs."

Flight Through Eternity saw Peter Purves make his debut in the programme, although not as his regular character of Steven Taylor. Martin cast him as Morton Dill, an American tourist on top of the Empire State Building when the Daleks land there, but he was brought back at the end of the serial to play Taylor when the decision was made to make the character a companion.

Purves said in 1972:

"The whole *Doctor Who* set-up was amazing. Making that show from week to week was a killer. I actually auditioned to play a giant butterfly in one (*The Web Planet*), and the director said 'Thanks, but no thanks', but promised he'd use me in a later one if anything came up. He kept to his word and that's how I got to travel through time for a year."

The Doctor is cornered by Frankenstein and Dracula robots in **The Chase**.

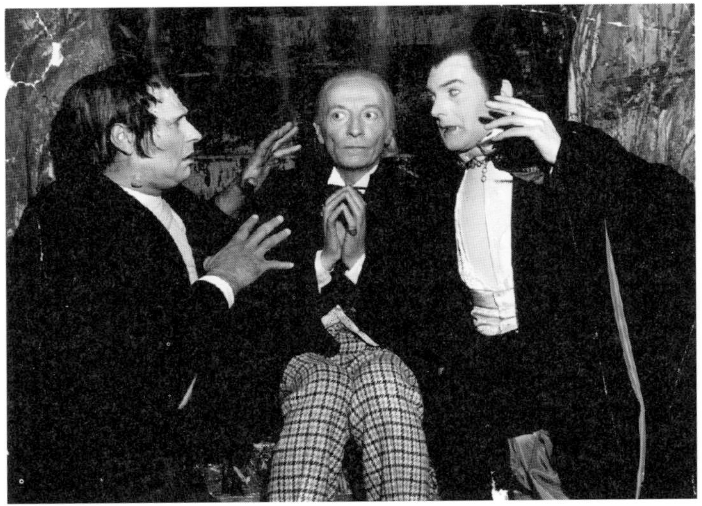

THE DOCTORS

On 21 and 28 May, *Journey Into Terror* and *The Death Of Doctor Who* were recorded. It was not a story that Hartnell remembered with any affection when he spoke in 1967.

"The story where my friends left the Tardis was a long-winded bore. I had no time for the story, no time at all. I felt it was a poor way to have them go after so long. I felt that it was not a suitable departure for such a fine pair of actors."

Donald Tosh, fresh from completing a long stint as the script editor on *Compact*, arrived to take over from Spooner, working extensively with him on the rewrites of *The Time Meddler*, which Camfield returned to direct in the first few days of May.

The four part story had been chosen to bring the second series to an end, although production would continue on two further stories which would be held over for the now confirmed Season Three.

Spooner:

"I went to join Terry (Nation) on *The Baron* (One of ITC's many adventure/thriller film series made in the 1960s), as one of the main writers. Before I left, I'd asked him to come up with another Dalek story, which was certainly no more than six parts long, but something went on with Huw Wheldon..."

Wheldon, then the Director of Television for the BBC, was an admitted fan of the programme, but his mother was a total addict. He specifically asked Lambert to commission a 'mammoth' Dalek story, so Nation's six became twelve episodes.

Spooner continues:

"Suddenly, he had to come up with double the number of episodes and as I was moving over to join him, I offered to help write them. I thought I'd left *Doctor Who* behind, but once you've been there, you never break free."

The principal 'villain' of *The TIme Meddler* was the first character introduced to the series who came from the same planet as the Doctor, which was then still unnamed, as was his race, the Time Lords. All that was clear was that the Meddling Monk also owned a Tardis. Camfield cast the role carefully, and somewhat surprisingly.

"I was looking for someone with the kind of comic energy that would stand up against Bill's, and I quite literally thought about the *Carry On* films, and whether there was anyone there who would do. Peter was an immediate idea, and he said yes as soon as we asked."

Peter Butterworth relished the chance to play a 'Doctor Who Baddie', as he called it, and said on the set of *Carry On...Follow That Camel* in 1967, when asked if he would be returning to *Doctor Who*:

"I'd love to. The old Monk has a score or two to settle with Doctor Who, and I know Pat Troughton (he was well into his first run of stories by that point), so it would be fun. Bill Hartnell was actually in one of the early *Carry On* films (the first, *Carry On Sergeant*), so we had a fair bit in common.

"He always got a bit jealous and complained to one of the writers about my Time Machine working when his didn't. I overheard him doing this, caught his eye and huffed on my hand and polished my knuckles on my cowl, smiling at him. He threw up his hands and said it was a conspiracy. He was fun to work with."

Butterworth made his proper debut in the story with the second episode, *The Meddling Monk*.

ABOVE: Peter Butterworth.

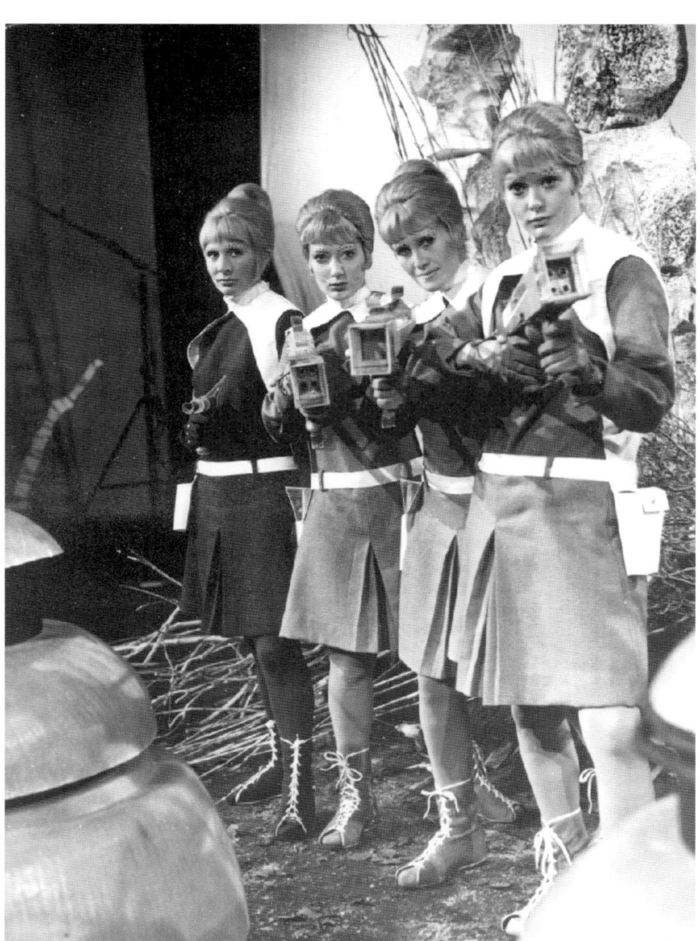

RIGHT: The Darhvins from **Galaxy Four**.

"Bill wanted me to have a name, but Douglas Camfield wouldn't let him, so he called me 'Hieronymous' behind his back."

Dennis Spooner:

"Hartnell was beginning to get a bit disheartened with *Doctor Who* towards the time I left, because everything was changing around him. I'd actually left, but when I came back for the big Dalek story (*The Dalek's Master Plan*), it was certainly far more tense.

"Donald Tosh told me that the final blow was when Verity told Bill she was leaving, which was quite late in the day. He just couldn't accept she was off as well, that was too much for him, and the protests soon followed."

Hartnell in 1965:

"Of course, I was upset when Verity Lambert left. She had been with *Doctor Who* as long as I had, there was never a more considerate producer, and I could not have asked for a more skilled one. She epitomised everything that was good about the programme then. She asked me what I thought on countless matters, and even let me make suggestions as to whom we should ask to be guest artists.

"Today, things are rather different. I have to contend with directors of little experience or tact, who say they know better, but have yet to prove this to me. This is my third year as *Doctor Who* and I do it for the children. They respect *Doctor Who*, they believe in him, and that makes it worthwhile."

There is an extraordinarily bitter tone to Hartnell's words, illustrating how he did not see eye to eye with either Lambert's successor, John Wiles, or Spooner's (Tosh). He makes slight exaggerations about having cast approval and being sought for advice on production matters, but the fact of the matter was that he respected and liked Lambert and never felt as settled in the series again.

The cutting of an episode of *Planet Of The Giants* meant that an extra episode was allocated to the production schedules. The second season ended after thirty-nine weeks, so an additional one-part story was planned for the beginning of the third season. After William Emms' *Galaxy Four*, a single part prelude to the Dalek epic was written by Nation with *Mission To The Unknown*, the last story Lambert would oversee.

John Wiles arrived to trail Lambert during the latter stages of *The Time Meddler*, where he formed an instant rapport with Douglas Camfield, which would lead to him being asked to come back to direct *The Daleks' Master Plan*.

The general opinion was that everything would settle back into the normal routine when the production team came back together after the annual holiday. Hartnell needed a break, he had only had two official weeks off (During the third episode of *The Space Museum* and the second of *The Time Meddler*), and as Spooner said:

"Bill always got rather tetchy towards the end of a run. He looked forward to his fishing trips. It was just the right tonic for him and he always came back re-energised."

Mervyn Pinfield returned to direct *Galaxy Four* at the beginning of June, making several radical changes to the scripts. For example, the Drahvins were originally a race of cloned men but Pinfield cast them as women.

Filming began with insert shots at Ealing during the fourth week of June, when it became apparent that Pinfield was not at all

A gathering of alien delegates at the United Galatic Headquarters in **Mission to the Unkown**.

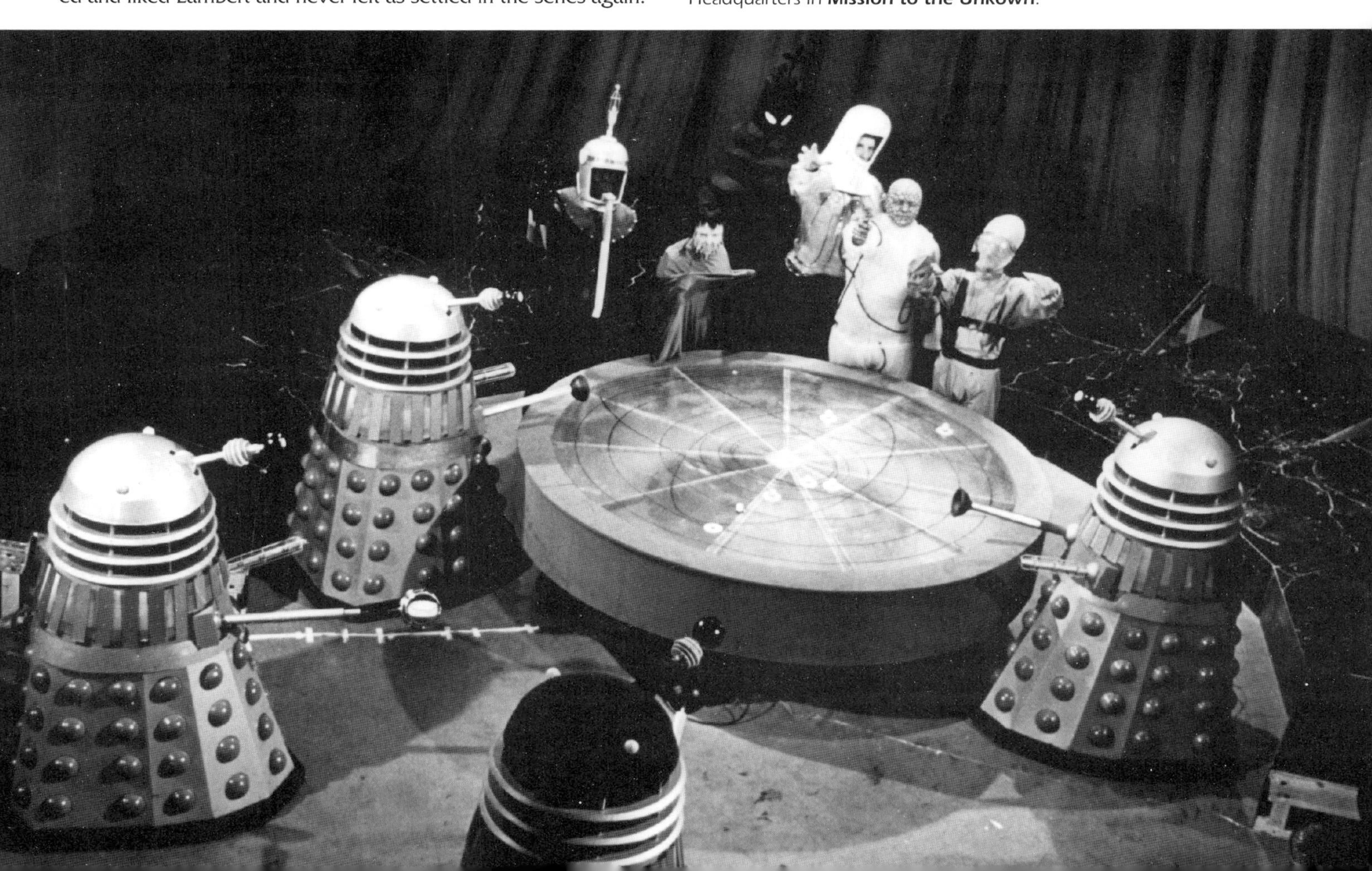

well. Lambert took the decision to have a second director standing by, hiring Derek Martinus, in case Pinfield had problems. By the time *Four Hundred Dawns* went into studio in TC4 at TV Centre, Pinfield was no longer with the production, and Martinus had taken full charge on this, his first TV assignment as director.

Martinus:

"*Galaxy Four* was strange in that we had to hire midgets to play the Chumblies. I think they were meant to be another set of Daleks, or whatever, by they couldn't do much apart from shuffle around a bit and go 'blip'."

The Chumblies, which Hartnell is reputed to have called 'beehives on wheels', were the robotic servants of the Rills. Hideous creatures who, like the Drahvins, were stranded on the planet in Galaxy Four.

The script was not popular with the cast, as it was a leftover from when Ian and Barbara were travelling with the Tardis, and it had not been changed to accommodate the fact that it was now two entirely different characters.

After eight months solid work, completing thirty six episodes, the main cast broke up, while the production team kept going. Richard Hunt stayed on from designing the sets on *Galaxy Four*, to share credit on *Mission To The Unknown* with Ray Cusick, who returned to oversee the use of the Daleks for this one episode.

Derek Martinus also stayed on, directing a cast which, for the only time in the programme's history, featured none of the main principal characters. As recording finished in TC3 on 6 August, it marked the end of Verity Lambert's tenure as the producer. She would go on to work on *The Newcomers* and oversee another fantasy/ adventure series with Sydney Newman, called *Adam Adamant Lives!*, before moving to ITV.

She left the series on a high. *The Web Planet* had been the biggest ratings success, and a third Dalek story maintained the highly respectable figures *Doctor Who* was getting, with an average of over nine million viewers tuning in for each episode of *The Chase*.

Season Two finished broadcasting on 24 July, and there was little over a month before *Galaxy Four* started on 11 September. There were several casualties along the way as far as scripts were concerned, as Spooner's notes reveal. Three stories were turned down, failing even to be commissioned, included works by future *Doctor Who* regulars.

Firstly, there was *Doctor Who And The Dark Planet*, by Brian Hayles. The story concerned a world where the fall of night turned the adults into savages, attacking any strangers, and where only the children are immune to this effect. The Tardis crew met a group of young warriors, defending their village from their parents. Spooner noted that this was tricky to do as it could influence some of the younger viewers in the wrong way.

Britain AD 408 was by Malcolm Hulke, and dealt with the Roman occupation of Europe, with Spooner turning it down noting that it would be too close to his own story, *The Romans*, which had been made shortly before.

The Space Looters has only the surname of the author noted, Holmes, leading to the conclusion that it was probably an early piece of writing by Robert Holmes, who would have his first of many *Doctor Who* stories broadcast during the Troughton era. This dealt with a band of space traders floating icebergs across space to planets where there was a water shortage.

Season Three started out with a tongue-in-cheek historical saga, *The Myth Makers*, when recording resumed 31 September, with Hartnell, Purves and O'Brien returning for *Temple Of Secrets*.

Adrienne Hill.

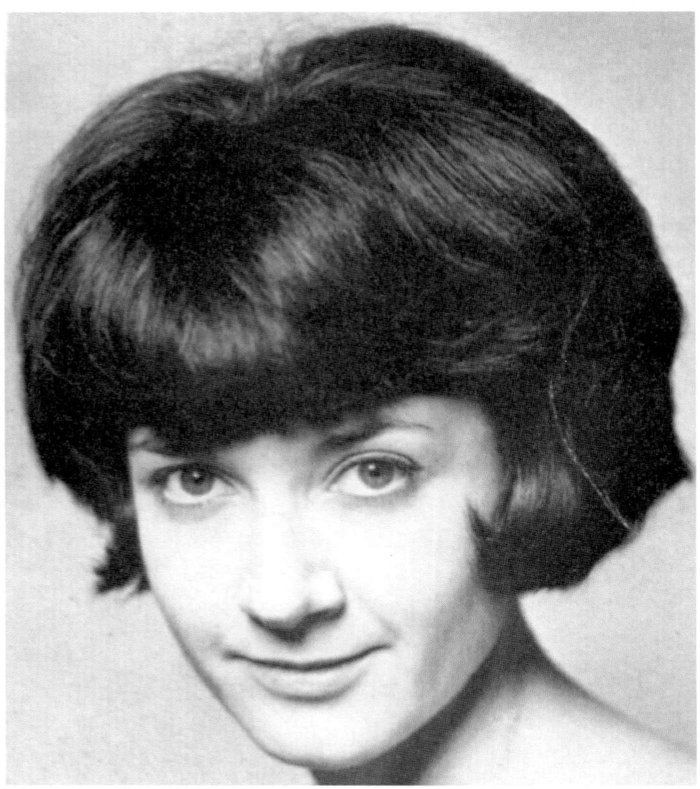

Douglas Camfield and wife Sheila Dunn during production of **The Daleks' Master Plan**.

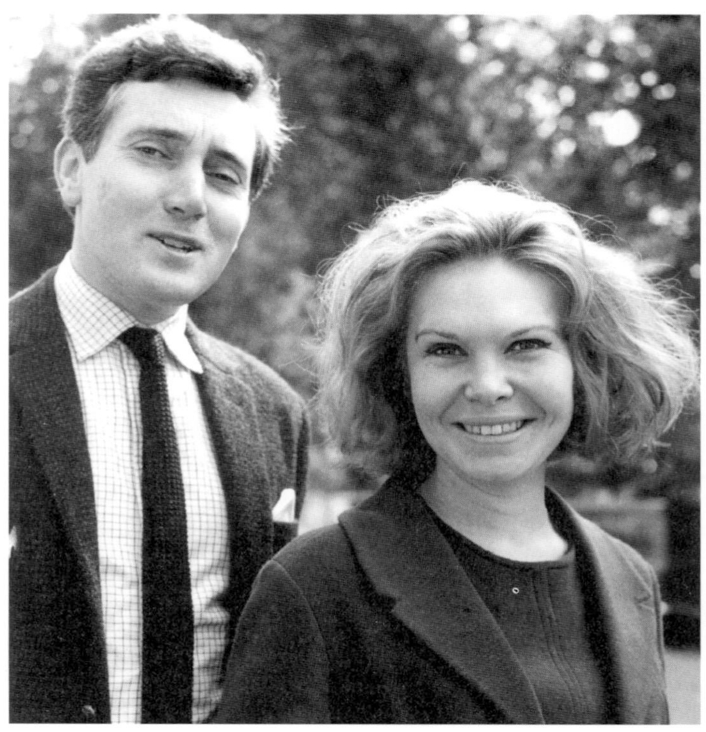

Michael Leeston-Smith was directing with Wiles now producing full time, having trailed Lambert on her last three stories. John Wood was brought in as designer.

Maureen O'Brien had expressed a desire to leave at the end of the second season, having grown increasingly dissatisfied with the development of her character. This came to a head with *Galaxy Four*, and Wiles agreed to let her go after the first story when they returned from their break. Donald Cotton had written a minor character as a serving girl called Katarina, played by Adrienne Hill, who had auditioned for a part in *The Crusades* during Season Two.

"I was asked to stay on and become part of the Tardis crew, so what could I say, other than 'Yes, please!'. It was always planned that Kastarina wouldn't last long, I knew all along that I'd only be there for a few weeks.

"William Hartnell took me under his wing and was very protective towards me. Maureen O'Brien had told me before she left that he tended to forget his lines now and again, and that you had to keep on your toes with him. In that respect, we looked after each other."

Douglas Camfield was now back once again, preparing the considerable task of planning out *The Daleks' Master Plan*, which was of such interest to the press that they even went so far as to cover Camfield's wedding (to actress Sheila Dunn) shortly before filming began. Ray Cusick and Barry Newbery had joined forces to share out the episodes between themselves, with Cusick concentrating on the Dalek spaceships and the creatures, while Newbery dug up information on ancient Egypt – one of the stories main settings.

Horse Of Destruction featured the main set piece of *The Myth Makers* when it came to recording on 21 October, with the use of Wood's impressive reconstruction of the famous 'Wooden Horse'. Built in miniature, it was intercut on film footage with location work that was carried out in Frensham Ponds, near Surrey, in the week before the studio work began.

Camfield was hard at work on the sequences for the first block of six episodes that needed completing on the Dalek story before studio work could begin. The first five episodes were by Nation, the sixth by Dennis Spooner, who comments:

"It was pretty much a fifty-fifty situation. Terry had commitments at ITC, he had enough time to do the first batch of *The Daleks' Master Plan*, then he passed the baton to me to round it all off for the last few, using the basic plotlines he'd drawn up.

"My major input was to bring Peter Butterworth back, giving it a bit of a lift midway. The last thing you expected was for him to turn up in the middle of a Dalek story, so it was a little twist."

The villain working alongside the Daleks, Mavic Chen, was quickly cast with Kevin Stoney, whom Camfield had known for years and would later use again as the main villain (Tobias Vaughn) in the epic Troughton Cyberman story, *The Invasion*.

Spooner:

"Stoney was brought in to counterbalance the Daleks. Twelve weeks of Daleks ranting to themselves would have been mind-numbing, so he was put there to rant along with them. As it turned out, Douglas got a very suave and sophisticated performance out of him and he stole the show from under everyone else's feet."

The schedule was a nightmare, with only 15 days between completion in the studio and broadcast. Camfield ran the whole operation like a military campaign and as Newbery recalls:

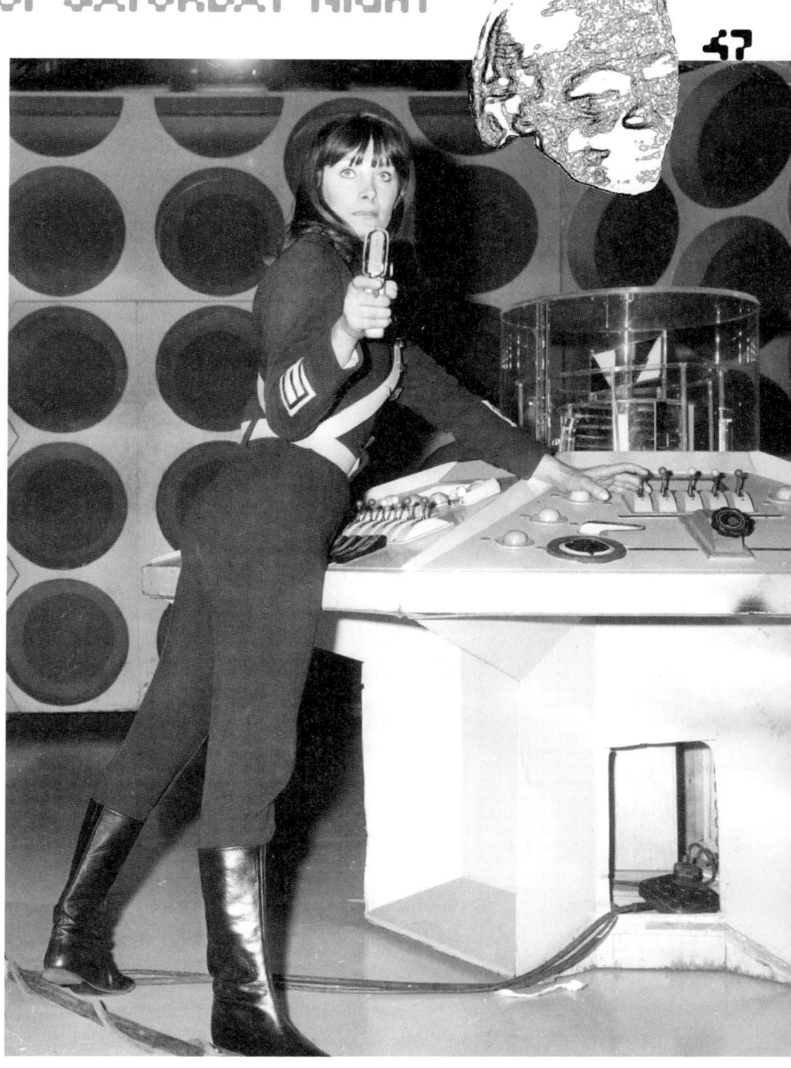

Jean Marsh as Sara Kingdom.

"He used to call me 'Major', and when I asked why, he said, 'That's the rank you'd be, if this was a war!'"

The Traitors marked the departure of Katarina, who sacrificed herself to save the lives of the Doctor, Steven and Bret Vyon, who was also killed at the end of the episode.

Camfield:

"There were some accusations that the big Dalek story was overly brutal, but that was only from the watchdogs outside the BBC. Anybody inside was asking me all the time about what was going to happen next, and of course I said, 'Watch it and see!'"

Dennis Spooner:

"There were apparently complaints about the number of deaths in the episodes, with companions dropping like flies, and I brought this up with Douglas. His attitude was the one I adopted, which was to be totally realistic. The Doctor and his group were actually trying to save the universe, not a planet, but the universe itself – and when the job's as big as that, as Douglas said, 'People get hurt'."

The Feast Of Steven was recorded on 3 December, the only time that a special Christmas story has ever been staged within the programme itself, with the bulk of the episode revolving around a silent film studio. This particular part of the production is notorious for another reason.

Dennis Spooner:

"That was the Christmas Day episode where they had a bit of a lull at the end where the Doctor toasted the two companions with him. Well, Bill took the opportunity, and nobody ever thought he'd do it, to turn to the camera and wish the viewers a 'Happy Christmas'. John Wiles blew his stack in the control gallery, and Dougie's jaw hit the floor. There was nothing they could do about it, and there was no time for a remount, so there it stayed. I thought it was quite a bit of fun, to be honest."

Volcano, an episode broadcast on New Year's Day 1966, saw Spooner taking over as the main script writer. Recording took place every Friday and the run concluded with *Golden Death, Escape Switch, The Abandoned Planet* and *The Destruction Of Time* which featured the graphic death scene of Jean Marsh's character.

Barry Newbery:

"We had an extra, heavily made up, crawling through the sand as she aged to death. Douglas did a wonderful job with that scene; it looked really quite disturbing."

William Hartnell commented on the use of the Daleks, midway through recording the story:

"The Daleks have now become part of the show, part of its history. I don't mean to undermine their success in any way, but I don't think they could survive on their own. They need Doctor Who to outwit and confound their every move, he is a continual challenge and a continual frustration to them."

The Daleks' Master Plan came to an end on 14 January, with the final episode completed on schedule. Totally exhausted, Douglas Camfield, according to Dennis Spooner, vowed that he'd had enough of Daleks for keeps.

"I think Dougie preferred monsters who were more mobile. He couldn't stand the logic that running upstairs floored your average Dalek completely. I think he'd had enough of *Doctor Who* as well. There was a hell of a lot of pressure on him to get it done. John (Wiles) basically left him to it, because he was not exactly what you could call, 'happy with his job'."

Wiles acknowledges that he was a reluctant Producer, much preferring his career as a writer, and felt restricted in what he could do with the *Doctor Who* format.

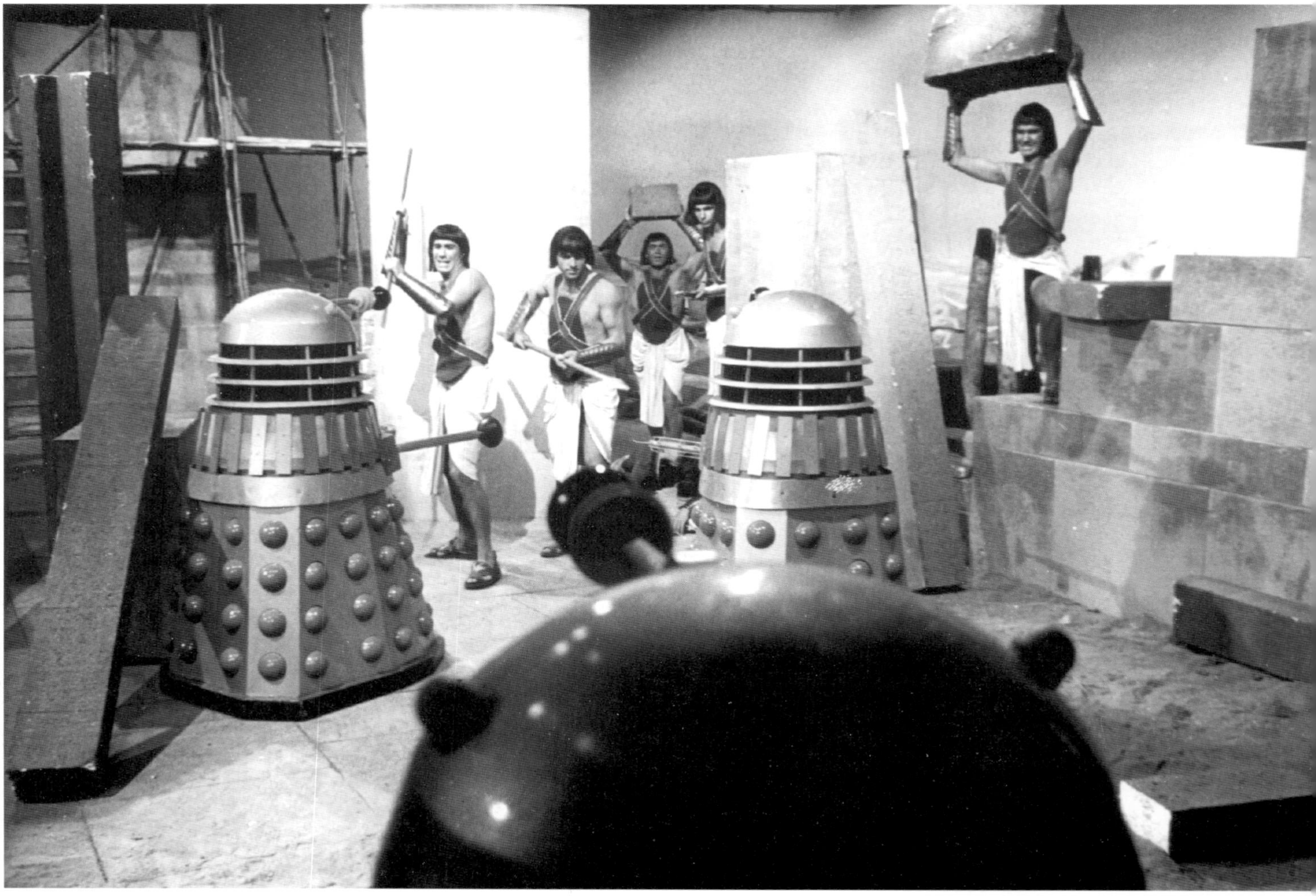

The Daleks battle with Egyptian slaves in **The Daleks' Master Plan.**

It was during production on *The Massacre*, which came directly after *The Daleks' Master Plan*, that he made it clear he intended to leave – a move that inspired Donald Tosh to leave at the same time. Sydney Newman stepped in to find a replacement producer, as Innes Lloyd explains:

"I was dabbling with the odd play here and there, having spent a hell of a long time with O.B. (The Outside Broadcast Unit),

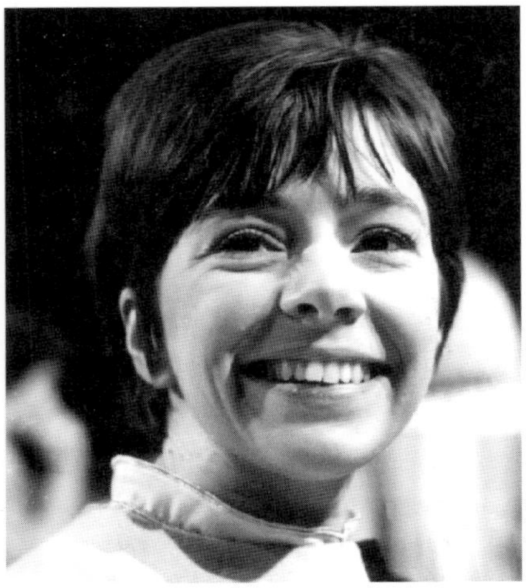

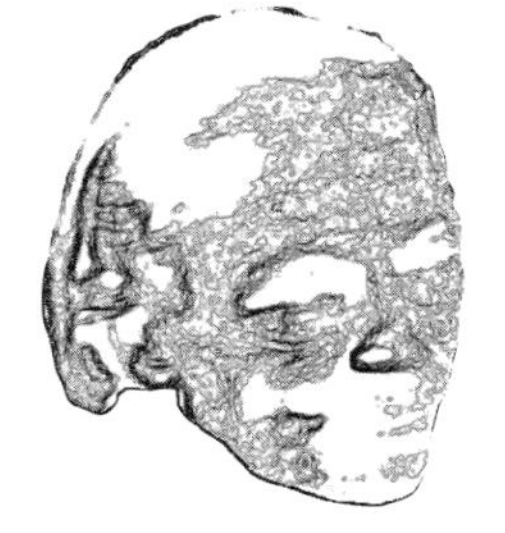

Jackie Lane.

and Sydney gently said it was time for me to make the move to production. I said, 'Thanks, but no...', as I wanted to get into the Plays Department.

"Sydney basically said, if I took *Doctor Who* on for a while, that door would open far more easily when I was through."

After missing out on *Inside The Spaceship*, Paddy Russell finally made her directorial debut with the series, bringing Michael Young with her as the designer. Tosh was planning to leave with Wiles on the completion of the following story, *The Ark*, so Gerry Davis was brought in to trail him as his replacement script editor, having spent some time working on the football soap, *United!* Davis.

"Bill Hartnell was overjoyed with that one, because he got to play two roles. One was a monk (The Abbot of Amboise), and the other was the Doctor. I basically had to learn the ropes off Donald Tosh, who told me what was what."

Hartnell commented on the story in 1967:

"I remember with great affection, the story where I doubled up as the Abbot. I have to confess that I was growing tired of playing the Doctor for such long periods, but that story offered originality and a great scope for me as an act."

Priest Of Death was followed by *Bell Of Doom*, which was the only part of the story that actually called for any location filming. The original idea was to introduce a new companion in the story with Anne Chaplette and this created an interesting dilemma. The Ark was actually a gigantic spaceship housing the entire human race and examples of all forms of life on earth. According to the scripts, the Tardis would land in the Ark at the beginning of the adventure and then travel 700 years into the future to see how the situation on board the Ark had developed. Tosh and Wiles felt that there was only so far you could take *Doctor Who* in manipulating history. Taking the Chaplette character out of the past would obviously have an effect on the future.

Spooner expounds on the point:

"There comes a point where you had to start to respect the viewers' intelligence – it wasn't beyond the average viewer to guess that if you remove someone from the past, all the ancestors on that particular time line cease to exist at that instant. *Doctor Who* would never do anything so reckless, so that's why you had to be careful where you took the travellers from. When it's the present or the future, people don't think of the same point."

The ending of *Bell Of Doom* was quickly reworked to include an introduction for Dodo (Jackie Lane) on present day earth, with a hint in the dialogue that she was a descendant of the Chaplette character, thus showing she survived the massacre of Saint Bartholomew's Eve.

Wiles had wanted to do a story set on a giant spaceship for some time, and The Ark was the realisation of that idea, although it was actually completed as he left the programme. Paul Erickson

Lane, Hartnell and Purves on the set of **The Ark**.

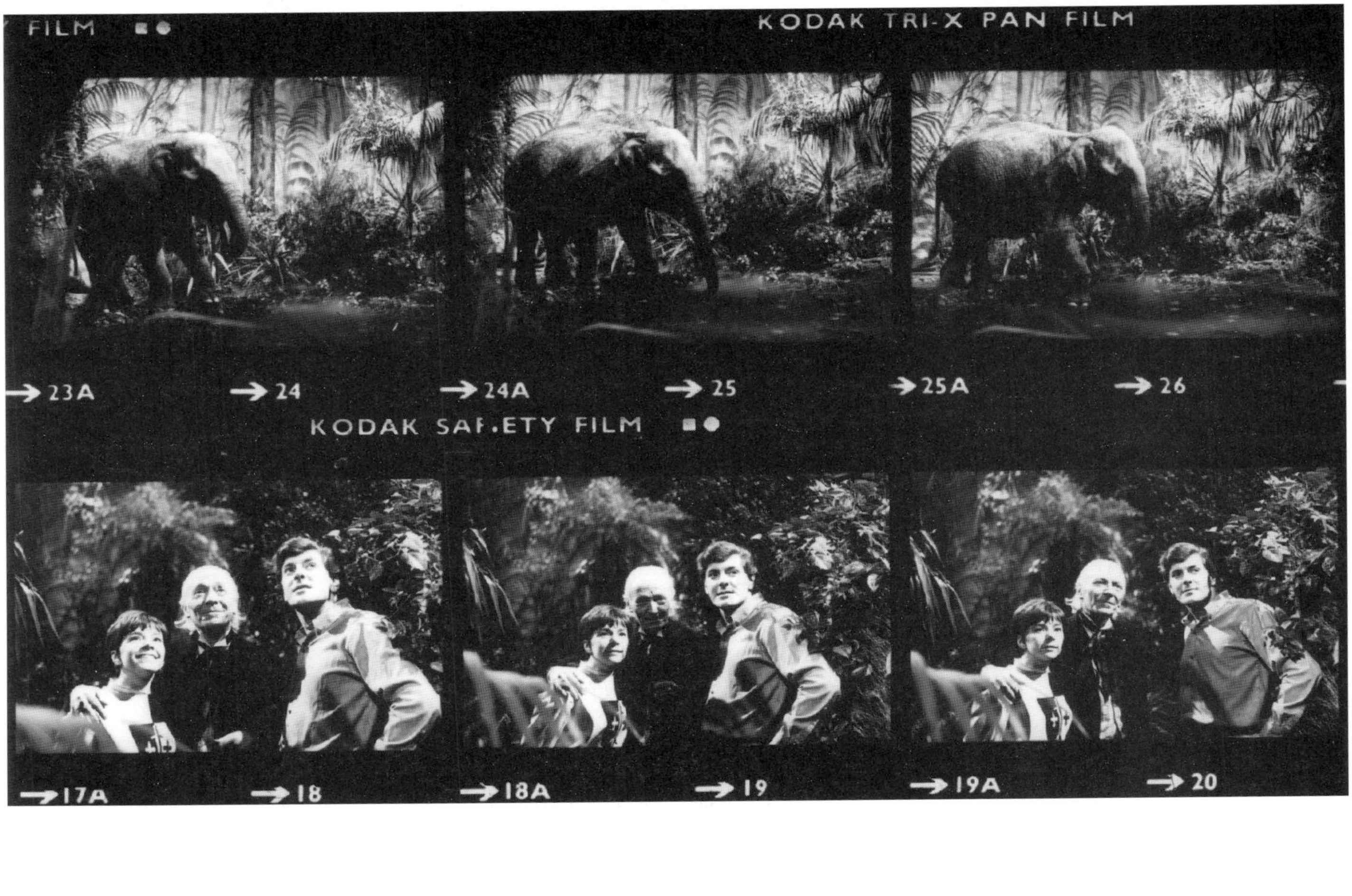

and Lesley Scott took on writing the four part story, although Erickson later admitted that Scott had no input into the finished product.

"Lesley was my wife, and we worked as a team but *Doctor Who* was a bit beyond her. Not an area she was altogether keen on, so I ploughed on by myself and just left her name on it with mine."

Michael Imison took on the directorial chores, with Barry Newbery returning once again. Cusick's last serial for the programme had proved to be *The Daleks' Master Plan.*

"I'd been on the show for about three years of continuous work and to be honest, I felt like it was time for a change. It was beginning to give me severe headaches towards the end, and I could do without that kind of thing, so I moved on."

The intricate plot involved two basic stories on the same location. The first two episodes, *The SteelkSky* and *The Plague* dealt with the human population on the vast space ark, with their one-eyed alien slaves, the Monoids.

The second half was set with the Tardis returning to the ark seven hundred years later, when the Monoids are at war with the humans, having revolted against their slavery. (*The Return* was completed on 4 March and *The Bomb* on the 11th at Riverside Studio One). Chris D'Oyly John remembers the Monoids, having worked on the series with Imison.

"The poor actors wearing that get-up had these ping pong-balls in their mouth, that had been cut in half with an eye painted on the front. They were pegged to the tongue, so they could move them around, with the lips acting as eye-lid. They were quite painful to wear and it was my job to clip them back when they fell out."

Innes Lloyd:

"I remember there was an elephant on set. Not a prop, they got a huge Indian elephant on set, and everyone was a bit worried about what Willie (Hartnell) would say about this, but they got on like a house on fire.

"Nobody could figure it out, because this elephant was all over him, and I asked him about it a couple of months later. He didn't say anything, he just took one of the peanuts he had in his pocket out, cracked it open, popped it in his mouth and smiled."

The Celestial Toymaker represented the first credited production to Innes Lloyd in his new job and the first story, at last, by Brian Hayles who had been sending in plotlines for years.

Innes Lloyd:

"One of the things I wanted to do with *Doctor Who* was populate it with good actors. Not just jobbing actors, but faces that people would see and recognise in an instant.

"That first episode of mine started the ball rolling because I managed to get Michael Gough and as far as I know, he actually turned down a film to come and do it. He was very enthusiastic, and he made the Toymaker this odd, enigmatic character... a very good performance."

The Gunfighters.

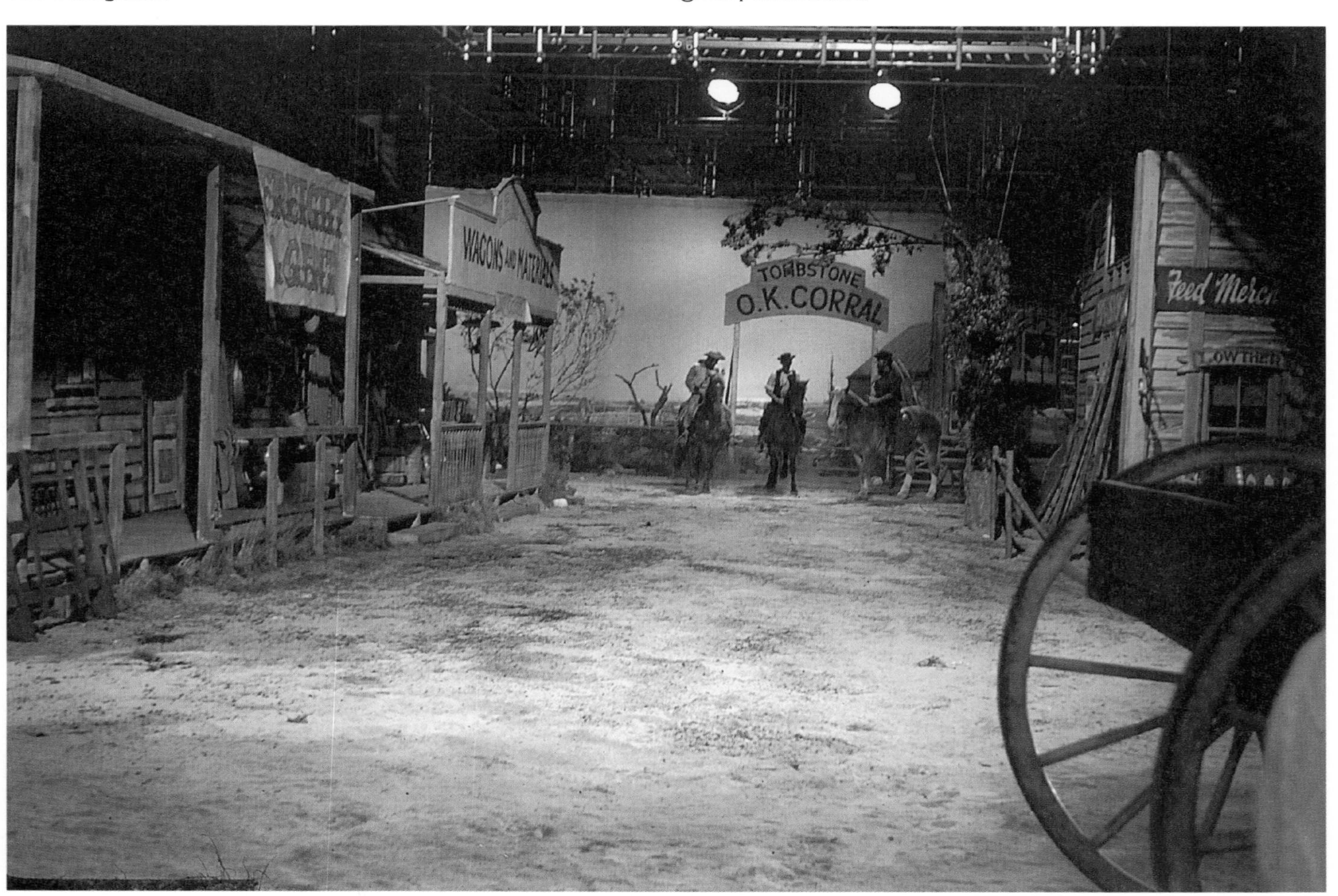

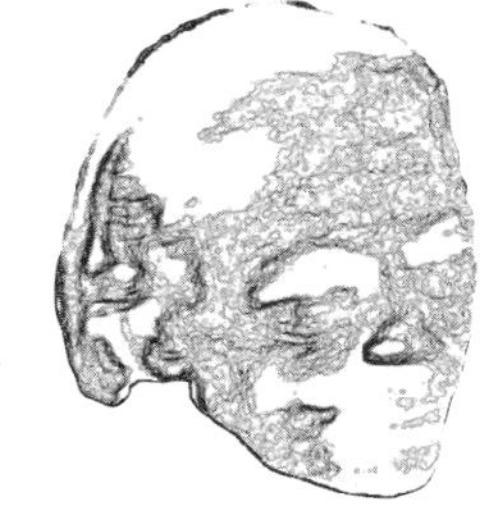

The Celestial Toyroom went before the cameras on 18 March, with the programme still based at Riverside Studio One. William Hartnell took his regular two-week break for episodes two, *The Hall Of Dolls*, and three, *The Dancing Floor*, with the Toymaker making the Doctor invisible and silent for the duration of these installments. The only time Hartnell was heard, it was via pre-recorded tape inserts he had made before he left for his holiday.

He returned for *The final Test*, recorded on 8 April. Lloyd is full of praise for the story:

"The Toymaker had a certain charm and was quite a heavy fantasy-based story, which was not something I was keen on, but I felt this one worked. In contrast, *The Gunfighters* was not something I was over-keen on."

The Gunfighters brought the original producer, Rex Tucker, back to the programme some three years after his last formal involvement. He recalls:

"I was not keen on getting involved with *Doctor Who*, but the whole idea of making one set at the OK Corral had a certain appeal, and was a challenge to mount in the studio. I certainly remember staging the shoot-out, and thinking 'what on earth am I doing?', but it was a job."

The script was by Donald Cotton, and Barry Newbery created the western street that was erected in TV Centre. Research material had come from America.

"There were invaluable books on the wild west, and on the town of Tombstone itself. We had the most wonderful backdrop at the end of the street and with the cameras pointing at the right kind of angle, it genuinely looked as though we had a huge set, when the reality of it was that it was really quite cramped. The right kind of backdrop could create a wonderful false illusion."

TC4 housed Tombstone for *A Holiday For The Doctor*, on 15 April, and the cast and crew moved back to Riverside Studio One for the following week with *Don't Shoot The Pianist* (22 April).

Gerry Davis:

"*The Gunfighters* was nothing to do with me. I think Donald (Tosh) was responsible, though it was actually the kind of thing that Dennis Spooner would have commissioned, now I think about it.

"Innes took one look at it and said it was not *Doctor Who* as far as he was concerned and I agreed, but there was nothing we could do about it. There was no time to get a replacement in, so we gritted our teeth and went for it as best we could. Rex Tucker did try hard, but the whole thing was a bad idea from the start."

The Gunfighters also marked the last time that the stories would have individual episode titles. Each adventure would now have a general title that covered it throughout its run, no matter what the length.

It was a policy that Lloyd introduced:

"I couldn't quite see the reasoning behind calling each one by a different name. If it had an overall title, fine, but splitting it up like that confused things, so Gerry and I agreed to stop that as soon as we could."

Some quite extensive location filming was done while *The Gunfighters* was in rehearsal, with Purves being one of the main members of the principal cast needed at a gravel pit, near Buckinghamshlre and another one (more sand than gravel) near Oxshott in Surrey.

Innes Lloyd:

"I remember going down to the quarry, and seeing these ancient old men round the honeywagon (the canteen) and thinking, 'Why on earth have we hired such decrepit actors?', with thoughts of the insurance risk racing in my mind in case any of them got hurt. Then I saw it was just make-up, and that's honestly

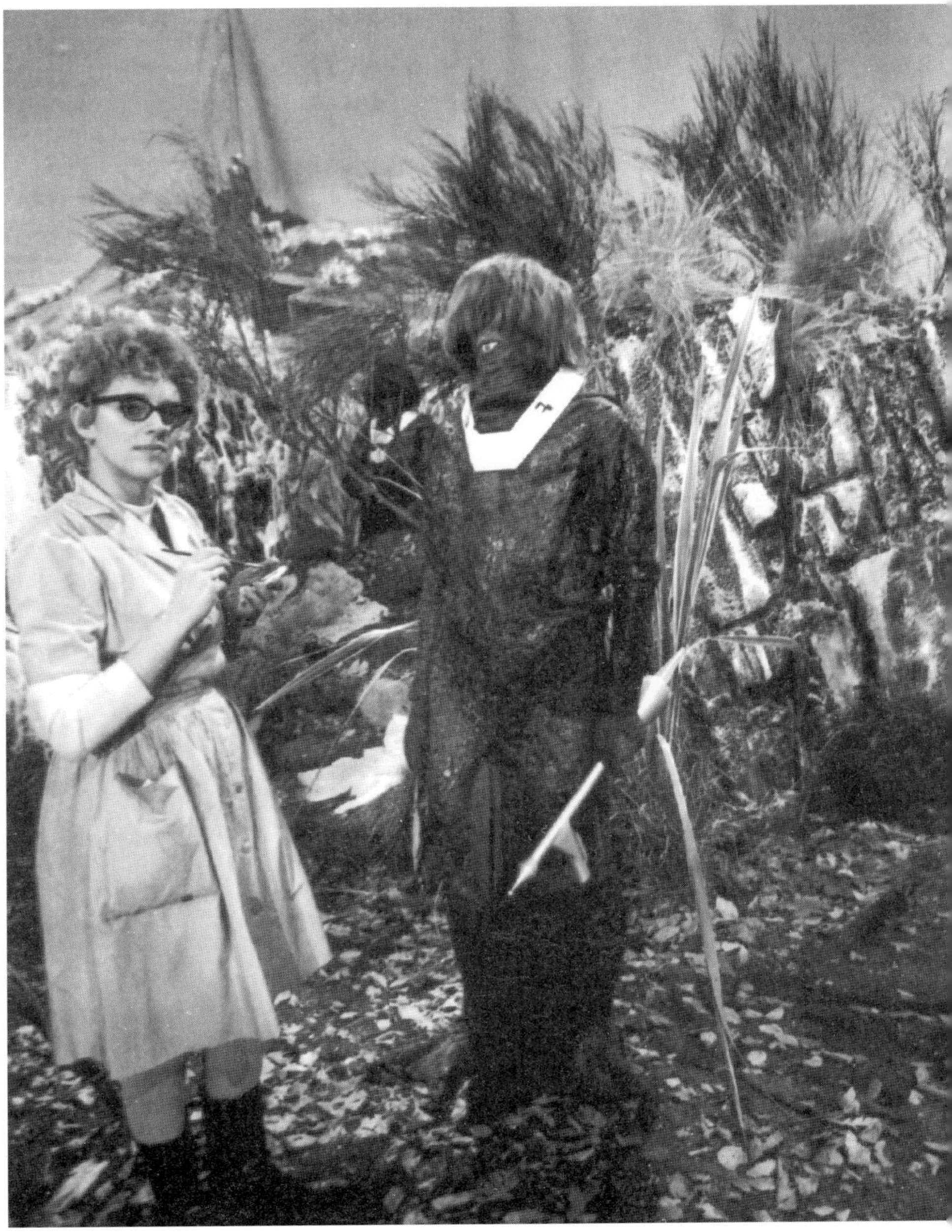

Monoid and make-up artist.

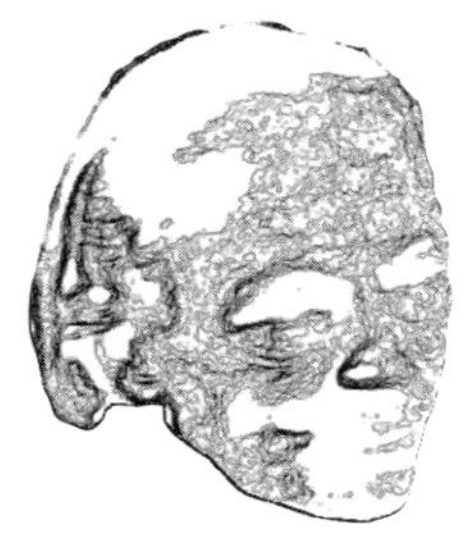

the first time that I began to realise the kind of magic you had to bring to *Doctor Who*. You had to suspend your sense of reality and leave it at the door as you came in. It was as simple as that."

Doctor Who was beginning to lose in the ratings. It was not drawing the audiences anymore, with the initial peak of over eleven million with *Galaxy Four* slipping to as low as just over four million with the next story, *The Savages*.

Peter Purves had grown tired of the series and complained to Lloyd that he wanted to be given more adequate parts to play in the storylines. This was not resolved, and Purves elected to leave.

Lloyd:

"Peter's character was just an average anybody as far as I could see – there was nothing that special about him, and there was very much a habit of making him a 'Yes' man. 'What a good idea, Doctor', 'Gosh, Doctor. I'd never have thought of that', making him just stand there pointing out how clever Willie was.

"It was when Peter left that we brought Mike Craze and Anneke in. They were far more in line with the age of the audience we were trying to attract."

Purves made his farewell appearance in *The Savages*, with Christopher Barry returning once more, and Stuart Walker acting as the designer. Ian Stuart Black had been asked to write the story, initially under the title of *The White Savages*.

The Savages moved into Riverside One on 13 May, and recorded an episode a week until 3 June, when the story was completed.

Lloyd and Davis were searching for an unofficial scientific advisor to work on the series to bring the extra edge to it that Lloyd was after. He takes up the story:

"I went back to O.B. and said, 'Have you got anyone here who has a flexible knowledge of science and has the kind of mind that would be able to turn it into drama?' They said I ought to talk to Dr Kit Pedlar who was around at that point making some programme on eye surgery (he was an ophthalmic specialist). I got in contact, and asked him to pop up to Union House."

Gerry Davis:

"We were talking to people like Dr Alex Comfort and Patrick Moore, who was intrigued but didn't want to leave *The Sky At Night* (which he's presented for over thirty years on the BBC). Innes found Kit, and arranged for him to come and see me. We bounced ideas around, and we started talking about how an 'intelligence' could overpower London.

"The GPO tower had just been built, and it was a bit of an eyesore, and I said what about using it as a base? What could dominate the capitol from there? And Kit said it would have to be a computer, which immediately sparked an idea for a story. It was hammered out between us that there would have to be robots under its control that it would kill on its command and herd people around the place. That's where *The War Machines* came from.

"Kit was the first to admit that he wasn't a scriptwriter, although he wanted to have a go at an idea of his own, so we gave it to Ian Stuart Black to draft up."

The War Machines saw the departure of Dodo from the series. Lane had never been fully utilised as a character and she left with only five adventures to her credit. Michael Craze was cast as Ben Jackson, a young cockney sailor, and Anneke Wills as Polly, a secretary and subtle love interest for Ben.

Lloyd:

"Ben and Polly were your everyday people of the street. They just happened to find themselves in an extraordinary situation when they walked into the Tardis, and their reactions were meant to be the same as the viewers at home. They were there for them to relate to and share the adventures with more effectively than, say, someone from the 25th Century."

Michael Ferguson was brought in to helm the extensive location filming that the finished scripts for *The War Machines* required, with Raymond London as his designer. Shooting began during the fourth week of May, with the unit moving from Fitzroy Square to Battersea power station, to old Covent Garden and Cornwall Gardens, making it the most extensive location work done on the programme since *The Dalek Invasion Of Earth*.

Although there was meant to be an army of twelve war machines on the loose, only one was completed. It had a number plate on the side that could be changed to create the illusion of it being different .

The War Machines started recording on 10 June, with all episodes being shot at Riverside Studio One. Episode two followed on the 17th. This actually involved the final appearance of Dodo, who was not to be seen in the rest of the story.

Part three was completed on 24 June and episode four on 1 July. Hartnell, Craze and Wills were not, however, present for the rehearsals at the beginning of the week. On Saturday 25th, they left for Cornwall, where Julia Smith shot location footage with them for the next story, *The Smugglers*. They returned by the Tuesday, and everything resumed as normal.

Once again, a backlog of material was created for the confirmed fourth season. *The Smugglers* was held over and *The War Machines* was chosen as a suitable finale for the season.

The season finished on 16 July, with a steady audience of between four and a half and five million now watching regularly. Lloyd and Davis were determined to revitalise the programme in the new season.

The Smugglers was written by Brian Hayles, possibly a redrafted version of a pirate story he had submitted earlier under the title of *War Of The Cut-Throats*, which was far too B-Movieish, according to Spooner.

Julia Smith was working with designer Richard Hunt, and brought the cast and crew back to Riverside Studio One for the studio recording after a week of filming in and around Cornwall.

Innes Lloyd:

"The pirate story had a rip-roaring quality that had a cracking pace behind it, but it was then that I really began to notice how tired Willie was beginning to look. His features were drawn and he was beginning to get very difficult."

Gerry Davis:

"He once got incredibly annoyed over a chair that was in the wrong place and I had to go all the way down to Riverside and carefully explain that it had always been there, and that it was the Doctor's favourite chair. He accepted that because he regarded the script editor as having more authority than the director."

Shaun Sutton:

"It got to a point where things were a bit frantic all round. There were arguments left right and centre and I think Billy was using this blustering attitude he had to cover up how ill and how difficult it all was for him. As far as I can recall, there just came a point where he was gently being pushed, saying it was time to go."

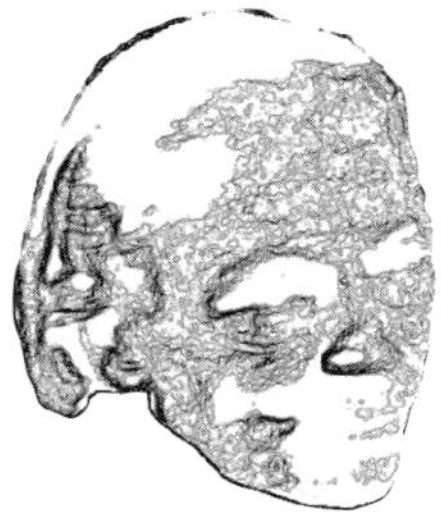

Lloyd:

"Willie came to me and said, 'Is it possible for the show to continue without me?' It wasn't ego, or anything like that. He genuinely felt responsible, as though it was his duty to keep the series going. I explained that we could change the Doctor, make him someone else, as he was such a magical character.

"He said, 'But, it will keep going? I'd hate to be the one who kills it off!' I said it would. It was then that he said he'd like to move on. I won't say that people were telling him to go, but it was clear to him that the situation would be easier for everyone if he did."

Hartnell agreed to return after the annual break, and leave 'in style', so Lloyd and Davis now had the task of taking the show in a totally different direction. Sydney Newman came back to help supervise, as did Shaun Sutton, who was now Head of Series.

Michael Craze and Anneke Wills would stay with the 'new' Doctor and plans were underway to introduce a new race of robots for Hartnell's swansong – The Cybermen.

It's perhaps fitting to include Hartnell's thoughts on the matter, as part of his life came to an end:

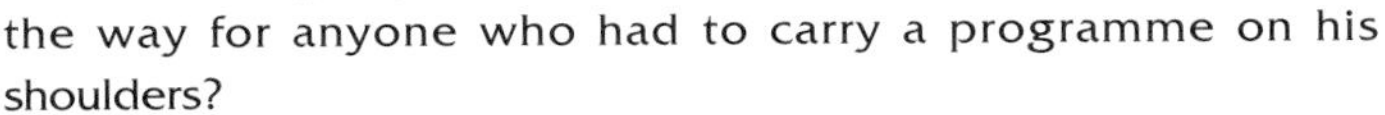

"I was heroic, something that'd I'd never been. I was the friend of all children, no matter what the age. Yes, I was difficult and I fought over any point I saw as being unjust... but wasn't that the way for anyone who had to carry a programme on his shoulders?

"The beginning was an adventure. Nobody had ever done anything like *Doctor Who* before; we were part of Saturday nights for the nation. Everyone knew who we were. We had the most inventive directors and designers, so many faces, all there and willing to help to make me the centre of attention. I needed them, but I never knew how to say thankyou.

"My health was not what it could have been and I am the first to admit now, although I could not face the fact then, that the lines were never easy to learn. But as it came to an end I knew that the viewers would not forget. I would always haunt the memories of those who were there and be one of the ghosts of Saturday night..."

The Doctor and the elephant.

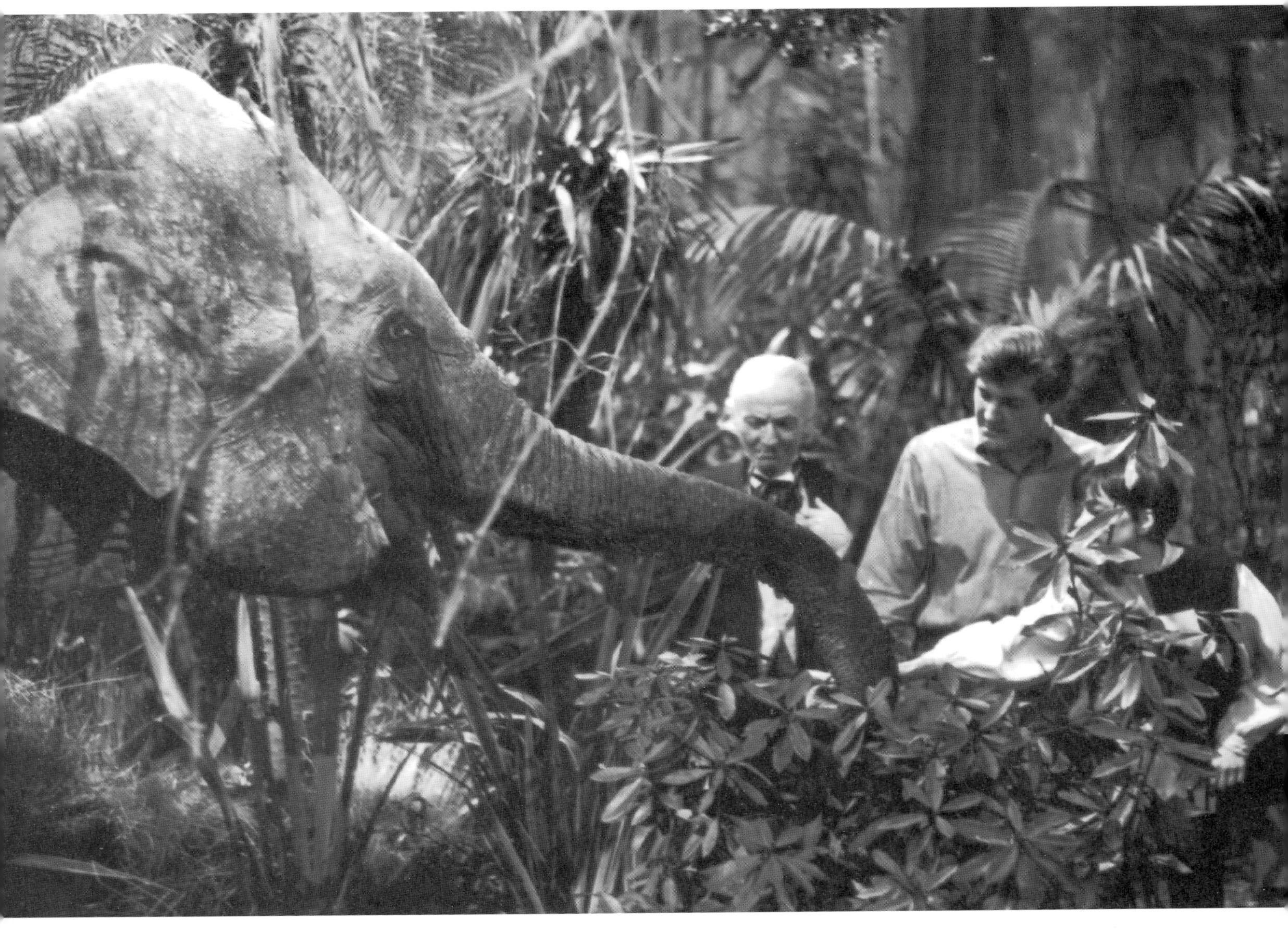

CHAPTER 3

(INNOCENT WHEN YOU DREAM)

INNOCENT WHEN YOU DREAM

(INNOCENT WHEN YOU DREAM)

"Pat will be a hard act to follow… he's proved that *Doctor Who* can keep going with other actors… that can't have been easy…"

JON PERTWEE unpublished interview – July 1969

"Cybernetic surgery is by no means a way of prolonging life forever. There comes a point where questions must be asked over how much of the body can be augmented in such a way. At what point does a patient stop being human and become a robot?"

Kit Pedler's basic theory intrigued Innes Lloyd and Gerry Davis to such an extent that they asked him to write a story about a race which had become robotised through such circumstances. Pedler had an idea for an adventure where Earth's twin planet suddenly arrived back in orbit alongside the moon after many centuries of moving through the universe and a race of human 'Star Monks' were found to be its only inhabitants.

Gerry Davis:

"Kit was never happy as a writer, and the Star Monks idea was not working. He asked me to co-write the story with him but this was difficult. There are only so many hours of TV drama a year that a BBC staff script editor is allowed to write for himself. So, it was basically done in secret (Davis did, however, get an on-screen credit for writing parts Three and Four with Pedler), and I helped draft in the Cybermen."

It was commissioned as the first story that would go into production with the fourth year of the series and Lloyd felt the race of cybernetic-humans had the potential to be a popular *Doctor Who* monster, but there was a huge problem to overcome before even rehearsal began.

Lloyd:

"Willie had agreed to leave the programme, as his health was becoming more and more of a problem and we decided to take him out on a high with a new race of monsters (The Cybermen) but we couldn't figure out how to explain that there was going to be a new Doctor."

Shaun Sutton, then in position as Head of Series:

"Sydney Newman wasn't going to let it die. He was too close to it and, being a huge science fiction fan, he was keen to use Hartnell's departure as an opportunity to bring some fantastical element to the show, to give a reason behind Billy changing into someone else."

This was nearly attempted earlier on in *The Celestial Toymaker*, using the device of making the Doctor invisible and simply having a different actor reappear, with an explanation that the Toymaker had caused this to happen and that the Doctor now simply had a different body. Nothing was going to be that simple with *The Tenth Planet* (a title thought up for the story by Pedler's wife).

Davis:

"We needed something unique – Doctor Who was, after all, meant to be an alien. It had to be something that could be done in the studio and with little cost. My line of thought was that if he was from outer space perhaps when his race die, they are instantly reborn as new beings."

Innes Lloyd:

"He had to be the same man, but somehow totally different. I had the idea about having him run on a life cycle, with his body rejuvenating as soon as it got too old for him to cope with. Once every eighty years or so, he would become a younger man again."

Many names were considered for the role of the new Doctor. Ron Moody (who later stated how big a mistake he made in turning it down), Sir Michael Hordern (Sutton: "Michael would have been like a general, but basically the same as Billy"), Patrick Wymark (Lloyd: "*The Plane Makers* – a series starring Wymark – was a great favourite of mine but Patrick was committed to a new show with ITV and couldn't do *Doctor Who*), Peter Jeffrey (Lloyd: "He didn't want to be held to a series at that time, though he did come and do *The Macra Terror* for us.") Film star Trevor Howard was also approached. Lloyd: "I can't think whose idea that was, but he *was* asked, and said no because of all the film work he was getting."

One name came through the lot of them as a firm favourite – Patrick Troughton.

Shaun Sutton:

"Everyone knew that Patrick would bring an energy to the programme that would revitalise and re-energise it. It was a wonderful idea. Pat was a good choice and a very good contrast."

Hartnell:

"Of course, I knew of Patrick Troughton's work and of his background in the Navy. I have to say that I was worried they would bring in one of the American stars from all of those ghastly American programmes they were showing but I was more than happy to know that Patrick would be filling my shoes."

Troughton recalled the approach made to him by the BBC:

"I was working on one of those Hammer Films where they had a few fur-lined bras and called it a Viking epic. We were in Ireland (making *The Viking Queen* from June to July 1966) and I had a phone call making this offer, saying 'Would you come and play Doctor Who?'

"I thought it was a joke, believing that it was Bill Hartnell's job for life. They reassured me that he was leaving and that the offer was genuine. I said 'No'. And I said 'No' when they rang again, and again, until it was becoming really silly.

"I asked my wife about it, and she asked how much they were offering. I asked for a ridiculous amount of money, and they came back and said 'Yes', so, I thought what the hell and agreed to do it. I thought we'd be taken off after a few weeks, but the money would pay a few bills."

Derek Martinus came back to the programme to Direct *The Tenth Planet*, with Peter Kindred as his designer, and began shooting some of the extensive sequences that had to be filmed at Ealing by the end of August.

William Hartnell was not needed for any of these sequences. A double, Gordon Craig, was called in for the brief shots needed of the Doctor leaving and entering the Tardis as it landed in the arctic.

The Cybermen costumes were designed by Sandra Reid. Seven basic suits were made, consisting of a bodystocking with black holes in the face the represented the eyes and mouth. The body was covered with a clear plastic suit, over which metal plates and tubes could be fixed and the chest unit clamped to the front of the actor. The 'handle-bar' headpiece was precariously held in place with a mixture of glue and sellotape!

Lloyd had changed the basic plan for the season, with rehearsals now starting on Tuesdays and recording being done on Saturdays.

The work in Ealing was completed by 2 September and rehearsals began with the full cast. Hartnell arrived for his final rehearsal on 13 September.

Lloyd:

"Those final rehearsals with Willie were strange. He'd become very picky, complaining if people coughed, or if they were breathing too heavily. I put it down to his nervousness about making his last *Doctor Who*."

The first episode was completed at Riverside Studio One on 17 September and part two followed on the 24th. There was an incident during the recording on that day, as Innes Lloyd recalls:

"It was a strain for Willie and at one point he collapsed in the studio and missed out for a week. It wasn't a happy time for him. He had agreed to go and he was beginning to have doubts as it came to an end."

The third episode was recorded on 1 October. Craig once again doubled for an unconscious Doctor and Hartnell returned to work a week later when *The Tenth Planet* part four was shot.

Lloyd:

"We laid out Willie and Pat on either side of the Tardis set when it came to phasing one in and the other out. I directed that bit. Pat was sitting up and shouting to Willie on the other side, 'Hello, Dad!'

Patrick Troughton prior to accepting the role of The Doctor.

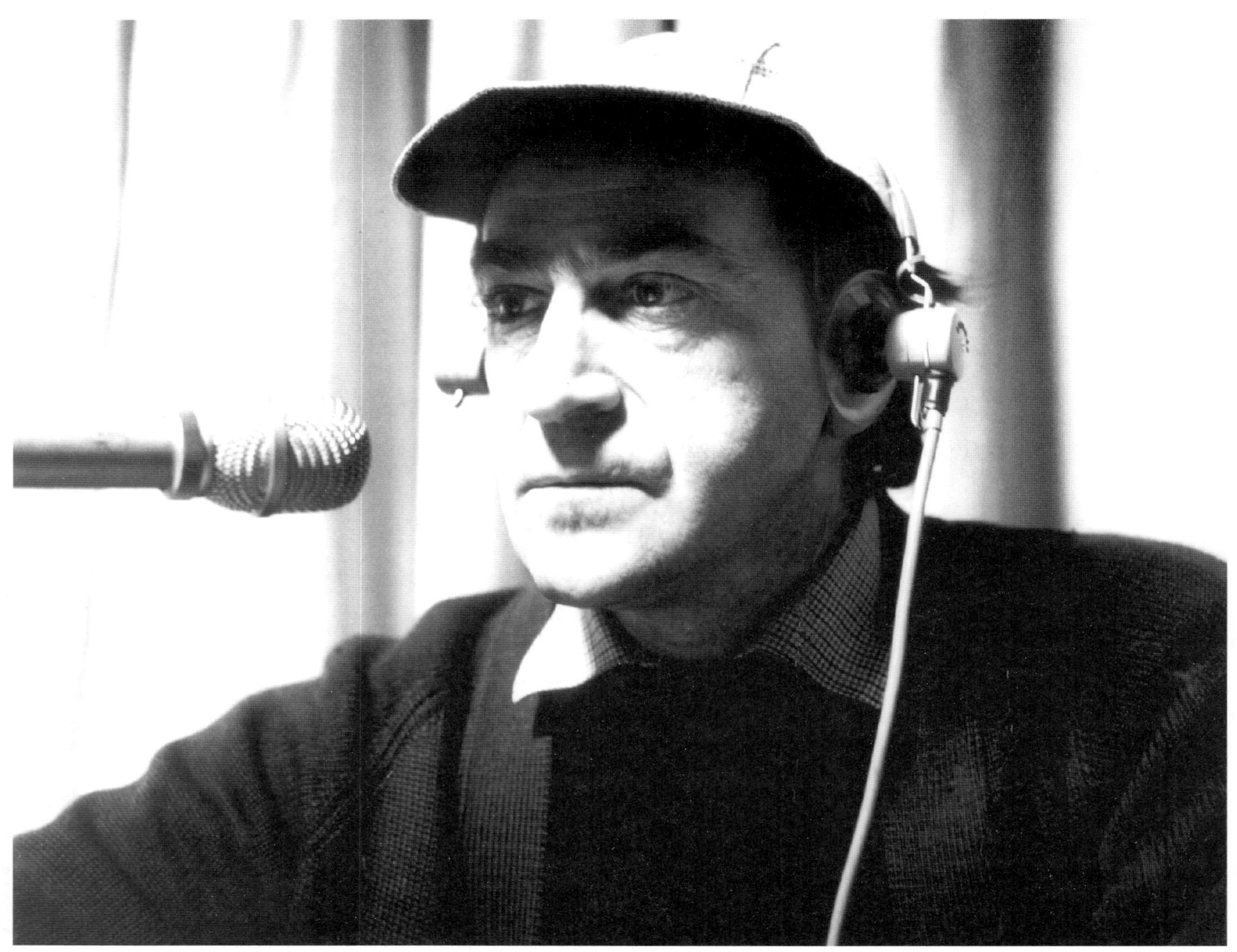

"We mixed their faces in using two cameras and did a slow mix and dissolve through. I never wanted Pat to do an exact copy of Willie. That would have driven him mad and held him back, which was not his way of doing things. His character sort of came together as soon as we'd found the right costume...the right look for the new Doctor."

The start of the fourth season began with an all-time low in the ratings but as soon as word got out that William Hartnell was leaving, curiosity began to bring the viewers back. Compared to the start of *The Smugglers*, with under four and a half million, *The tenth Planet* rose to seven and a half million by i's final episode and the figures would continue to rise as the adventures of the second Doctor began.

The 'look' of the Doctor had been established through a series of costume tests which were supervised by Innes Lloyd and Shaun Sutton, until someone else intervened...

Shaun Sutton:

"We had one or two tests and the one that Pat favoured was a sort of river pilot from the Mississippi, looking rather like a 19th century ship's captain. We knew that Sydney Newman was going to come down, because he wanted to be invloved. When he saw Pat in costume there was a terrible pause, and Sydney said, 'Could I have a word with you outside?'

Innes Lloyd:

"Sydney went off and told Shaun that he hated it. He came back in and took one look at Pat. 'Make him Chaplin! Make him a goddam hobbo of the skies!' So we found that baggy black coat, the bow ties and the braces. Pat found some pixie boots and that was it...apart from that damn hat!"

Patrick Troughton:

"I found this tall black hat, like something out of a Dickens story. The kind of thing Mr Quilp would have worn. I think I kept Billy's cape, and with the recorder, that was my Doctor sorted."

The stove-pipe hat to which they referred featured in the first three Troughton stories before it mysteriously vanished.

Lloyd:

"The hat went into the waste bin, because everyone thought it looked pretty ridiculous – except Pat, who never took it off. He loved his hats."

Shaun Sutton:

" We also used to hide the recorder. Innes stood at the side of the set all the time, watching to make sure that Pat behaved. Pat used to cover up forgotten lines by suddenly picking up the recorder and playing it. That had to stop."

Gerry Davis had gone to Terry Nation to see if he would write the first story, featuring the Daleks, as Lloyd explains:

"I thought Pat would need some support to make sure that people got used to him and that his Doctor was not pre-judged. The best way to get people to watch was by bringing the Daleks back."

Nation was committed to *The Baron* at ITC. David Whitaker explained what happened next:

"Terry suggested I should write Pat Troughton's first Dalek story, as I'd practically overseen the creation of *Doctor Who* as it was. He was very flattering about me and after Gerry Davis commissioned me, I seem to recall chatting to Terry about one or two ideas.

"I was working on other pro;ects, trying to come to terms with the difficulty of writing books (Whitaker had written the first *Doctor Who* novelisations – *The Daleks* *The Crusades* which, along with Bill Strutton's adaption of *The Zarbi,* made up the first trio of *Doctor Who* books), and the general discomfort of facing blank pages of glaring white in my typewriter each morning. I just didn't have time for any rewrites."

Having had no indication of how the 'new' Doctor would be played, Whitaker, understandably, underwrote the basic character of the Time Lord.

Dennis Spooner:

"I was between jobs, actually waiting to start up *The Champions* (a series he devised for ITC), when Gerry Davis gave me a frantic call. The scripts David had done over-ran horrendously. They needed tightening up and some characterisation added for Pat Troughton.

"I met Pat, got a few tips on the kind of things he wanted to do, and practically did the whole lot in a weekend. David always said that the art of editing *Doctor Who* was to trim away the meat, but always leave a taste of it on the bone... and there I was, having to do it to his scripts!"

Davis had no time to do any work on *The Power Of The Daleks*, which it became after initially being handed in by Whitaker as *The Destiny Of Doctor Who*.

He explains:

"Those early days with Pat were chaos because the people we were getting in to writethe scripts started to drift away. Elwyn Jones had written a draft of *The Highlanders* but he had to go and start editing *Softly, Softly* (the second season of a popular 'cop'

Michael Craze and Anneke Wills as Ben and Polly.

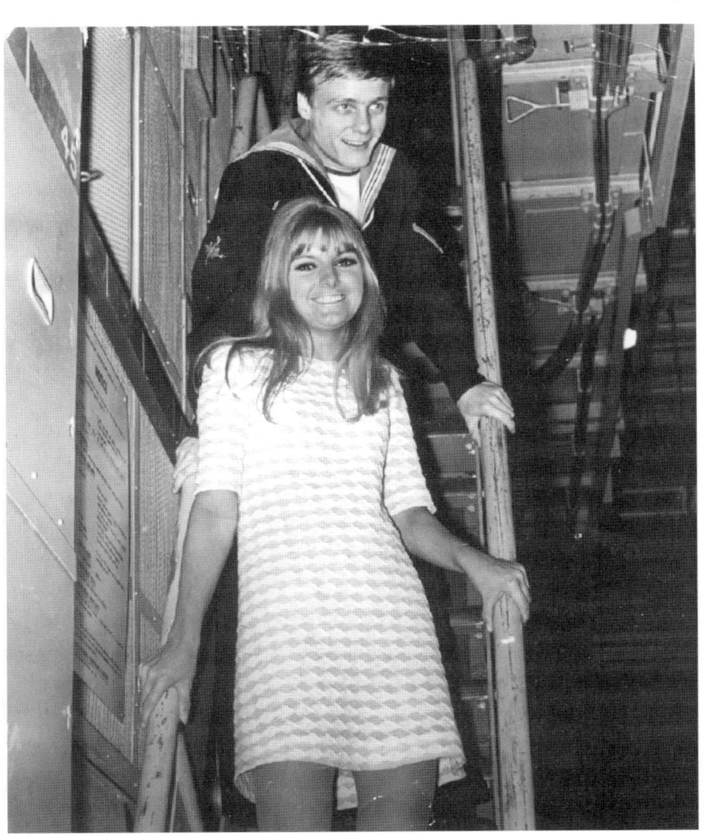

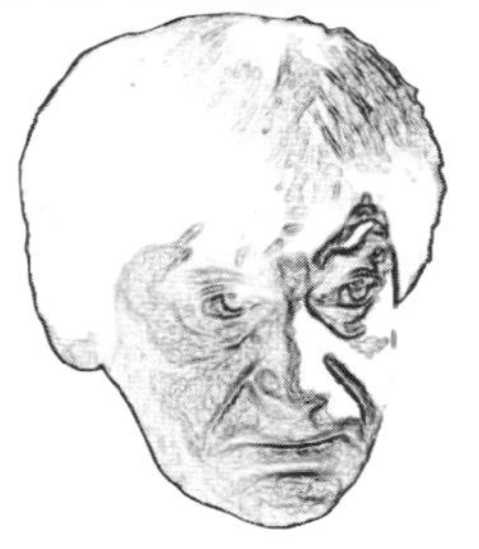

show, that was the follow-on from *Z-Cars*.), so I had to sit down and finish the whole thing off properly before Hugh David (the assigned director) arrived."

Under Christopher Barry's direction, the cast started rehearsing for the first episode on Tuesday 18th, before entering Riverside Studio One on 22 October. Episode two followed on the 29th, as the viewers saw the unthinkable happen. Hartnell departed on-screen in *The Tenth Planet* part four.

Troughton:

"I remember my first episode because we had a wonderful villain in Bernard Archard (Bragen). We knew each other from working in rep and I think we were in one or two of the old Children's Department serials together. It was nice to have a familiar face around because I was scared to death about the whole thing."

Episode three was recorded shortly after Troughton made his television debut on November 5th, with most of the cast watching in their lunch break on set at Riverside.

Lloyd:

"We had one or two television sets wheeled into the studio and Shaun and Sydney came down to watch. Pat couldn't face it and went and sat in the canteen. I remember because when he came back in, everyone stood up and applauded. That made him fluster like mad. He was very unsure and I think we gave him an inkling that he was going to be a hit."

Episode four was completed minus Anneke Wills, who was on holiday but returned in time to accompany Craze and Troughton as they left for Frensham Ponds in Surrey, to shoot outdoor scenes for *The Highlanders* with Hugh David Directing.

The fifth episode saw the famous 'Dalek Production Line' sequence where the creatures were seen being mass produced on a conveyor belt. The upper half of their casings were lowered onto the lower, as the creature inside (seen as a blob of tentacles) was lowered in to control the machine. Michael E. Briant, later one of Pertwee's directors, was the production assistant on the story.

"Chris Barry complained that the Dalek innards looked like strained cabbage, so we hurtled down the road to Woolworth's and bought a load of shaving foam, which we doused the things with so they looked as though they were oozing something unmentionable."

Episode six wrapped on 26 November. Sutton and Lloyd's faith in Troughton had paid off. The story hit a high of eight million viewers and the figures were set to rise even further for the next story, *The Highlanders*.

ABOVE: Patrick Troughton with his recorder.

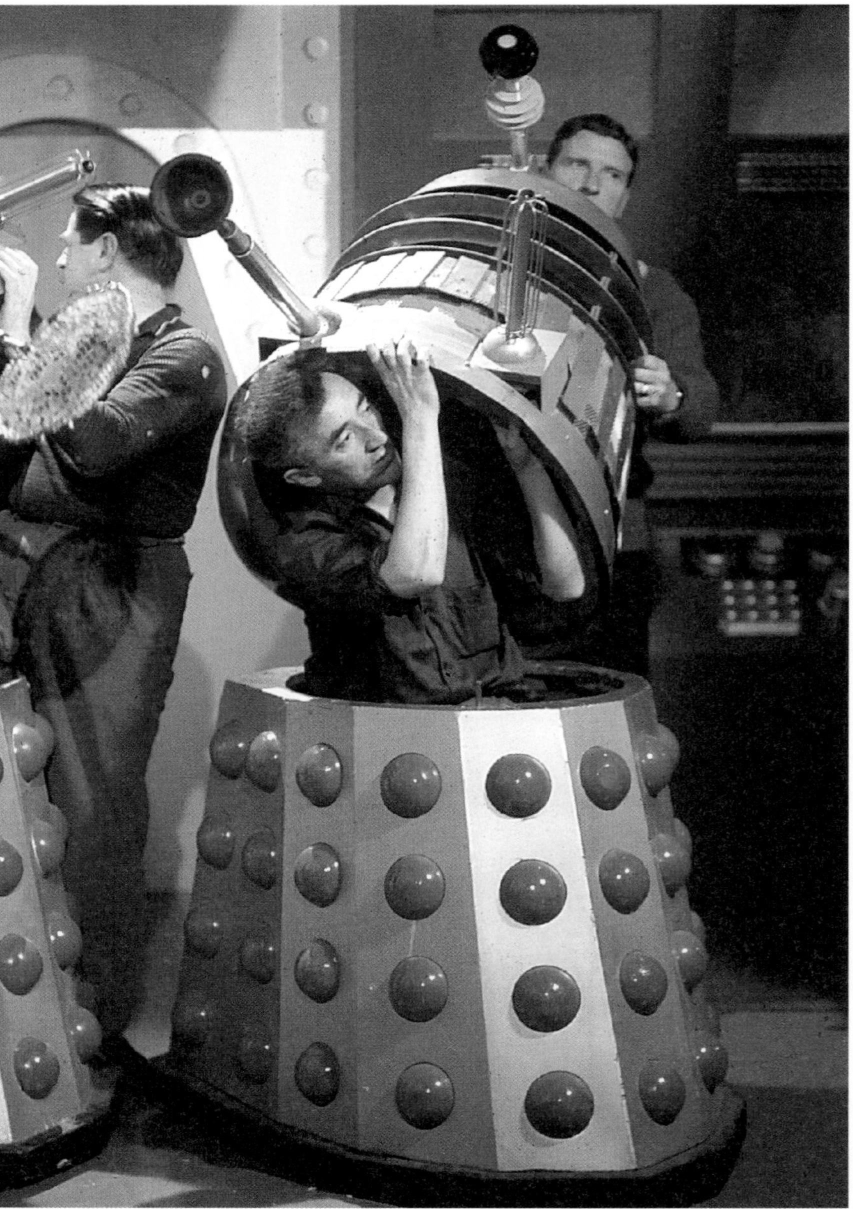

RIGHT: John Scott Martin being helped into a Dalek casing.

Hugh David:

"Innes was an old friend and grabbed me in the corridor of Union House and said he'd just taken over on *Doctor Who*, and would I like to come and direct one? I explained how I very nearly was the Doctor and he slapped me on the shoulder, and said, 'All the more reason to direct one then!'. Before I could say another word, he'd gone."

Davis had completed Jones' rewrites with little time to spare, as he recalled:

"Things were pretty much nightmarish, because the minute I'd finished with Elwyn's story, Geoffrey Orme's scripts were arriving (for *The Underwater Menace*) which were pretty unworkable.

"Kit had come back to me with an idea for a Cyberman story which was on the moon with a weather control station being attacked by them and I thought 'Great!', because we needed a monster back pretty quick or we'd start to loose the viewers again."

The production team now busily reworking all future episodes due to the performance of one of the actors on the location shoot for *The Highlanders* at Frensham Ponds. The character in question was Jamie McCrimmon, played by Frazer Hines.

Hugh David:

"Frazer was an old pro at that time. He'd been in films since he was a kid and knew the business backwards, so when I cast him I knew he'd be good. Innes and Gerry were so impressed that they showed Shaun Sutton the rushes and he agreed with them that Frazer should become a companion."

The production team went on location again from Monday 12 December to Tuesday 13th around Portland Bill in Dorset to shoot the main sequences involving the entrance to Atlantis, using a vast cave mouth, for *The Underwater Menace.*

When the main cast returned, work resumed on *The Highlanders* with episode three going into the studio on 17 December, while the rest of the week leading up to that Saturday was spent at Ealing where *The Underwater Menace* crew utilised the water tank facility there.

Hugh David:

"We had one long sequence where Mike Craze got keel-hauled, which was a hell of a torture. I did a load of research into it because I was curious as to whether people actually survived. A few did and they became rather wierd. It seems that the changes in pressure made their brains go funny as they were dragged under the boat and back up the opposite side. A lot of them seemed to become murderers, so I called Mike 'Killer' from that point on."

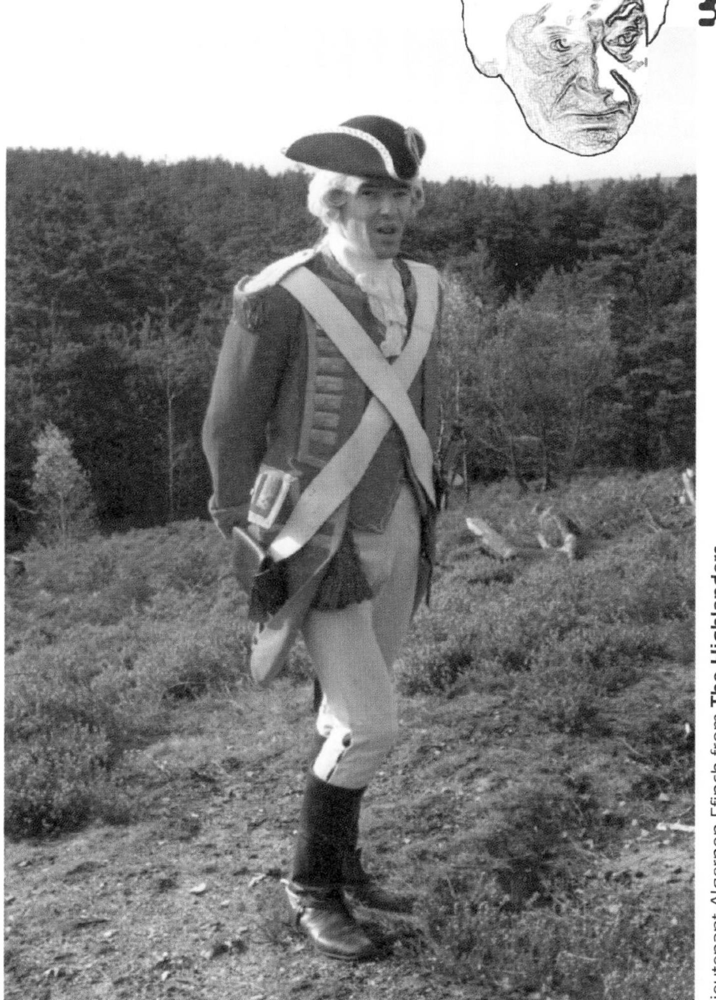
Lieutenant Algernon Ffinch from **The Highlanders.**

The final episode of *The Highlanders* was wrapped on Christmas Eve, with the cast moving on to a party thrown by Shaun Sutton afterwards, celebrating the renewed success enjoyed by *Doctor Who*. The second episode of the same story went out on the same day.

Hugh David:

"I thought that Innes wouldn't want to know me after turning down the Atlantis story, but at Shaun's party he came over and said he'd like me to come back. I was a bit tired and said could I leave it for a year. He smiled and said he'd hold me to that, which is exactly what he did." (David's next story, *Fury From The Deep*, started preproduction almost exactly a year later.)

The cast got back together on 3 January, following a week off during which Patrick Troughton began to experience what it meant to be Doctor Who.

"The letter box needed taping up, there were all these Christmas cards coming through and I just couldn't understand what was going on. My wife pointed out that the children who watched the show were sending them to Doctor Who... me!"

Episode one of *The Underwater Menace* caused problems for the production office when it was broadcast.

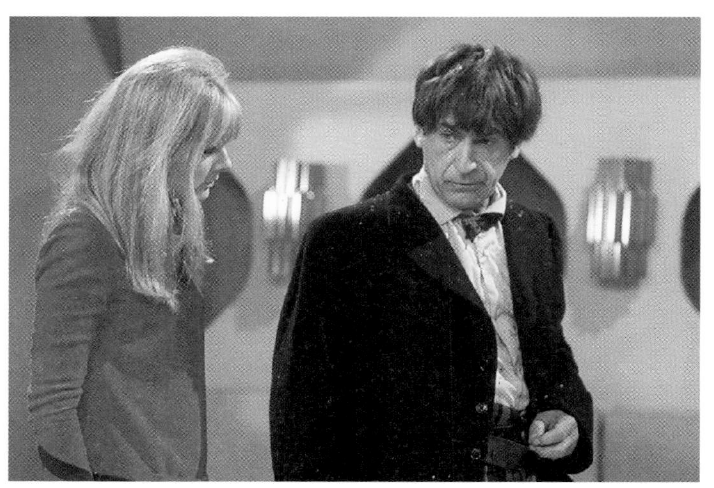
Patrick Troughton and Anneke Wills.

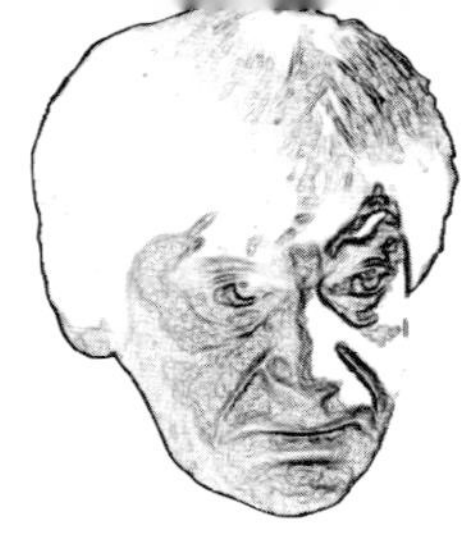

Innes Lloyd:

"I had some angry letters and phone calls because Anneke was injected by one of the villains. There was a Nurse who went spare because all her school children were due to have a jab during the following week, and she though they'd be terrified of having one after watching *Doctor Who*.

"A couple of days passed and my own Doctor rang up, asking whether I knew what I'd caused. I was about to rattle off an apology when he stopped me and said, 'Why are you saying sorry...I've had a queue of about twenty kids here this morning, all wanting injections because they saw your show!' Looking back on it though, I think we did make a blunder with that one."

Following on from Geoff Kirkland on *The Highlanders* and Jack Robinson on *The Underwater Menace*, Colin Shaw had arrived to work as the designer on *The Return Of The Cybermen*, with Morris Barry as Director. The story underwent a title change to *The Moonbase* during the early stages of production.

Shaw had erected a vast lunar landscape at Ealing where Morris Barry assembled the cast, cutting into two days of rehearsal on *The Underwater Menace*, to film the scenes of the Tardis landing, the travellers' ensuing weightless escapades and the trek to the moonbase of the title.

Patrick Troughton:

"We went to Ealing to film all the moon bits and they had us like *Thunderbirds* puppets on wires. You had to tell them your exact weight, so they could judge how hard to yank you to get you airborne. One or two of us told a few white lies on that point, mentioning no names, but let's just say she collided with me and her bottom ended up on my face!"

The Underwater Menace episode two was shot on 14 January and three on the 21st. The episodes were now only being completed in studio a week before broadcast, creating one of the tightest schedules the programme had ever had to face.

The 'monster' element of the story came in the shape of the Fish People, the results of medical experiments carried out on humans to create a slave worker capable of working underwater.

Lloyd:

"Ah, the Fish People. What can I say? Seemed like a good idea on paper, looked like a good idea in the design, looked horrendous on screen. If I remember correctly, the cost of doing the Cybermen on the moon cut into the money on that one and the result was like something from one of those old movies they made in America in the 1950s. *Attack Of The Nasty Ocean Creatures*, that sort of thing!"

The Cybermen were heavily re-designed with the more familiar 'metal' figure being seen for the first time. The main body was covered with a vinyl boiler suit sprayed silver and the chest unit had been made far more compact. The actor's head was concealed inside a mask that was bolted into place. The effect was startling.

Lloyd:

"The new Cybermen worked really well. I wasn't at all happy with the thought of bringing the cloth versions back because they always reminded me of rag dolls. When Morris directed them, they'd become a force to be reckoned with. I was delighted."

The vast set of the weather control centre housed a heavy, working prop that had to be supported from the roof of the studio.

Patrick Troughton:

"They had this thing called a Gravitron. I know, because it nearly killed me. When I played Doctor Who, I used to potter around the set on the Saturday afternoon in the tea break, just to get used to everything and see what was what. I was looking at this thing from underneath, the sides and all round the place and just as I started to walk away...BANG!...the whole bloody lot had fallen from the roof! If I'd been underneath, I'd have been squashed as flat as a pancake. Morris Barry nearly had a heart attack when I told him!"

The main cast were again taken away for location work on the next story, a rubbish tip in Brighton being the venue for *The Macra Terror*, with John Davies directing. A building sight nearby was also utilised in the day or so of shooting that was required.

The cast returned to rehearse the fourth episode of *The Moonbase*, due to record in studio on 25 February. The Cybermen voices had changed dramatically since their debut story. Just like the Daleks, their voices could be produced by the actors using

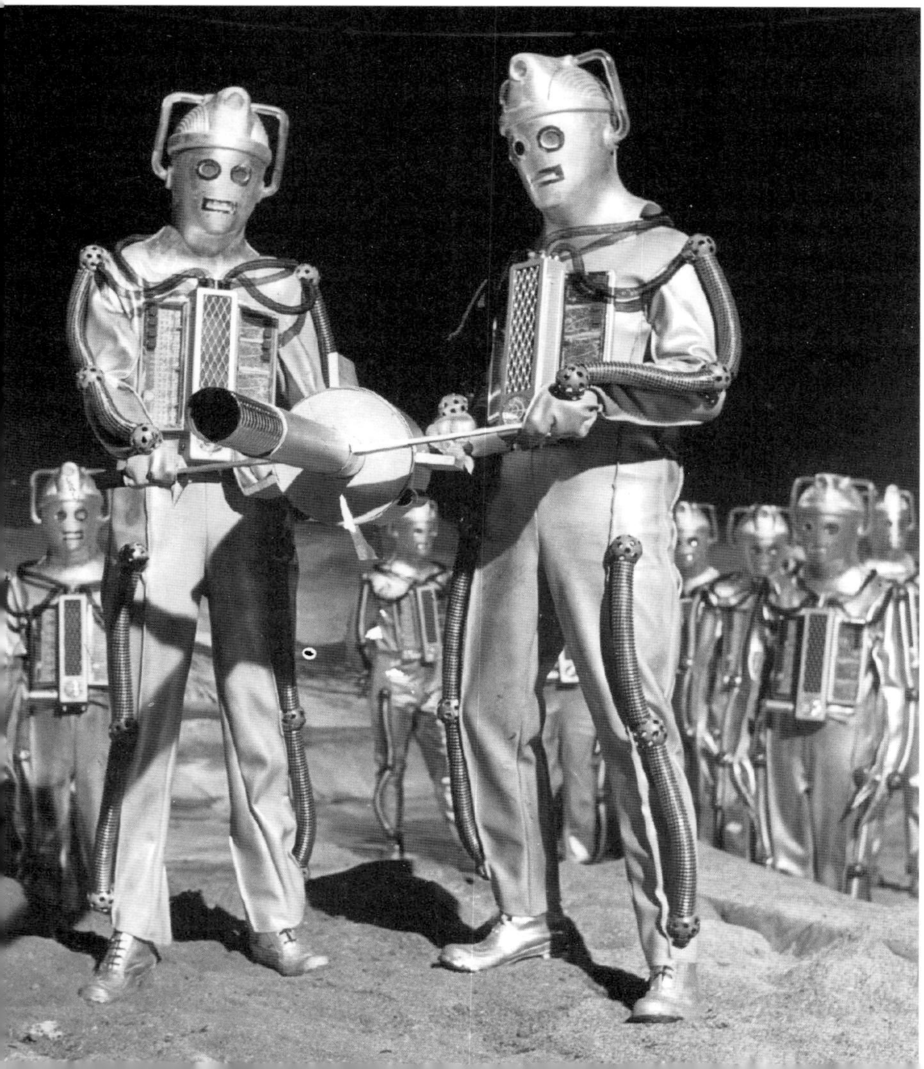

The Cybermen prepare to attack **The Moonbase**.

distortion on the microphone set with which they were working. With the first Cybermen, the actor in the costume had to open his mouth on cue, to match the dialogue of the men behind the Cybermen's voices, actors Roy Skelton and Peter Hawkins. The new costumes had a 'letter-box' mouth flap, that could be opened by the actor's chin inside, making it slightly easier to get the dialogue in sync. Hawkins was again involved as a Cyberman and had to use a dental palate.

"I had this lead plate in my mouth connected up to some batteries that made it hum continually. By mouthing the words in the script, it came out as a cyber-voice. It was the same kind of thing that people who loose their vocal chords use to speak but it gives you a hell of a headache with the continual pulse of electricity going through your skull."

Additional filming sequences at Ealing for *The Macra Terror* were now complete and the creatures of the title were brought to life on the back of a small van.

Gerry Davis:

"Ian Stuart Black had written a story where gigantic spider-crabs were using humans to mine gas for them. Innes loved it. He liked things where nature was distorted and the Doctor had to fight against it.

"They only had one of these crabs and they had to get it into the studio on the back of a van because it weighed so much. When they got it on the studio floor, it looked like one of those wierd suits you used to see the contestants in on *It's A Knockout*.

"As soon as the lighting went down, the mist was pumped through the pipes surrounding it and this awful roar came belting out over the speakers. The crab's eyes started to glow as it chased after Frazer. I couldn't believe how frightening it looked. That just went to prove how you can never underestimate the designers."

Designer Kenneth Sharp and John Davies had gone round various museums' Natural History departments in their quest for a 'look' for the Macra and eventually favoured a kind of crab as opposed to a spider.

Patrick Troughton:

"I remember when we had this damn great crab in the studio, and it was quite hysterical because as soon as they called 'Stop Recording', there would be a pause, and the rear end of this thing would suddenly flip up and a little man would get out lighting up a cigarette."

As of episode four of *The Moonbase*, *Doctor Who* moved back to Lime Grove Studio D, where episode one of *The Macra Terror* was recorded on 4 March.

Innes Lloyd:

"I made it my personal quest doing *Doctor Who* to get as many of *The Plane Makers* cast as I could into the series, and Peter Jeffrey was one of them. I aimed to get well known actors, and succeeded to a certain degree, but when Peter and Marius (Goring, who appeared in *Evil Of The Daleks*) came in for a few weeks, we were suddenly legitimate and not a nasty kids' show any more. Agents actually began to come to us with their 'name' clients after that point"

Lloyd had decided by this time that the characters of Ben and Polly were no longer working, and that the show had to bring in 'new blood' to survive. Wills and Craze were informed of this shortly after work had begun on *The Moonbase*. Lloyd recalls:

"It was time for a change and I felt we needed to bring in someone new. My other thought was that the Tardis was beginning to look a bit overcrowded. It was fine having Mike and Anneke there when Willie was the Doctor because he was a lot older and they brought colour and energy to the stories.

"Patrick was not that much older and he was lively and dancing about the place all of the time, so I told them I felt it was best if they moved on. I didn't want them killed off, or anything like that. As far as I and the viewers knew, they were a couple and they had to leave together. It was as simple as that."

Gerry Mill had arrived to direct the next story, *The Faceless Ones*, in which the characters would leave and Geoff Kirkland returned as the designer, having previously worked on *The Highlanders*.

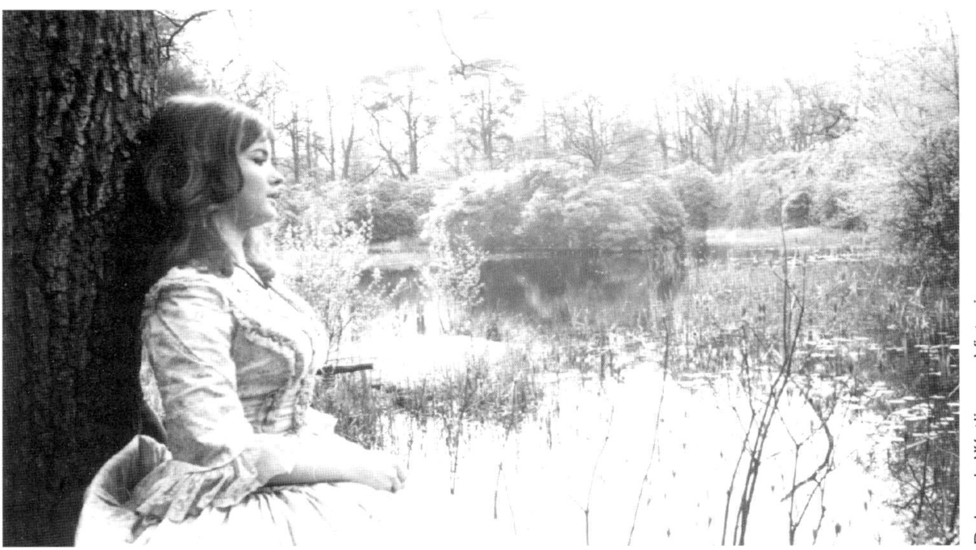

Deborah Watling as Victoria.

Lloyd:

"I was keen for some filming to be done at a location that would be immediately recognisable – a landmark or a point of industry or travel. Gatwick Airport seemed an idea and when we approached them, they 'ummed' a bit and said 'Yes' eventually.

"We had a script that was set somewhere else (*The Big Store*, set in a department store), and Gerry came up with the idea of reworking that one. He was actually in the process of leaving when all that happened. I had wanted Gerry to take over from me as producer, but he didn't want to know."

Davis:

"I wouldn't have felt comfortable in the same position as Innes. I was a writer then, as I still am, and I didn't want to be that trapped. As a script editor I could still do the odd bit of tinkering with stories here and there but producing would have taken that one thing away. That was too much to ask."

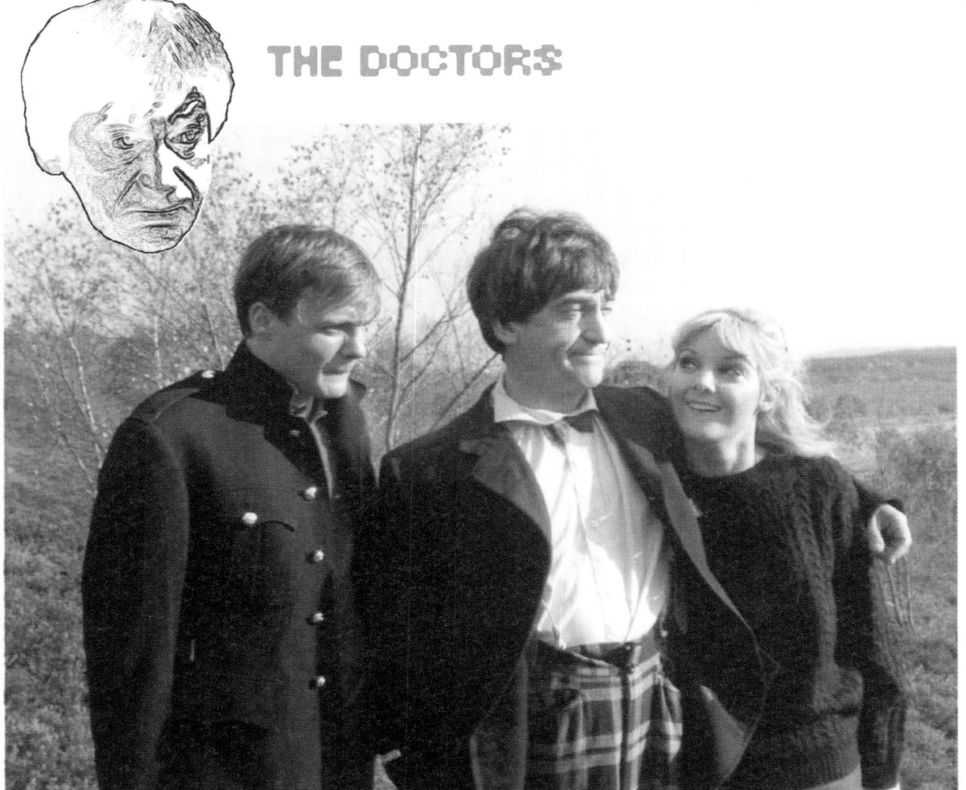

The Doctor with Ben and Polly.

Former TV and Radio actor Peter Bryant was trailing Davis, having joined the team as a story associate as far back as the latter episodes of *The Moonbase*. Lloyd formally offered Bryant the job to take over from Davis, which he accepted.

The new Gatwick story, *The Faceless Ones,* was written by Malcolm Hulke (who had had many ideas rejected on *Doctor Who* in the past) and David Ellis (who had also submitted several plotlines in the past). Peter Bryant is credited as the associate producer for the first three episodes. As he explains:

"Innes was showing me the ropes, as I was being groomed to take over from him when he finally left."

The Faceless Ones was a dry run and Bryant would be given his own story to produce. *The Faceless Ones* went into rehearsal on 28 March, and went into studio with episode one on 1 April. Episode two followed a week later, marking the last work that Craze and Wills would do on the programme.

The actual farewell scene shared between Ben, Polly, Jamie and the Doctor had been shot at Gatwick, and they were not needed for the studio work beyond episode two. Patrick Troughton was sad to see them go.

"Mike and Anneke had been there when I arrived, so we'd been through a lot. They'd wet-nursed me through my initial terrors of being Doctor Who, and kept me going in the run up to my first story. Anneke used to keep an eye on me to check I was all right. We were a family, but Innes Lloyd wanted to see a wider variety of faces moving through the Tardis, so it was time for Mike and Anneke to go. I was very sad, but I still had Frazer with me, and Debbie was waiting round the corner."

Around mid-April, work began on David Whitaker's *Evil Of The Daleks.*

Whitaker:

"The story of *Alice In Wonderland* had always been of great fascination to me and I had an idea about setting a *Doctor Who* story in the same kind of mystical Victorian landscape. I never thought that the idea would come to anything but Gerry Davis contacted me with a view to writing a 'final' Dalek story, and that's what *Evil Of The Daleks* became."

Terry Nation had been planning to make his own series featuring the Daleks with his production company producing the finished shows. A pilot script was written after he completed work on *The Baron* at ITC, and it was sent to the BBC only to be rejected. Nation then planned to take his creations to America, and make the show there effectively taking the rights to use the characters in *Doctor Who* with him. As it turned out, the Dalek series was never filmed but it would be a matter of five years after *Evil* before they were seen again in *Doctor Who.*

Evil Of The Daleks ran to seven episodes. Derek Martinus returned as the director, with Chris Thompson as his designer. The first of the locations he selected to be used was the Grim's Dyke Hotel, in Middlesex, and filming started on 20 April. Troughton and Hines were shooting on that day and the 21st, before returning to *The Faceless Ones.* Kendal Avenue in London was used to double up as Gatwick for the pick-up from the previous story where the Tardis is stolen from the airport.

Evil Of The Daleks also saw the debut of a new companion. Victoria Waterfield, played by Debbie Watling, had been selected after extensive auditions but this had not always been the plan.

Lloyd:

"Pauline Collins was in the Chameleon story shot at Gatwick, and she was very much meant to be a kind of *Avengers* girl, very strong and fashionable. I even asked her to be the new Who-girl but she said no, as she preferred stage work to TV. It was a shame, as the character (Samantha Briggs) would have worked well with Pat and Frazer but Debbie came into it and she was wonderful."

Lloyd was impressed by the Chameleons, who were seen as featureless humanoids, with their arms and heads blistered to the point where you could clearly see their veins, thanks to heavy latex make-up.

Lloyd:

"The creatures we had on that were very striking, and they represented an element I enjoyed bringing into the show, where the most horrendous threats come from beings that are very similar to our own race. As with the Cybermen, as Kit always pointed out, we could end up like them..."

Evil Of The Daleks started recording on 13 May and the following week marked the arrival of Marius Goring as Theodore Maxtible.

Lloyd:

"Marius was a huge star, a big film star and for a while I think that everybody felt slightly intimidated by that fact. After a couple of weeks, however, they were all like old friends. I think Patrick must have known him already, having been in an awful lot of films himself."

Evil Of The Daleks saw the BBC Visual Effects team become actively involved with the programme for the first time. From this story onwards, they would handle all the effects work, following problems with the freelancers used on *The Faceless Ones.*

Patrick Troughton:

"The effects guys always struck me as being one yard short of a mile. You have to be slightly dotty to be able to stand in front of an explosion just to test if it will burn you. They knew their job inside out."

The grand finale went before the cameras on 24 June, with the climax being the destruction of the Emperor Dalek.

Derek Martinus:

"The Emperor was a huge prop, sitting in its own throne room – it was sort of the King of the Daleks. It didn't have a gun or anything like that, just this damn great eye stalk waving around with tubes connecting it to the roof. It really looked quite incredible."

The creature had already been destroyed during the filming at Ealing, under Timothy Combe's supervision.

"We had this damn great Dalek packed with explosives. We had cameras all over the place, so that I had every angle covered when we blew the thing up. I gave the nod and hid, and KABOOM! The rafters shook, doors blew open, the explosion was heard right down on the Ealing Broadway (some quarter of a mile away), and dust and splinters showered down from the roof.

"I thought, 'If those cameras didn't work, I'm a dead man!', but they did. Derek Martinus was delighted and when he cut it all together, it looked unbelievable. I'm surprised we didn't cause any damage, to be honest."

Gerry Davis finally left the production team midway through *Evil Of The Daleks* and Peter Bryant formally took over for the final four weeks of the story.

Lloyd:

"We gave him the next Cyberman story, because they were a sure-fire thing. They were popular and you'd have to make some pretty horrendous errors to go wrong with them. We got Morris Barry back as well because he knew how to cope with them."

Barry had joined the team by episode four of *Evil* to start work on *The Tomb Of The Cybermen*, which was jointly written by Pedler and Davis. Victor Pemberton, who was working as assistant script editor on *Evil*, took over from Bryant for*Tomb* while he got on with producing it.

It was decided early on that the sequences that showed the Cybermen emerging from the Tombs of the title had to be shot at a film studio. Martin Johnson, the designer, wanted to utilise the concept to the full and present something that would not let the idea down. Ealing was selected and work began there from 13 June.

For the rest of that week, the main filming for the 'awakening' sequence was shot, revolving around a 29 foot high scaffolding rig with honey-comb like cryogenic compartments housing a Cyber-actor on each of its multi-levels. The compartments were sealed with a sheet of clear plastic film stretched across their front. On cue, the actors inside forced their way out through the sheets and climbed down to ground level. One of the most famous sequences in the programme's history had been created.

The fourth series drew to a close on 1 July as *Tomb* went into Lime Grove studio D for recording of its first episode. As with the previous seasons, material recorded at the end of the year was held over for the next series. *Tomb* would open the fifth series.

Apart from *The Smugglers* at the beginning of the run, the fourth season had maintained an average audience of between six and just over eight million viewers. The second episode of *The Moonbase* reached a high of just under nine million.

Patrick Troughton:

"The end of that first year had settled any doubts I had. I have to admit that there were one or two thoughts going through my head about leaving within six months and letting them get

BELOW LEFT: On location in Wales for **The Abominable Snowmen**. Innes Lloyd can be seen on the right wearing a camel-coloured duffel coat. BELOW: A yeti receives assistance.

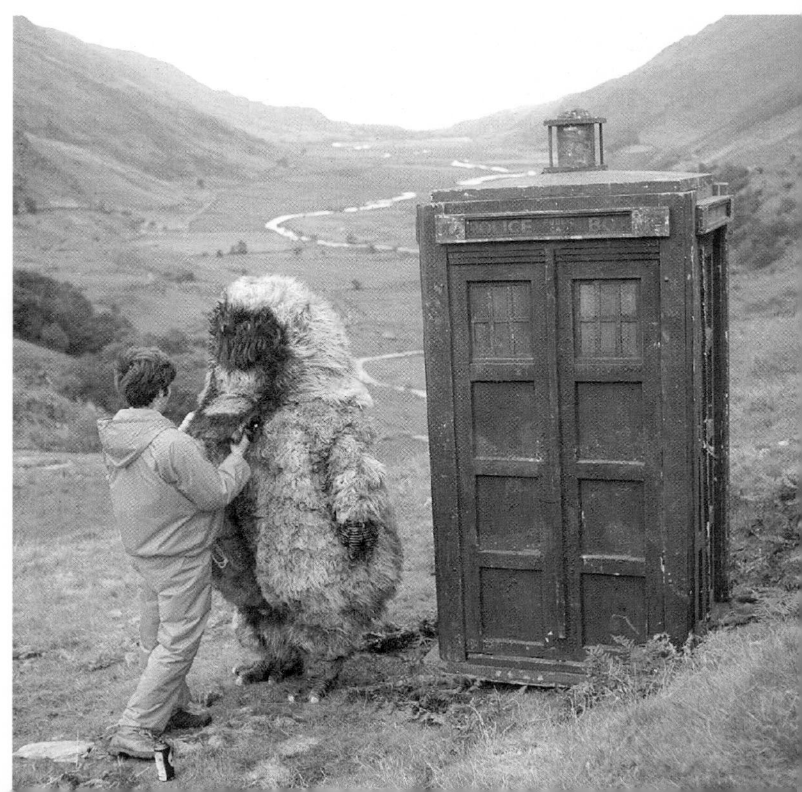

someone better in, but I actually began to enjoy myself.

"When Debbie came in, and with Frazer there already, we had the feeling of being a real team. We socialised together, played jokes on each other, and generally had an awful lot of fun. I was happy to go on for another year."

The annual holiday began as *Tomb* wrapped and the production team reverted to their normal routine with Lloyd back as Producer and Bryant as the Script Editor. Pemberton left a few weeks later having been commissioned to write his own story for the end of the fifth series, *Fury From The Deep*.

Lloyd realised that as Terry Nation had taken the Daleks to America to try and get their own show started there, he was left without *Doctor Who's* most popular monster. There were the Cybermen, certainly, but little else.

Lloyd explains:

"I was never a fan of science fiction as such, but of strong narrative drives with interesting characters. If science fiction was presented to me in that form, fine, I was happy to be involved. I wanted monsters who had a real background written in, ones with a past... not ones who had nothing to do for an afternoon and decided to invade the Earth, but creatures with a past, with a culture."

There had been stories for years about sightings of a strange race of creatures in Tibet which the press had christened 'The Abominable Snowmen'. That kind of reality also appealed to Lloyd.

"The Yeti story came about because I wanted the odd story where *Doctor Who* confronted Earth's mythology and found that it had an alien presence behind it. I didn't want to disprove the Yeti myth, which is why we had a real one spotted by Jack Watling at the end. I think I asked for a Loch Ness Monster story as well, but we didn't get anywhere with that idea."

Mervyn Haisman and Henry Lincoln were commissioned to write a six-part story called *The Abominable Snowmen*.

Lloyd:

"By lengthening the stories to six episodes, we saved a bit of money, allowing us to do a bit more work on location. The Yeti one was a big step, because we went away for a week, which was unheard of up till then."

Director Gerald Blake was given the story to helm, with Malcolm Middleton working as his designer. Blake explained about the scheduling of the location filming.

"We couldn't go down to Surrey and pretend it was Tibet, that would have looked awful. We had to go big and actually go to a mountain. Innes wanted snow, so we thought of Ben Nevis, which proved unworkable, so we went down to Snowdonia in Wales. We actually ended up filming in exactly the same spots where they did *Carry On Up The Khyber* a couple of years later."

The Yeti themselves were designed by Martin Baugh and were incredibly bulky. The shape of the creatures was achieved by creating a framework with bamboo canes which was supported across the Yeti-actors shoulder with braces and covered with a thick layer of rubber-backed fur. There were no visible features on the face area; the fur was just a shade darker than the rest of the body. A cavity was left in the chest area to house their 'control spheres' and the claws and feet were made of thick rubber, courtesy of the visual effects department.

The spheres were vac-formed and painted silver. These enabled the 'Great Intelligence', the shapeless entity and villain of the story, to send orders to the robotic creatures. The actors vouched for the fact that the finished suits were very comfortable, and, as Blake explains:

"There was a plus and minus to the Yeti. When we got to Wales the rain literally came down, and we lost a couple of days shooting because of it. The mud was really slippery and the Yeti went flying whenever they tried to walk across it because they couldn't see a thing from inside the fur.

"The plus side, and it was revenge for the Yeti when people laughed at them falling around the place, was the fact that the actors were as warm as toast inside, while the rest of us got our nuts frozen off!"

Filming finally got underway on 6 September. Scenes revolving around the Tardis arriving in Tibet and the sequences involving the attack on Professor Travers' encampment were the first to be shot.

Travers was an explorer intent of discovering the truth about the mystical creatures and was played by Jack Watling, Debbie Watling's father.

Innes Lloyd:

"There was only a slight degree of nepotism behind that but Jack was a good actor and I'd known him for years. I seem to remember it led to a considerable degree of corpsing amongst the Watling family on set but that happened anyway with Pat being around the place."

Patrick Troughton:

"I loved the Yeti. I've always had a soft spot for them. The idea was good, and the costumes were so cuddly. I've always said that I'd be quite happy to come back to *Doctor Who* for a day, totally uncredited, and be a monster as I'm sure it's a hell of a lot of fun. I secretly wanted to be one but Innes would have none of it and said a quite catagoric 'No!' when I asked him.

"The thing that I found amazing was that the children loved them. Absolutely adored them. We were followed by a gang of kids in Wales and the Yetis used to wander towards them, and they just stared at them and stroked their fur. Didn't scare them in the slightest – but when they were brought back, that was a different story altogether."

Innes Lloyd:

"The decision was taken in the first couple of weeks we were working on that first Yeti story to do some sort of sequel. We asked Mervyn and Henry to do it then and there because we knew that the Yeti would be popular, judging by the reaction we had on location (The result of the second commission was *The Web Of Fear*). We toughened them up when they came back. It was the last one I had any input with, and I know I wanted them to look rougher, a bit nastier."

Gerald Blake:

"You haven't lived till you've seen two make-up girls fussing round a Yeti in the middle of the Welsh mountains, fluffing up its fur with a hairdryer. The monsters got the full star treatment in those days."

The trip to Wales cut into the plans for the studio work quite considerably, and the only way to get everything back on line was to record the material needed for episodes one and two over two consecutive days. The general routine for the fifth series would be to have a readthrough on the Saturday folowed by rehearsals Monday to Thursday and recording on Friday night.

For *The Abominable Snowmen*, episodes one and two went into Lime Grove's Studio D on Friday 15 and Saturday 16 September. Insert filming for the rest of the episodes was finished of at Ealing following that with episode three going into studio on Friday 22nd. After that, things were back to normal. *Tomb Of The Cybermen* had started transmission on 2 September, so there were now only three weeks between recording and broadcast.

Derek Martinus was now back, some three months after finishing *Evil Of The Daleks*, to direct Brian Hayles' new six-part story, *The Ice Warriors*. This submission had won a commission because Lloyd was fascinated with the idea of having an intelligent race of alien soldiers come up against the Doctor.

Lloyd:

"We managed to get Peter Barkworth, which nobody could quite believe when he said 'yes', but I was delighted (he was in *The Plane Makers*), and we had Peter Sallis and dear Bernard Bresslaw as the head monster. I remember Shaun Sutton saying, 'When are Olivier and Ralph Richardson going to play Daleks, Innes?'"

Episode four of *The Abominable Snowmen* went into the studio on 29 September, the day before the first part of the story was broadcast. As episode five started rehearsing, Martinus borrowed some of the regular cast every so often for the filming that was underway that week at Ealing, where Bresslaw first experienced wearing his Ice Warrior costume.

A huge body shell fitted over the arms and legs which were encased in thick latex skins, held up with braces and across the shoulders with straps. The chin of the actor was made up with reptilian skin and the head was covered with a helmet which had red gells across the eye holes. Make up was applied around the eyes underneath to conceal them.

Bresslaw recalled:

"Derek Martinus had described this character to me, making it sound as though I was going to play some Norse God that comes up against Doctor Who. I thought the scripts were good and I turned out to be a huge, armoured soldier. No furs or metal helmets at all!

"We had an awful time getting into the costumes, as it was rather like a jigsaw, with bits going on to make the other bits fit. I think it must have been made of fibreglass, or something just as itchy, because the skin that was bare underneath got rubbed raw."

Derek Martinus:

"We had to supply boards at an angle, so that the Ice Wariors could lean against them and get their breath back when they weren't needed on the set. They got very hot and tired, and there was no way they could sit down and ever be able to get up again in that costume, so the boards were the only way we could figure out the help them."

Rehearsals for the fifth episode were affected by the filming which was now starting on the next story, David Whitaker's *The Enemy Of The World*.

Whitaker explains:

"Bunny Webber had wanted to do a story where there were two Doctors, one bad and one good, so that there could be a climax at the end of the story where the two met up, and nobody could tell which was which. I sent in a plotline which was eventually dusted down and used. I had a fascination for Australia, and I've been here for a few years (this was 1978), and I just thought it would be an interesting setting for a *Doctor Who*. Not a normal, run-from-the-monsters-and-scream story, but one with a political edge to it's narrative."

The director was future *Doctor Who* producer Barry Letts, who took a film crew to Littlehampton in West Sussex for sequences intended to look like a beach on the Australian coast. Villiers House in Redhill was used as the exterior of the headquarters for Salamander, the Doctor's doppleganger in the story.

In retrospect, Letts now admits that the story was technically very demanding.

"During the season, they were doing one every Friday, and that's a real killer for anybody. If you were doing a six-parter, trying to keep up with the camera script and trying to work out what's happening next, especially if the script's late, you found yourself working a sixteen hour day."

The Ice Warriors was completed on 24 November.

Innes Lloyd:

"We had the Yeti, and the Ice Warriors, and then there was the Australian one with the two Patricks, which was when I left. Sydney kept good to his promise, and gave me *Thirty Minute Theatre* to move onto, which was just the kind of thing I'd wanted to do all along.

"Don't get me wrong, *Doctor Who* was a baptism of fire and I enjoyed every minute of it. Of course, there were the highs and lows, but that's the same with anything you do in television."

Episode One of *The Enemy Of The World* was recorded on December 1st, with part two following on the 7th, again at Lime Grove Studio D. Troughton was having to deal with playing two characters, and as he recalled:

"I had a ball with that one. The baddie was this gruff mexican-type, very dark and brooding, while the Doctor was his normal self. It was a bit of mental swings and roundabouts to get through it but it worked because I remember a woman coming up to me and asking how they found someone who looked so much like me for the part. Quite a compliment, really."

Barry Letts:

"Patrick was a very experienced character actor. Once he'd rehearsed what he was doing, he'd be able to snap in and out of character at the snap of a finger. He was superb, both as an actor and technically too."

The story finished recording on 5 January 1968 and Troughton expressed his concern to Letts during this period about how he was growing tired of the extreme, unrelenting work schedule on the series.

Letts:

"We'd been colleagues and friends since 1950 and worked together a lot, and we were chatting in his dressing room when he said, 'Look, I want your advice. They've asked me to go on to another season, and I don't know whether to or not, because this is a killer. Also, I don't want to get known as Doctor Who, and never work again.'

"So, we talked about it a bit, and I said, 'Well, I'll tell you what I'd do', and I suggested that the sensible thing would be to say he'd like to do it again, but as a shorter season. A six month season would leave enough time to do proper filming, instead of the killing schedule of having to do a seven-day week."

The changeover came into effect when *Doctor Who* moved into colour towards the end of 1969 and Jon Pertwee took over. Patrick Troughton never saw the benefits of Barry Letts' idea.

At the beginning of January, Hugh David took the principal cast down to Margate for location filming on *Fury From The Deep*, with Peter Kindred as Designer.

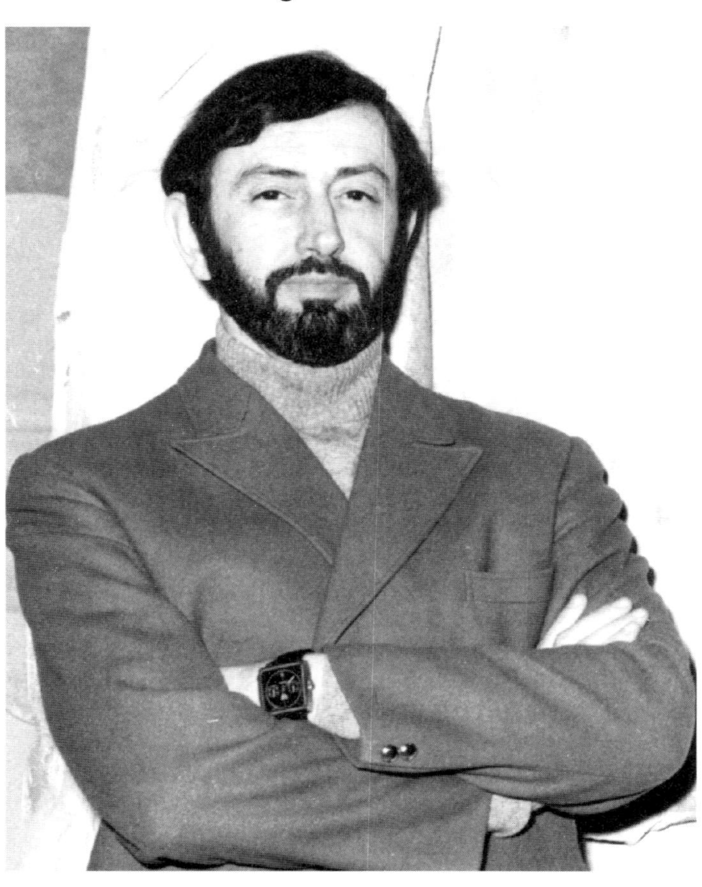

Brian Hayles, creator of the Ice Warriors.

Hugh David:

"We were there when it was Debbie's birthday, and Pat and Frazer had a word in my ear, asking me to go for an extra take after I'd got one I was satisfied with. They wouldn't tell me why, but I guessed it had something to do with all the foam we'd sprayed onto the shoreline.

"I gave Pat the nod to let him know I was happy and he winked, and they went for it again. Suddenly, the two men grabbed a leg and an arm each, picked her up and threw her into the foam. Everybody was howling with laughter and poor Debbie was spitting this stuff out, saying how 'perfectly horrid' she thought we all were, and then she started to laugh as well."

Episode One of *The Web Of Fear* went into studio D on January 13th. Haisman and Lincoln had brought back Professor Travers in their scripts, with Jack Watling having been forewarned about the return of his character towards the end of work on *The Abominable Snowmen*, allowing him to book his time in advance so that he would be available for the recording dates.

"The Yeti came back after I'd gone," remembers Watling, "but I couldn't resist going and having a look. I was surprised because they'd gone from looking like 'Teddy Bears', to being 'Angry Teddy Bears'. They looked as if someone had attacked them with a razor!"

The Yeti costumes were the same basic suits that had been constructed for *The Abominable Snowmen*, with adaptions so that they were a lot thinner and their eyes now glowed. The addition of having them carry web-guns, which sprayed a lethal jet of the substance at their victims, altered their appearance quite dramatically and the production team was worried enough to have Troughton record a warning for younger viewers about the Yeti's return. This was screened after the end of *The Ice Warriors*.

The main setting for the story was the London Underground system, which the production team thought London Transport would be happy to let them use.

Douglas Camfield:

"We hit a brick wall when London Transport said it cost two hundred pounds an hour to film there. That would have meant spending practically the entire year's budget on one episode. We built our own in the studio, copying the original designs, and using the odd altered angle here and there. We got away with making it look as though it was far more than just twenty feet of tracks.

"When the episodes were screened, Peter Bryant had these furious officials write to him saying they were going to sue the BBC for every penny they had, for filming on their property without their permission. I thought that was the best compliment David Myerscough-Jones was ever likely to have. I mean, if we even managed to con them?"

A footway tunnel in Greenwhich had doubled up for an entrance to the Underground system, and the battle between the Yeti and Colonel Lethbridge Stewart's troops was staged in the early hours of the morning in and around Old Covent Garden. David Langton, later to find fame in *Upstairs Downstairs*, was cast as Lethbridge-Stewart by Camfield, but he backed out at short notice.

Camfield explains:

"I'd cast Nicholas Courtney as the Captain of the Paras in *The Web Of Fear*, having worked with him already on *Doctor Who* with the Dalek story (*Master Plan*). When Langton pulled out, I did a rethink and decided to make the character younger and more of a 'Mad Mitch' of the Argyles sort.

"I think we played around with the name a bit, and came up with the full Alistair Gordon Lethbridge-Stewart title. Nick gave a hell of a performance and it was the first of many. Whenever we've seen each other, Nick's always bought me a drink to say thanks. He's never forgotten."

While *The Enemy Of The World* was in production, Debbie Watling had gone to Peter Bryant and expressed a desire to leave the series in a couple of months. Bryant was very keen to keep her on but she was adamant, wishing to return to working on the stage. Victor Pemberton had been told to re-draft the ending of *Fury From The Deep* to accomodate her decision.

Meanwhile, towards the end of production on *The Web Of Fear*, more filming had taken place under Hugh David's direction for *Fury*. Michael E Briant was the production assistant on the story:

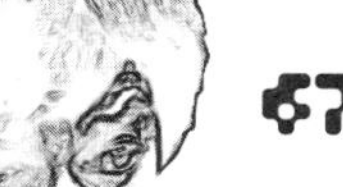

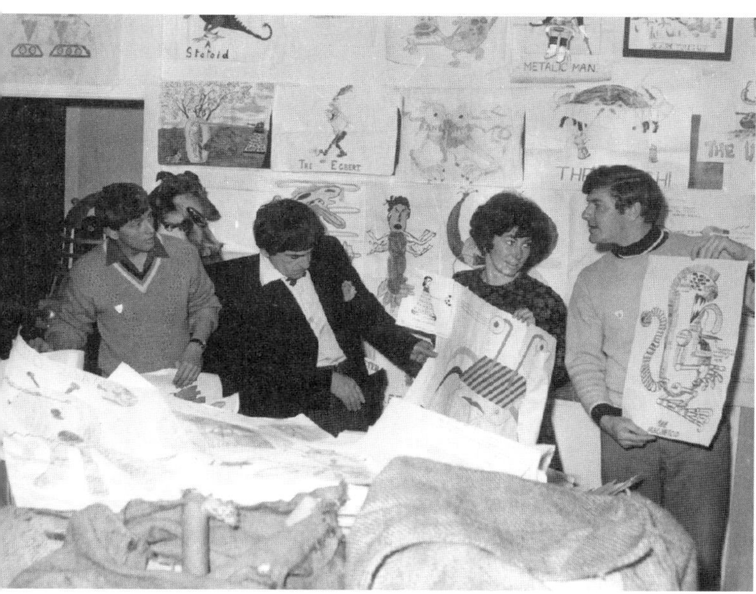

Patrick Troughton judging the **Blue Peter** 'Design a Monster' competition.

"We needed an oil rig but nobody in the North Sea or anywhere else would let us near theirs, so we ended up using an old sea fort in the Thames Estuary."

Episode one was recorded on 23 February, with over ten minutes of location filming, featuring the main scenes shot at Margate at the beginning of the year. With additional shoots at the sea fort, the other main set-up was at an airfield near Denham.

Hugh David:

"We wanted some heroic shots of Pat flying the helicopter, so we had a rig ready to make it look as if he was doing the piloting, while a stunt guy actually flew it. Pat took one look and went pale."

Troughton:

"Hugh David wanted me to go up and do a bit of 'Evil Keneval' stuff in a helicopter. The warning signs started to flash in my head and I said no, but he figured a way round it."

David:

" I put the cameraman in a child's pram, and had him pushed at awkward angles past the helicopter with the blades going and Pat at the controls. When I cut it together with the footage we had of the the helicopter actually flying, it looked as though Pat was an air ace in his spare time!"

Later episodes of the story featured the main appearances of the 'Weed Creature'.

Hugh David:

"We had this poor sod in a wet suit covered with bits of sea weed and strips of melted rubber. I thought, 'My God! How am I going to make that look frightening?' So, we flooded the set with foam and had the guy leap up in the middle of it with sea weed flailing around the place, and it looked terrifying. If the foam hadn't been there, however, it would have looked like one of Sooty's friends."

Episode six moved to TCI in TV Centre, the space at Lime Grove beinging too small to house the set for the main control room featured in the story. The control room had to be flooded with foam. While this was in rehearsal, work was already underway at Ealing on *The Wheel In Space.*

David Whitaker had produced the scripts from a storyline by Kit Pedler, as David was unavailable to work on the story.

Whitaker explains:

"I had always admired what I'd seen of the Cybermen and felt they were equally as menacing as the Daleks. When Derrick Sherwin (who was now the script editor, having taken over from Bryant when he became the producer) got in contact, asking me to write up Kit's story, I was delighted, although I was never happy with the way it went.

"It was a slightly disheartening experience as the work I'd put into the new girl was changed beyond recognition when it reached the television."

The 'new girl' was Zoe Herriott, a highly intelligent character compared to the vaguely naive victorian that Debbie Watling had been playing for the past year. The part was given to Wendy Padbury.

Fury From The Deep finished recording on 1 March and part one of *The Wheel In Space*, under Tristan De Vere Cole's direction, moved back to Studio D at Lime Grove for completion on 8 March. Having worked on *Power Of The Daleks*, Derek Dodd returned as designer.

Only two Cybermen costumes were made for this story, involving a delicate exo-skelaton over a new wet-suit design, which had a habit of falling apart as soon as the actors wearing them started to move.

Troughton:

"The Cybermen were my particular enemy, I suppose, because I kept bumping into them. I always found the idea of this race of automatons quite clever, but I could never tell which one was speaking. You had to keep an eye out for whose mouth-flap was open.

"After a while I cracked it. I got the actors to stoop forward slightly, or shift an arm whenever it was them in rehearsal, so that I had some idea where to turn. The Dalek's eye-sticks wobbled about a bit, the Cybermen shrugged – that was the routine I liked to work with."

Wendy Padbury joined the cast on **The Wheel in Space***, posing here on the incomplete Cyberman spaceship set.*

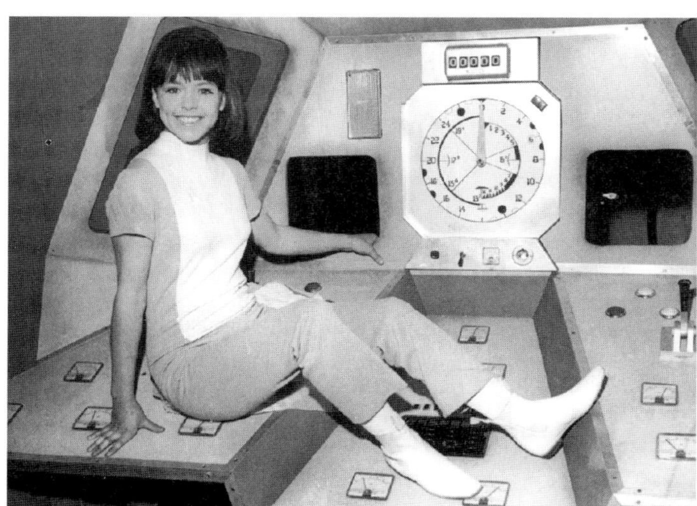

Everything was moved back to TC3 in TV Centre for Episode Two on March 15th, with Troughton absent for the recording, on one of his annual mid-season holidays. He returned for Episode Three, which moved to TCI on March 22nd.

Despite hisfondness for the Cybermen, *The Wheel In Space* was not a story that Troughton cared for very much.

"I thought the one where Wendy was brought into the show was dire. We were all getting tired, and people tend to get a bit prickly when they're under the kind of pressure that we were facing each week. After six months of making *Doctor Who* I think even the sturdiest Time Lord would get a bit whacked and I'm afraid I might not have been the most generous host to begin with, but she was soon part of the family."

Although the fifth season came to an end with episode six recorded on 12 April back at Riverside Studio One, production continued.

Shortly after *The Web Of Fear* had been written, Peter Bryant commissioned Mervyn Haisman and Henry Lincoln to write an adventure called *The Beautiful People*. This fell foul of rewrites from Derrick Sherwin and the two writers objected, falling out with the production team and demanding that their names be taken off the pro;ect. The story was retitled as *The Dominators* by Norman Ashby (a pseudonym for Haisman and Lincoln) and Morris Barry came back to direct for the series once again. Barry took the main cast to Wrotham Gravel Pits in Kent, where a couple of days filming was done during the rehearsals for *The Wheel In Space* part five.

The Dominators of the title used robotic servants called the Quarks, and the resulting costumes were so small that Barry decided to hire school children to operate them.

Barry:

"There was no way any adult could get inside one and live beyond a few minutes. They were built for small actors, so children seemed an ideal solution – and let me tell you, they were all too delighted to be *Doctor Who* monsters for a few weeks!"

The Dominators also marked the return of Barry Newberry to the series, after a lengthy absence, as the designer.

Sets included the war museum on the pacifist planet of Dulkis. The building's walls were a maze of crumbling octagonal brick work.

Newbery:

"The reasoning behind that was the argument that not everywhere in the universe uses square bricks to build with. It was an architectural exercise to see if it would actually hold together soundly, which it did, suprisingly."

There were problems for planned future episodes of the series as a result of Haisman and Lincoln's dispute with Sherwin. A third Yeti story was planned, set in a remote Scottish castle in Jamie's homeland when the Doctor finally managed to get him back to his own time. The Laird of the castle had been taken over by the Great Intelligence and the Yeti were once again roaming through the mists. The plan was for this to act as Jamie's last story but it was withdrawn from the schedules, and never saw production.

David Maloney was now with the production team, having been chosen to direct *The Mind Robber*, which was originally planned as a four part story called *The Land Of Fiction*, by Peter Ling. A gap had been caused by the cutting of an episode of *The Dominators*, and extra one was allocated to *The Mind Robber*, but Ling was unavailable to draft it. Derrick Sherwin stepped in and wrote the script instead but he faced a severe problem.

The production budget did not stretch beyond the money that had already been allocated, so the extra episode had to be drafted bearing in mind the sets and props that were available; The Tardis set, a white backdrop, and a few old robot costumes that Sherwin had found in storage.

Maloney took some of the main cast on a location shoot cutting into the rehearsals for part four of *The Dominators*. Hines was needed at Harrison's Rocks in Kent for half a day for the scenes where Jamie is menaced by one of the land of fiction's clockwork soldiers, and the others were needed for a sequence where the travellers are attacked by a Unicorn, which was staged in an empty aircraft hanger in Croydon.

Sherwin completed his problematic *Dominators* episode (which he subtitled *Manpower*) taking no on-screen credit and it was recorded on 24 May. A week later Frazer Hines caught chicken-pox and had to be replaced by Hamish Wilson (Hines' own cousin) for a complete episode and some scenes in the following one. The plot was quickly rewritten to have Jamie's face altered accidentally by the Doctor when he fails to solve one of the puzzles set for him by the Master of the Land of Fiction.

Troughton:

"The one with all the characters from the land of fiction was one of my favourite adventures. It was bizarre, yet totally in keeping with the series. I liked the way the Doctor had to use his knowledge of literature to battle the villain and bring all the great heroes to life. It was wonderful, and I'll always remember the opening episode with those strange robots. They were white on screen, but they were really puce yellow and green."

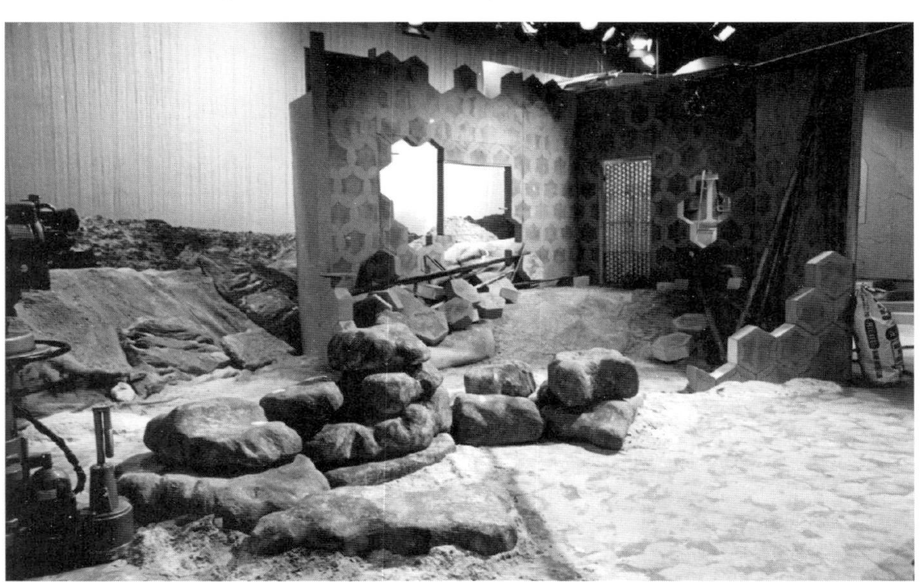

The crumbling octagonal brickwork at the War Museum in ***The Dominators****.*

Recording was completed for the fifth year on 21 June and the cast were released to have their summer break. During this holiday, Troughton made it clear to Bryant that he felt it was time to move on to other projects, and leave the series.

Troughton:

"I pretty much wanted to leave after the Land of Fiction story, but Peter Bryant persuaded me to stay on for another few months to get a replacement sorted out. I knew what kind of problems Innes had faced when he was trying to find the second Doctor originally, so I said I would stay until the spring."

The cast had been working, specifically Troughton and Hines, for fourty six weeks and the show was still on the air, even though *The Wheel In Space* had finished recording on 1 June. The final episode had been shot to lead into a repeat run of *Evil Of The Daleks.*

Troughton's Doctor was seen casting a mental projection of the adventure to show his new companion, Zoe, what kind of trouble she could end up in if she joined the crew of the Tardis. It neatly gave the series a continuous run and lead straight into the start of Season Six. The first episode of *The Dominators* began on 10 August.

Sherwin was lining up stories for the rest of the sixth series, working with his assistant, Terrance Dicks, who had been with the programme since the latter episodes of *The Web Of Fear*. He would formally take over from Sherwin towards the end of the season, and go on to act as script editor for JonPertwee's entire run as the Doctor.

The ratings were beginning to slide down again in the latter stages of season five, dropping down to below seven million. Throughout the next year, the series would struggle to maintain a steady audience, as problem after problem behind the scenes saw stories falling through in pre-production.

Sherwin's first new adventure for Season Six was *The Invasion,* based on an idea by Kit Pedler, and during the early stages of writing the story, Sherwin decided to bring back the character of Lethbridge-Stewart.

Camfield:

"We had Nick as a Lieutenant-Colonel in *The Web Of Fear*, and you couldn't really have someone of that rank in charge of a set up like UNIT (United Nations Intelligence Taskforce – an acronym for Pedler's international set-up, apparently devised by Camfield), so we promoted him to Brigadier."

Also planned to carry over from the Yeti adventure was a third appearance by Jack Watling as Professor Travers but the actor was unavailable for the filming dates. His daughter Anne Travers, played by Tina Packer, was also used in the original drafts but written out when Packer also proved unavailable. Professor and Isobel Watkins replaced them.

The Invasion gained two extra episodes midway through writing when *The Prison In Space* by Dick Sharples, the next story due to see production, was cancelled as the scripts were judged to be unsuitable.

Terrance Dicks quickly brought in Robert Holmes to rework a submission he'd sent in called *The Space Trap,* as a four part story, to make up the gap left by Sharples' story. David Maloney had returned to direct the second story for the new batch of episodes, and casting had already begun.

Holmes:

"I remember being told that my story had to replace one that Peggy Mount and Beryl Reid had been asked to do. I just couldn't see how two comedy actresses like that could possibly fit in with the 'house styles' of the show, but it was meant to be a comedy. Terrance (Dicks) just loathed it with a passion. I mean, he was desperate to get something ready in its place."

Retitled *The Krotons*, work got underway redrafting it while filming started on *The Invasion* in the first week of September. Technically, it represented the most ambitious location work on the programmeto date.

Camfield:

"There were some huge battle sequences at the end between the army and the Cybermen which needed heavy duty weaponry, and was the sort of thing that the BBC didn't really have access to. We got in contact with the Ministry Of Defence and told them what the problem was to see if they'd offer any help. The scripts were sent round and they saw that the soldiers were seen being pretty heroic, and to our surprise and delight they offered to lend us a complete platoon of guardsmen."

The main scenes of Cybermen 'invading' London were amongst the first to be shot, with locations moving from the Blackfriars Embankment to Saint Paul's Cathedral. Everything moved to the Guinness Factory in Acton for the main bulk of the location work, including the battle sequences.

Location filming at the Guinness factory in North Acton for ***The Invasion****.*

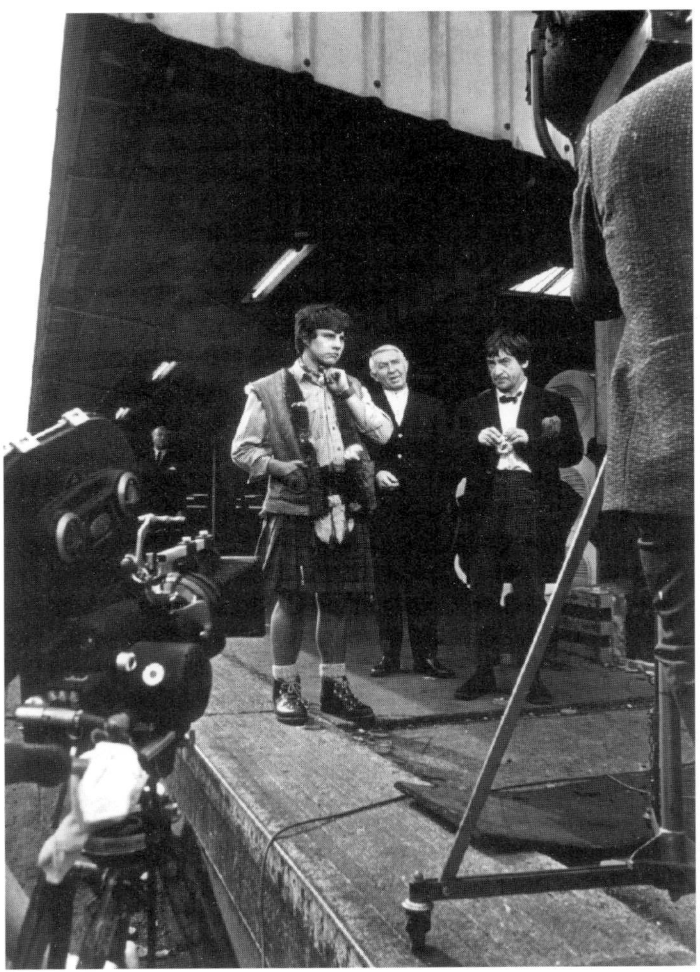

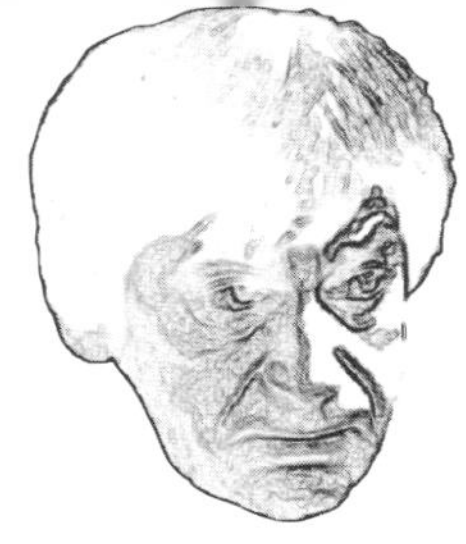

Camfield:

"Chris D'Oyly John (the proudction assistant) found this practically unused compound and the recce pictures made it look ideal. I've never known a production unit be more excited and enthusiastic in my life than when they found out what particular product was made there!"

Six Cybermen costumes were made using the same basic wet-suit design from *The Wheel In Space*, although the chest-units had now been made more compact and the heads redesigned, the more familiar 'ear-muff' style of the modern costumes making its first appearance.

A field in Ruislip was used to stage the opening scenes for the first episode when the Tardis arrives back on Earth.

Camfield:

"We went to Ruislip and we got hold of the O.B. Unit's helicopter for a day, but Frazer hated the idea of Jamie's kilt flying over his head when he climbed up its rope ladder as everyone could see his football shorts, so we had it weighed down. Nobody thought to do the same for Sally (Faulker – Isobel Watkins), so the wind got her skirt instead!"

The final block of location work was done at RAF Northolt, with a Hercules Tranporter provided to act as UNIT's mobile base. RAF ground crew, like the army, were happy to be involved in the shooting. Other shots were filmed at the BBC training centre at Wood Norton and the last sequences for which the film crew was needed were staged at Ealing, where the model work for the story was also done.

The Invasion – *Cybermen on location at St Paul's Cathedral in London.*

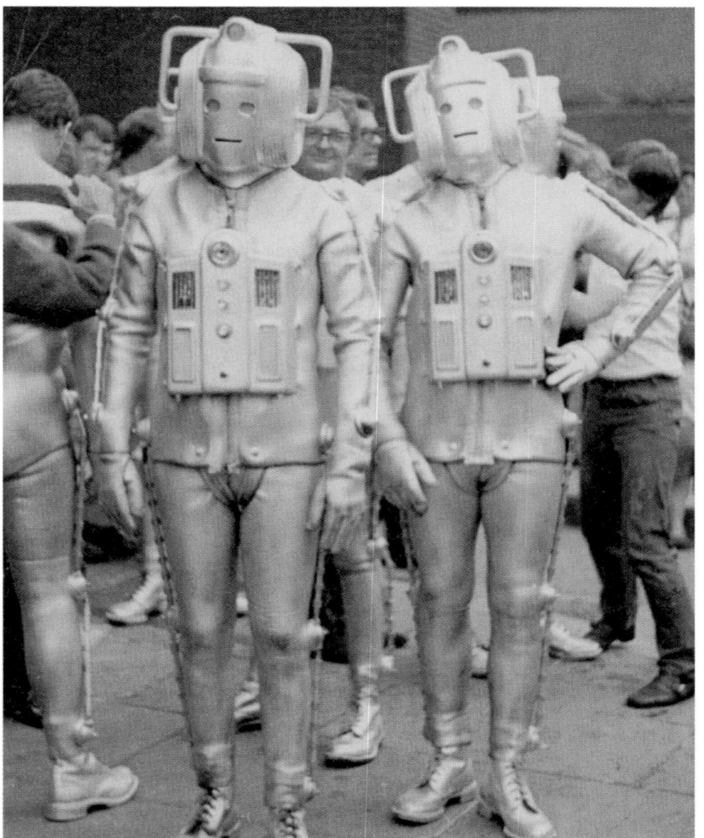

Kevin Stoney returned for his second *Doctor Who* story as the main villain, after playing Mavic Chen for Camfield in *The Daleks' Master Plan*.

Camfield:

"Kevin made Tobias Vaughn a superb villain. He brought the same kind of sneering superiority to it that he'd used in the Daleks story. I remember thinking that he and Pat made a good sparring team. Vaughn was the closest I ever think the programme's got to having someone as quick witted as the Doctor.

"The whole UNIT thing worked well for that first story and it was pretty clear that the format could be stretched out for another couple of adventures. Pat Troughton was keen to see them back but I don't think anybody on *The Invasion* anticipated what actually did happen."

The Invasion basically became the template for the first few years of Jon Pertwee's time as the Doctor, as the production team was keen to utilise the format of such stories to bring the invaders to earth, rather than take the Doctor to them.

The Krotons was next story in line.

Robert Holmes:

"The idea was to have these crystaline creatures that could be generated out of a chemical slime in a few seconds. They were meant to be big, powerful and very threatening. We ended up with a pair of angry egg-boxes!"

It was a problematic story to make. The money spent on *The Invasion* had cut into the budget for *The Krotons* and as a result there was not enough money available to create the monsters of the title.

Ray London had taken over as designer, following on from Richard (*Mission To The Unknown, The Smugglers*) Hunt who had handled *The Invasion*. Both he and the production team had their first experiences with the Krotons in a slate quarry near Dorking when Maloney took a film unit there with the principal cast during the week beginning 12 November.

Troughton:

"Those things were hysterical. Poor David Maloney stood at the bottom of this quarry and shouted for the Kroton to chase after Frazer and I, roaring its head off. We were cued in and went hurtling off, and all the Kroton did was make a sound like a muffled cough and fall over. It had to be helped around like an old man after that – the poor sod inside just could't breathe let alone move it!"

Robert Holmes:

"Apparently this made Peter Bryant go to the bosses and ask for more money to make better monsters, as the Krotons were so dreadful. They basically said something like, 'Well, as your doing so well with the money you've got, we don't see any reason why we should let you have some more. Now go away and make *Doctor Who*.' There were times, certainly in those days, when making *Doctor Who* was harder than trying to pee in the corner of a barrel."

Brian Hayles had been asked to submit a second story featuring the Ice Warriors shortly after their debut. While *The Invasion* was being made, he was working on *The Lords Of The Red Planet* and extending the hierachy of the race that Innes Lloyd had so admired. This was one of the few stories of that period that experienced no real problems during the scripting stage. It was pencilled in to follow on from *The Krotons* and Michael

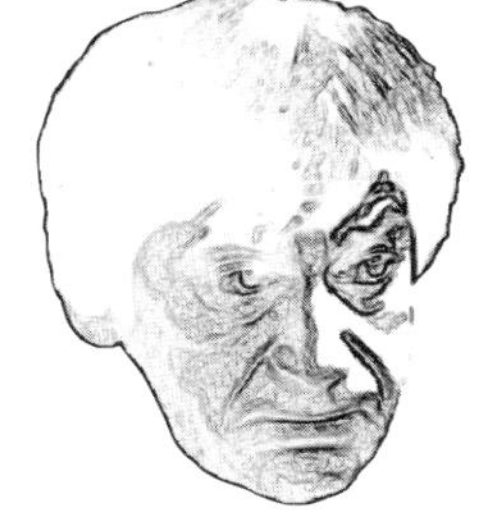

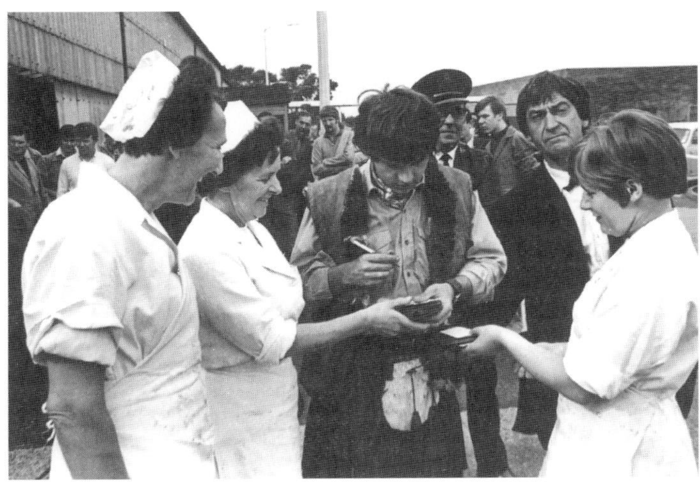

Signing autographs at the Guinness Factory.

Ferguson came back to follow on from *The War Machines* with this new story.

The cast left for their annual Christmas holiday on 13 December and it was made all the more merrier that year because of the filming of *The Invasion*.

Patrick Troughton:

"The people at the Guinness factory were so pleased at having us there that they gave us all 'Guinness' Christmas Puddings and sent us all a crate of beer for the holiday. I asked Peter Bryant if we could go back there, but we never did."

Troughton was now tired and wanted to move on as soon as he could.

"We were getting very silly for those last few stories. I mean, Frazer and I had been at it solid for close to three years and there's only so many Daleks a man can defeat before you start to get the giggles.

"I was also getting very edgy, the sheer pressure of doing *Doctor Who* week in and week out was making me angry at the smallest thing, for no apparent reason. I have to admit that there were one or two heated discussions, be it with the director or Peter and Derrick. I just felt that the show was beginning to go down. We weren't getting the quality that we'd had the previous year and I learnt a lot later that I had a bit of a reputation for being a monster myself towards the end."

Like Hartnell before him, Troughton worried about the possibility of the series ending if he went.

"I didn't want to kill it off and I knew that they had changed the Doctor once, into me, so I couldn't see why they just didn't do it again. I'd known Shaun Sutton since the 1950s, and as we were old friends and he was the Head of Series, I went and asked him straight out whether *Doctor Who* would die if I went.

"If that was the case, I wanted to go out with a big bang and end the thing in style, but Shaun said, 'Far from it, old chap. As long as I'm here, *Doctor Who* will be as well'. So I knew it was alright to go."

Hayles' script, *The Lords Of The Red Planet* underwent a title change and became *The Seeds Of Death*. With Paul Allen as his designer, Ferguson took the location filming unit out to Hampstead Heath for a day when production resumed on December 30th.

None of the principals were needed, as the sequences dealt with an Ice Warrior and a couple of human extras. Brian Hayles later related an incident that took place during the day in question.

"We only had one lone Ice Warrior wandering around and inbetween takes the actor inside (Sonny Caldinez) took his mask off. Shooting was taking place near the main road and one poor woman motorist nearly got killed.

"She must have been driving along quite happily, quietly minding her own business when suddenly she saw a man standing there wearing green scaly armour. She actually hit the kerb and came to a grinding halt and our Ice Warrior was amongst the first to get there to see if he could help. The minute she saw him... (clicks fingers)... she fainted!"

Extensive scenes where the Doctor is attacked by the foam created by the spore with which the Ice Warriors try to destroy the Earth were staged at Ealing. The same foam machine used in *Fury From The Deep* was dusted down, and as Troughton recalls:

"I had to hammer on a door for Frazer to let me in, while all this foam was flooding round me...I couldn't see a damn thing! The director kept shouting, 'Get up, Pat. Hit the door, shout and bellow for help!' and I kept skidding on the floor and disappearing. I was fighting to stay upright and I was told how convincing I'd made my struggle with the stuff look afterwards. Let me tell you, that wasn't acting!"

Episode one was recorded in Studio D at Lime Grove on 3rd January 1969, with the schedule now back to Friday nights. Episode two was shot on 10th January, with the new member of the Martian race being seen in full as the Ice Lord was introduced.

Brian Hayles:

"The Ice Warriors are meant to be a race of extraordinary nobility. I contemplated using everything from Ice Baron to Ice Captain, but Ice Lord had an authentic ring of authority to it that the other titles seemed to lack."

Episodes three and four were completed on the 17th and 24th January, with the other Ice Warriors featured in the story now fully active. Two of the costumes used in *The Ice Warriors* were worn, while the Ice Lord outfit basically consisted of a slender body suit, augmented with the familiar pincer claws.

The visible mouth area displayed the same reptilian flesh as the Warriors, while the head was covered with a high-domed helmet with red gel covering the eye holes. Alan Bennion played Slaar, and would go on to play Ice Lords in the two subsequent stories.

Episode five was recorded on 31st January, and the final installment was completed on 7th February. The Ice Warriors were more intelligent than the other alien races that had featured in the programme.

Brian Hayles:

"I didn't want the Ice Warriors to just lumber around with guns and blow things to bits – they had to be far more realistic. I thoroughly believe that on the day that mankind finally makes contact with outer space, he'll find that they have the same capacity for reasoning and rational thinking that we have.

"It's obvious that like the human race, they won't have been without the odd war, so they will have armour and weapons, just as we have. The Ice Warriors were my prediction, and I make no claim for it being an accurate guess."

Robert Holmes had quickly been called back after work was finished on *The Krotons*. Although the realisation had been flawed, the production team liked the scripts, and they asked him to come up with another six-part story, as there had been another casualty amongst the line-up that had originally been commissioned, *The Dream Spinner*, by Paul Wheeler.

Robert Holmes:

"There was a story that Terrance Dicks had, which was a bit too close to the one in the land of fiction (*The Mind Robber*), with a character, some old traveller I think, who could make people believe that their dreams had actually happened. Anyway, it didn't work that well, and Derrick made the decision to scrap it, leaving me about six or seven weeks to get *The Space Pirates* drafted up, which was not much time at all..."

The Director assigned to the story was Michael Hart, with Ian Watson as his designer. Episode one marked the last time that *Doctor Who* would be recorded in Lime Grove Studio D, with recording taking place on 21st February.

Prior to this, a week had been spent at Ealing, recording the extensive amount of model filming that was needed for the story. The timing of the story was quite apt, as the Apollo moon landing was in the news every day as the press charted its journey.

Holmes recalls:

"The big mistake that we made with *The Space Pirates* was to try and be too authentic. I did a lot of research into the reality of space travel, and how long it would take to get from point A to point B. Thinking I was breaking new ground as far as *Doctor Who* was concerned, by putting the sheer boredom of space travel across, I didn't realise until I watched the episodes themselves that I was boring the audience half to death as well..."

Episode two moved to TV Centre, where it was recorded in TC4 on 28th February, with episodes three and four following on the 7th and 14th March.

Troughton pondered the phenomenon:

"You began to wonder whether the people watching could follow some of the stories towards the end of my run, I mean, some were rather dull. There was one where we spent the first few episodes trapped in some spaceship. I kept thinking, 'Well, we'll be on some planet next week', but no. We just sat and twiddled our thumbs. That was when I really began to wish that the end would role on."

Malcolm Hulke had been commissioned to write a four part story to follow *The Dream Spinner*, with the finale for the series, and the Troughton era as a whole coming in the shape of a six-part adventure that Derrick Sherwin was writing. When Sherwin decided to scrap his own work, the only way to meet the production schedule was to extend Hulke's story from four parts to ten.

Hulke takes up the story:

"When I was asked to write a further six episodes on *The War Games*, my heart sank, as I'd just about drained the idea dry as it was. I made it quite clear that there was no way I could do it on my own, so Terrance (Dicks) came and joined up to help."

Dicks had to leave his post as script editor while he worked with Hulke, forcing Sherwin to return to his old job on *The Space Pirates*. Hulke and Dicks worked both night and day to complete the episodes.

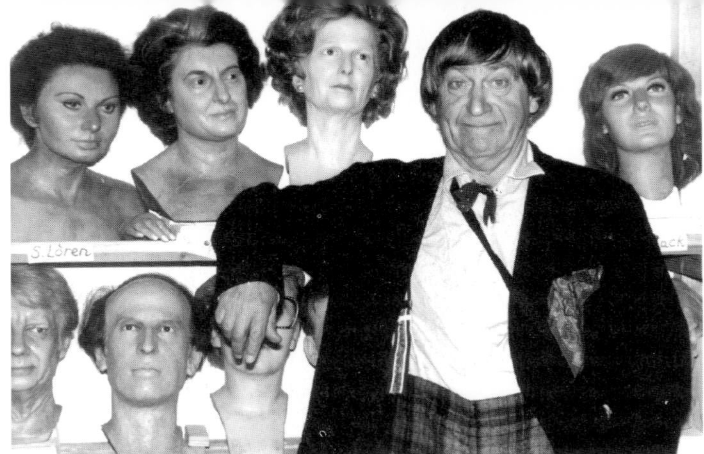

Troughton on location in **The Krotons**.

Hulke:

"I dread to think how much coffee went down our combined throats, but it was very much a case of 'Now Get Out Of That', with Terrance writing me into a situation, which I would have to get out of and set him up at the same time. We did it, but only just..."

David Maloney returned as the director for the epic story, while Roger Cheveley came in as the designer. Thanks to Troughton, Hines and Padbury pre-filming their sequences for the finale of *The Space Pirates*, it gave *The War Games* close to two weeks of location filming before the studio work had to begin. Hulke.

"We were told to set the first episode's location shoot in and around the battlefields of the First World War, as the location manager had managed to get the sets that were left over in Brighton from *Oh, What A Lovely War!* (directed by Sir Richard Attenborough in 1968/69). That's why the setting looked so good.

Other locations varied from the South Downs (for the scenes involving the Roman army attacking the travellers), to winding country roads (for the sequences where the World War I ambulance moves through the time zones) and an old farm in the heart of East Sussex (for the part where the Doctor faces the firing squad). The cast returned to go into rehearsal on 7th April.

Episodes one and two were recorded in TC4 on 11th April and 18th April. The broadcasts were barely over a week apart from being finished in the studio, with part one of the story going out the day after the second was completed.

The ratings were steadily going down. Having reached nine million viewers with *The Krotons*, some episodes of *The War Games* were as low as four point one million, which was an enormous drop. This fuelled the speculation that the series was to end.

The supporters who were there at the beginning were now gone – Donald Wilson was working on *The First Churchills*, and had distanced himself from *Doctor Who* completely. Sydney Newman was about to return to Canada, after leaving the BBC and trying to break into the film industry, working with a company which folded just as he had several projects ready to film, and Verity Lambert was about to move over to ITV and start work on *Budgie*, with Adam Faith, which would prove to be an enormous hit for her. Mervyn Pinfield had died not long after leaving the series, and Donald Baverstock was now setting up Yorkshire Television, where he would instigate another long-running series, *Emmerdale Farm*.

Shaun Sutton comments on the general mood surrounding the BBC Drama Department at that time:

"It was like the move from silent films into sound all over again – It was a case of waiting to see who would survive the transition, but in this instance, it was the move from black and white to colour. Some series actually came back, revitalised by the fact that they could now be made in colour, like *Steptoe And Son* for example.

"The dilemma over *Doctor Who* was that it would be more expensive in several ways, from the most basic fact that the sets and monsters would have to be more realistic in colour, to the cost of using colour stock for the location filming.

"Even if Patrick had stayed, there would still have been questions asked about moving into colour. With him going at the time he did, it gave the show an excuse for a total revamp, and that's what probably made it survive."

Episodes three and four continued *The War Games*, with studio recordings on 25th April and 2nd May in TC4. After this point, the production schedule altered slightly. The recording day was now set as every Thursday, to allow an extra day of editing for Maloney, who had to incorporate the film sequences that had been shot earlier.

Part five was recorded in TC8 on 8th May, with part six following on 15th May. Casting was now underway to find a third Doctor. Ron Moody was asked once again, but turned it down again while Bryant was keen to have a more comic actor for the role, to offer a complete change from Troughton's interpretation – as had been done before in the change to him from Hartnell.

The ideal choice in the producer's eyes was Jon Pertwee, who eventually accepted the part after finding it difficult to believe that he was suitable for the role. Bryant saw Pertwee using his talents to the hilt in his performance – he was renouned for his versatility, he could sing, dance (he'd had a big hit on the west end in *A Funny Thing Happened On The Way To The Forum*) and his funny voices were known through his radio work (*The Navy Lark* being but one series he worked on), but that was exactly the kind of thing that he avoided when he started filming, shortly after Troughton's departure.

Part seven of *The War Games* moved into the vast TC1 studio on 22nd May, while part eight moved back to TC8.

May 29th. The penultimate episode was recorded in TC6 on June 5th. Like Troughton, both Frazer Hines and Wendy Padbury had decided to leave the programme, and chose to go at the same time as their Doctor.

Troughton recalled:

"It was sad when it came to saying goodbye to Frazer and Wendy. I suppose I had been very lucky with the companions that my Doctor had, I couldn't fault one of them as either actors or friends.

"It made those three years really enjoyable. I'd say that apart from a television play I did a few years ago with Gwen Watford (*Reluctant Chickens*, broadcast in 1983), I'd say that *Doctor Who* really was the best working experience of my career."

The finale, as the Doctor was put on trial by his own race, was staged in TC8 on 12th June. Finally, the question that had remained unanswered for so long was dealt with, and the Doctor's origins were revealed.

He was a Time Lord, a race of beings who had mastered the ability to travel through time. They were neutral observers, going to any point in history they chose, but with a strict policy of non-intervention; a rule which the Doctor had broken, as he was unable to tolerate injustice of any sort while the others just calmly 'observed' it.

Troughton:

"I liked the idea of him charging off to battle all these horrific monsters and not really knowing what on earth he was doing at the same time. I'd always tried to play the Doctor as someone who was hiding his true purpose. If he met a madman or a megalomaniac, he almost wanted to push them forward to see how far they would go before he actually stopped them. It was quite nice to find I'd been steering him in the right kind of direction."

Malcolm Hulke:

"We wanted the Doctor to come across as a slightly rebellious character. His own society was incredibly tedious, and yet he was a born adventurer. The Time Lords must have seen him as some kind of Don Quixote figure, and they were totally unable to comprehend his continual battle against evil. He was an innocent dreamer who started to fight back."

There was always the thought at the back of Hulke's and Dicks' mind that the tenth episode of the story could be the last that was ever seen of the programme.

Hulke:

"There were an awful lot of ends to tie up. It wasn't just the climax of the story, it was sort of the climax to the series as a whole up to that point. If the series was never going to come back, we didn't want the question of who he was to remain unanswered, so that's why the Time Lord mythology was created. As it turned out, before we'd finished the series was given the green light to keep going, so we had to give it a slightly enigmatic ending as the new Doctor had not been cast at the time it was shot."

The War Games part ten was broadcast on 21st June 1969, with Troughton's Doctor last seen objecting to the way he was being treated as he was exiled to earth, with a regeneration being induced in the process.

Four days before transmission, the new actor stepped before the cameras of the press for the first time as Jon Pertwee was announced as the third *Doctor Who* on 17th June.

When asked what kind of epitaph he thought his Doctor should have, Troughton said, after careful consideration:

"At times, he was brave... but, he was never a coward. At times, he was clever... but, never a total idiot... and, at times, he played the recorder..."

Sadly, Patrick Troughton died in 1987 whilst attending a *Doctor Who* convention in America.

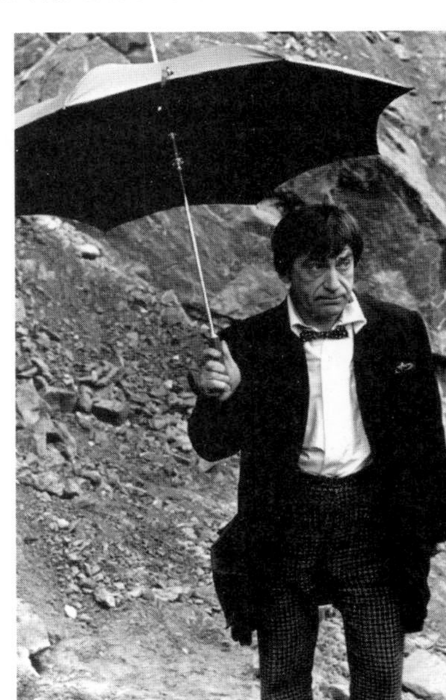

For many yeats after leaving the programme, Troughton was still happy to don his Doctor's costume for the occasional publicity appearance.

CHAPTER 4

JUST THE RIGHT BULLETS

JUST THE RIGHT BULLETS
JUST THE RIGHT BULLETS

"You can't just wipe the viewers memories of the other Doctors. You have to try and make as big a mark as your predecessor... and with Jon Pertwee that was quite a formidable task."

TOM BAKER interviewed – August 1975

"Plastic was everywhere. It was being hailed as the miracle of the modern age, something that could improve the lives of everyone. I started thinking along the lines of, 'What if there was some form of alien intelligence that could control and manipulate it?' When I started to look around my own home and count the number of things that this could apply to, the idea suddenly became quite frightening."

Robert Holmes had been approached to write a plotline for the 'revamped' *Doctor Who* towards the end of 1968 while he was still working on *The Space Pirates*. As the entire cast was leaving at the same time, it presented an ideal chance to rethink the format for the transition into colour.

By mid-April, Shaun Sutton had formally given the go-ahead for a new series to start production as soon as *The War Games* had been completed, although the run of episodes was now cut down to twenty five instead of over forty. This, as Barry Letts had pointed out during season five, would allow more time for location filming and take the pressure off the actors and crew with the studio work. As it turned out, season seven would need all the time it could get.

Although Peter Bryant was certainly around for the casting of Jon Pertwee, he had now effectively left the programme to take over on the second season of *Paul Temple*, which he had been asked to revamp. After attending a few filming sessions on Pertwee's first story, he left the series for good.

Derrick Sherwin was heavily involved in other projects, including plans for him to join Bryant working on *Paul Temple*, but he stayed to supervise the start of the seventh season. With the Doctor exiled to Earth by the Time Lords, the most logical step was to centre all the stories around UNIT and their battles against various invasion attempts. The Doctor would be made their unofficial scientific advisor but a companion was still needed for him.

Working with input from Terrance Dicks, Sherwin created a brilliant science-graduate in the shape of Liz Shaw and the part went to Caroline John, who had worked mainly on the stage up until then. *Doctor Who* represented a substantial break into television for her.

Derek Martinus was hired at the end of July 1969 to direct Holmes' script, which had the finished title of *Spearhead From Space*. Holmes admits that he was heavily influenced by the *Quatermass* serials of the 1950s when it came to drafting the four part story.

"It seemed an idea to try and recapture the spirit of having the army watching the radar screens as some meteorites crashed in the middle of Surrey, or somewhere like that, and then have the mystery of what exactly it is that's landed. Of course, the viewers know it's something nasty, but the suspense comes from having the military being totally oblivious to this fact. Some of the stuff we did with *Spearhead* was intended to be a sort of tribute to those old *Quatermass* serials."

With just over a week of location filming planned, to be followed by four consecutive studio recording days, production of the story was unexpectedly jeopardised by a scene shifters' strike at the BBC. The studio space that was available was allocated to 'more important' programmes.

The only answer was for Sherwin to ask for the facilities to shoot the entire story on location, a move which Martinus felt was workable. After initial reluctance, he was eventually given permission to use 16mm cameras. Meanwhile, Martinus scouted locations towards the end of August with his designer, Paul Allen, to find a suitable facility where basic sets for the UNIT offices and laboratory could be built.

Nicholas Courtney was now under contract for the entire season, as Brigadier Lethbridge-Stewart The only other character returning from *The Invasion* was Benton, played by John Levene.

The crew moved around between new and more familiar locations. The old manor house that the BBC had converted into an Engineering Training Centre at Evesham proved ideal as a facility for the UNIT offices. The Doctor's lab and the hospital ward scenes were all staged inside the building. The exterior doubled up as the cottage hospital to which the Doctor is taken, having been found in the woods in the opening scenes of the first episode.

The entrance to the UNIT Headquarters was, in fact, the old cargo station round the back of King's Cross railway station. Sherwin stepped in front of the camera to take over from an actor who had been dismissed, and played the security guard in the UNIT car park.

The woods around Evesham were used to stage the meteorite crashdown scenes and the first appearance of the Tardis, while a nearby cottage was subjected to an Auton attack.

Holmes explains the concept behind the 'new' adversaries:

"The idea of having dopplegangers replace high-powered officials is a standard plot device for thrillers. Things like those old Michael Caine spy films of the 1960s (The Harry Palmer stories, adapted from books by Len Deighton), and even the odd science fiction film used that kind of idea, so I did the same thing with *Spearhead From Space*.

"The Nestenes were like bits of a brain. Each one of the meteorites had a different brain cell in it and they worked as one mind, no matter how far you separated them. Because they could use

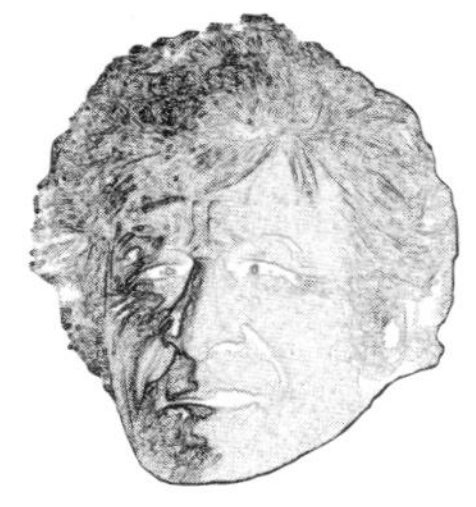

plastic, they made these facsimiles of human bodies which they could use, moving around totally unnoticed. It was a kind of secret invasion, because you'd never know who had been replaced by these Autons - the only give-away was that their skin looked a bit oily and smooth.

"I always tried to give an affectionate nod of appreciation to a favourite film or story with my *Doctor Whos*, and it would not be a million miles from the truth if you were to hazard a guess that that one was *Invasion Of The Bodysnatchers*."

The drone Autons were not as sophisticated as their brothers, being used to defend the Nestene base and hunt down lost meteorites. The costumes comprised of a featureless vac-formed head mask which concealed the actor's head completely. The eyes were hidden behind black gauze across the socket-holes and a dark blue boiler suit was worn with silver lace-up boots.

The Auton gun was a hand-shaped weapon with a hinge that caused the fingers to flip down across the middle of the palm, revealing the nozzle extending from inside. A simple powder flash indicated that the gun was firing and the actors on the receiving end of the blast had other charges sewn into their costumes, detonated by remote control.

For the sequence where the Autons emerged from the shop window of a department store, where they were disguised and dormant as shop window dummies, a Sunday morning was spent at 'John Saunders' in Ealing.

The main battle scenes at the story's climax were staged at the old Guinness Factory in Acton, where *The Invasion* had been shot. The complex was now leased to the BBC, who were using it in shows like *Mogul* and *The Troubleshooters*. The final sequences to be filmed before the actors moved on to start rehearsing for the next story were done at Madame Tussauds' wax museum, off Baker Street in London.

Because of the continual flow of visitors the exhibit attracted every day, the only time that the film crew could work without any interruption was at night.

Martinus recalls one of the incidents that took place:

"We were going through one scene when one of the make-up girls suddenly let out a hell of a shriek. She'd forgotten that at least five or six people were pretending to be dummies, so when I called 'Cut' and they started to walk towards her, it nearly frightened her out of her wits. She went quite red with embarrassment afterwards."

Doctor Who And The Silurians had been commissioned by Terrance Dicks and Derrick Sherwin as a seven part adventure at the beginning of 1969, with Malcolm Hulke writing the scripts. He had proved himself more than capable of handling lengthy stories when working with Dicks on *The War Games*.

Dicks now had a deputy script editor, Trevor Ray, who came up with the idea of bringing 'Bessie', the Doctor's yellow

ABOVE: The new Doctor – Jon Pertwee.

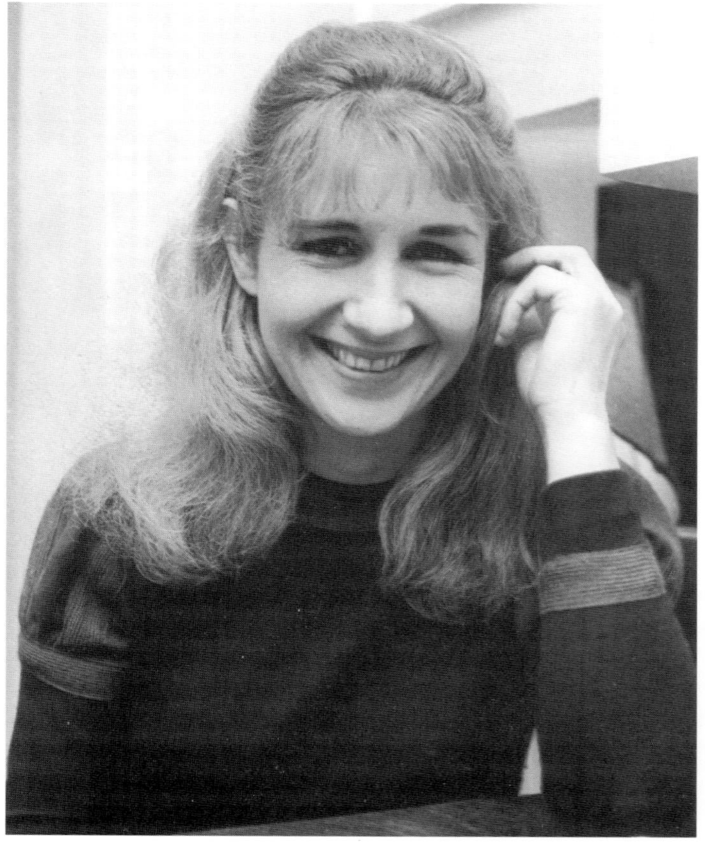

RIGHT: Caroline John was chosen to play Liz Shaw.

Edwardian car, into the series. Ray oversaw a lot of work on the second story while Dicks worked on the last two stories for the season.

Shaun Sutton was also looking for someone to come in and take over from Sherwin as the producer. Sutton approached Barry Letts who was then directing a children's drama series called *A Handful Of Thieves*.

Letts:

"I've got a strong suspicion that Shaun touted the job around, offering it to various people, and they said, 'What? *Doctor Who*? You must be joking!' There is no question that at that time, it was going down, down, down in the ratings."

Letts was reluctant at first, and made it clear that he had not given up his career as an actor to become a producer He wanted to direct. Sutton offered a compromise with an open contract that would allow him to both produce and direct, so Letts accepted the job.

The problem was that he had not actually produced any shows before, although he had taken the BBC director/producer course. He basically had to learn from scratch, and he was thrown in at the deep end.

"I arrived at the office on 20 October and said, 'Here I am.' Derrick and Peter said, 'Oh, great. If you need us, we'll be at TV Centre,' and off they went to make *Paul Temple*. I was left with Elaine, our secretary, Terrance and Trevor Ray.

"I always used to say to Terrance, 'You should never make a crisis into a confrontation', and the first thing that happened was that I inherited an enormous crisis, with the show that was in production, *The Silurians*."

Timothy Combe, who had already worked on *Doctor Who* as an assistant floor manager and a PA, had been hired as the Director for the story. Barry Newbery returned as the designer. The location filming, over a period of five days, started at the end of October, a few days after *Spearhead From Space* was technically meant to have finished. The main setting for the exterior sequences in Hulke's scripts called for a windswept moorland.

Combe remembers:

"I wanted to go up to Derby, or the salt flats up on the Yorkshire Moors, but the budget was tight as a heck of a lot of money had been spent on the story Derek (Martinus) was doing. We ended up at an MOD Base (in Farnham, Surrey) and all over Frensham Ponds."

For scenes involving UNIT searching the moors for an injured Silurian, Combe wanted to film a large scale military operation.

Combe:

"I wanted to see if we could get some of those all terrain vehicles, a couple of helicopters and possibly even a tank. Derrick said he'd see what he could do. In the end, we had the old BBC O.B. Unit Helicopter, and a Land Rover for Nick Courtney to drive around in."

The reptilian Silurians were played by non-speaking extras who had, nevertheless, to learn the lines to be able to move on cue. Peter Halliday was brought in to provide the voices. Sherwin remembered him for his work on *The Invasion*. Apart from playing Packer in that story, he did the Cyber-voices as well, using the same kind of voice modulator he was to use in *The Silurians*.

The Silurian costumes were body-suits with a suitably scaly texture, clawed gloves and clawed boots. The most elaborate feature was the head mask. Cast in vulcanised rubber, they were hand painted and fitted with a battery operated light in the creature's third eye at the centre of the forehead. Whenever a Silurian attacked someone with its mental energy projections, the actor could make the light flicker.

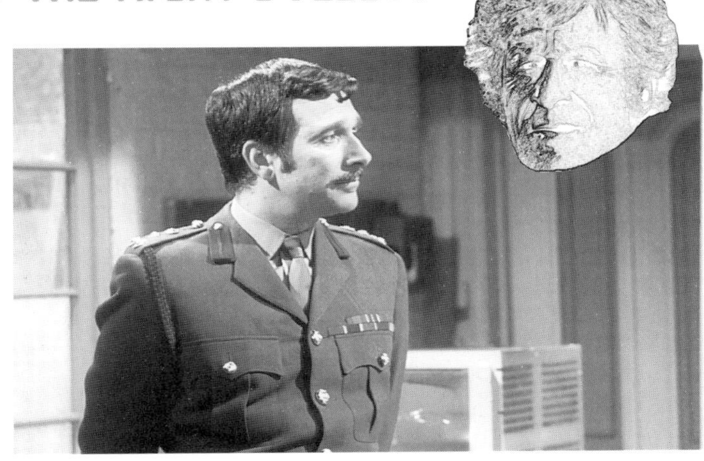

Nicholas Courtney as Brigadier Lethbridge-Stewart.

Spearhead From Space made its debut on 3 January, with a lot of advance press interest and a full-colour cover on the *Radio Times* to herald its arrival. The public were curious to see what the new Doctor would be like and the ratings picked up considerably compared to the end of season six. Over eight million viewers tuned in for each of the first four episodes.

Doctor Who And The Silurians finished recording on 26 January. Immediately after this, the next story into production started location filming. *The Ambassadors Of Death* was submitted by David Whitaker as a story for Patrick Troughton's Doctor, under the title *Invaders From Mars*, shortly after he'd finished work on *The Wheel In Space* during the spring of 1968.

As Whitaker explained:

"I had heard quite a lot about what Peter Bryant had done with the second Yeti adventure (*The Web Of Fear*) and I quite fancied the idea of doing a contemporary thriller with science fiction roots. The thought of a powerful military figure trying to manipulate a race of aliens, very much like the kind of thing Quatermass would have come up against, was the basis behind the idea.

"I had very little to do with the finished product as Terrance Dicks persuaded Malcolm Hulke to do a rewrite of the whole thing. I cared very little for what I saw, as it really wasn't my story any longer."

Dicks brought Hulke in to expand the six-part story into seven episodes and in the process bring in all the new regular characters. The director, hired by Bryant before he left, was Michael Ferguson and the designer working with him was David Myerscough-Jones.

Some of the first sequences to be filmed were shot along country roads in Uxbridge, near Buckinghamshire, with the hijacking of the escape pod of the Recovery Seven space craft.

Barry Letts:

"As a director, Mike (Ferguson) apparently used to say, 'I will go on till the producer tells me to stop'. So he was always expanding on the script. When it came to the hi-jack, which was done with two men on motorbikes in the script, he had

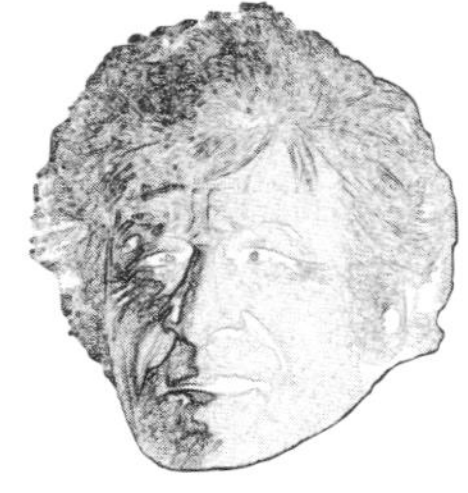

helicopters and practically the whole of the HAVOC stunt team!"

HAVOC was effectively an agency for stunt men and could supply a full team with the appropriate skills to realise any action sequences that a TV show needed. They were used throughout the Pertwee era.

The hi-jack was completed over a couple of days and location work continued, moving to the Southall Gasworks and back to the Guinness Factory in Acton once again for the battle between the UNIT troops and General Carrington's men. A gravel pit near Maidenhead was also utilised for an afternoon's filming.

Rehearsals began for the studio recording during the second week of February. The story would feature a lot of work with the relatively new effects system of Colour Separation Overlay, which allowed model shots and live action to be combined. The model would be filmed by one camera, which would mix the image of the actors working against a blue background on another, and combine the two in one shot.

Barry Letts:

"We had the fascination of playing with CSO. Mike and I were both enormously keen on it and the BBC wanted us to experiment with it and gave us a studio for two whole days to do just that. We had the facility to do whatever we liked and we did all sorts of things, including using model sets.

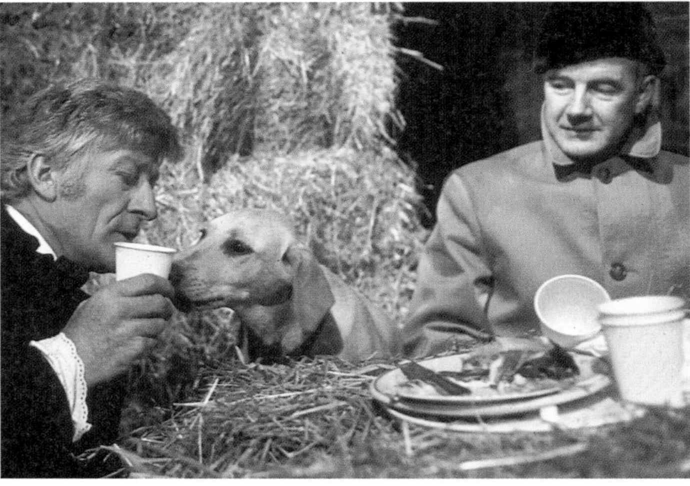

Lunch break on location for **Doctor Who And The Silurians**.

"We had Margot Hayhoe, one of our assistant floor managers, walking in and out of a model house which we got the visual effects department to bring down to the studio – all done with CSO."

Ambassadors saw the return of John Levene as Letts set about establishing a regular group of characters within UNIT to avoid having the Brigadier as the only recurring role alongside the Doctor and his companion.

David Whitaker was growing disillusioned with the current version of the series:

"That story just illustrated how far the series had left our original premise. The beauty of *Doctor Who* was that it was a continual mystery; you didn't know who he was, or where the next story would take you as a viewer. When they decided to start answering all the questions, a little bit of the magic inside quietly died."

By mid-March, Douglas Camfield was back with the production team starting pre-filming work on *Inferno*, with Jeremy Davies as his designer. Don Houghton's scripts ran for seven episodes and had a whole subplot, added in the early script editing stages by Terrance Dicks, taking the Doctor to a parallel universe. Camfield worked out a tight four day filming schedule for all the location work, which would need a futuristic industrial setting. Recce's were carried out while *The Ambassadors Of Death* was being completed. Camfield took the cast and crew to Berry Wiggins and Co. Ltd. in Kent. The team had to work under stringent safety conditions as the complex was partially an oil refinery. Smoking was strictly forbidden.

Both 'real' and 'alternate' characters were needed for the parallel universe encounters, and the costume team created a fascist-style uniform for the 'other' UNIT soldiers. The make up department created suitably different looks for Caroline John, giving her a brunette wig, and Nicholas Courtney, with an eye-patch and scar running down the side of his face.

One shot involved Camfield having to persuade Pertwee to climb up onto a gigantic gasometer and the actor was far from happy about it.

Camfield:

"I pointed out to Jon that he would look incredibly heroic and that the cameras would give the game away if we used a double.

That seemed to swing it, and he actually got up there. I have the greatest admiration for him being able to overcome his doubts and do that, but I think if I'd made a joke of having to go for it again, it would have killed him rather than made him laugh."

Filming was completed on 3 April and rehearsals for the *Inferno* studio work began the following week. Letts wanted to do a trial run with this story, using a different system of recording two episodes over two days once every fortnight. To this end, Camfield meticulously planned out his camera scripts so that day one would be spent on camera rehearsals for the two episodes in question, while day two was spent actually shooting them... but it was not destined to work out so easily.

Letts:

"I was in the office and I had a phone call from Jon Pertwee who said, 'Barry, you must come down here. Dougie's very ill but insists on going on, and nobody will ring you up and tell you.'

"I went straight down and there was Dougie, sitting with a cup of coffee, absolutely ashen white. I got him off to hospital and told him not to worry, as I'd carry on, which I did, working from his camera scripts."

Camfield suffered from a mild heart flutter and was unable to return for any further work on the story, although he would come back to direct two Tom Baker stories.

Inferno had a philosophically intriguing storyline.

Letts:

"*Inferno* had a very, very grim idea behind it - the philosophical idea that the only way to make time travel possible is to have an infinite number of parallel universes, where everything that could possibly happen has, somewhere in one or other of these universes, already happened.

"Philosophically this is very, very disturbing, because it means that no choice is of any value, that there is no morality, and that you are just making this choice in this universe at this moment. In story-telling terms, it means that nobody ever wins, because even if you win in this world, you'll loose in another. And that's what happened in *Inferno.*"

Season seven drew to a close with twenty five episodes completed. The final episode was broadcast on 20 June. After peaking with a ratings high of over nine million viewers midway through *The Ambassadors Of Death*, the figures for the series had gone down, but it had proved popular enough for a new series of twenty five further episodes to be commissioned.

Letts continued to develop the format of the programme, adapting it so that season eight would take on a style that would remain throughout the rest of the Pertwee era. Several important changes took place before production began.

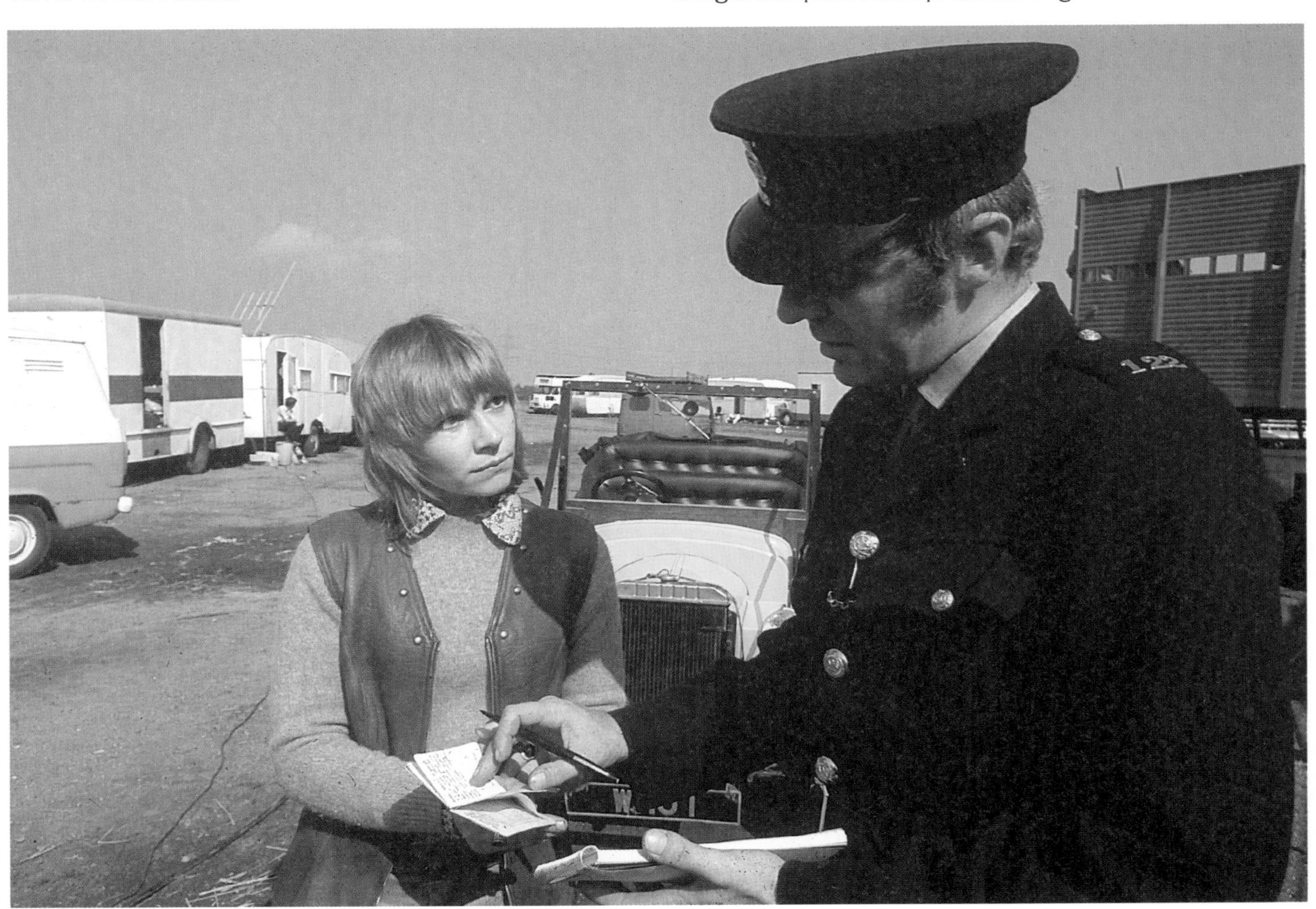

The Doctor's new campaign, Jo Grant (Katy Manning) in **Terror Of The Autons**.

Firstly, Caroline John left the series, her character of Liz Shaw effectively disappearing without any farewell scene between her and the Doctor. The problem with Liz was that she was an incredibly intelligent scientist, which led to narrative problems.

Letts explains:

"I thought Caroline gave a very good performance. She's a good actress and it was a great shame that we had to say, 'Sorry, but your character's disappearing'. Whether she would have liked to have gone on or not never came into it.

"It wasn't so much that we needed someone to scream, we needed someone to say to the Doctor, 'Doctor, I don't understand, will you please explain'. He would explain to the character, and the audience would get the explanation as well. As it was, you had to fake it some way in the scripts, because Liz and the Doctor would have exchanged a few cryptic, scientific terms and understand exactly what was going on, which was no good for the story...

"Also, you needed someone for the younger audience to identify with. You see, Liz was supposedly a little older. One felt she was about thirty. Perhaps we went a little too far the other way in making the new girl, Jo Grant, so naive and rather silly in terms of intellectual achievement, but that was deliberate."

Letts auditioned around two hundred actresses for the part of the new assistant, eventually boiling that number down to two. The final phase of the process involved them working with a group of actors Letts had brought in including regular *Who* actor, Michael Wisher. They spent two hours going through the entire rehearsal process, using a script they'd had time to learn, to see how they coped with the kind of routine they'd face with each story.

Katy Manning was awarded the role and Richard Franklin won the part of Captain Mike Yates. Letts had wanted to expand the UNIT ranks, and create a more senior right hand man for the Brigadier. He and Dicks created the part of Yates. The character was incorporated into the audition piece for Jo Grant and out of the actors he saw, it was down to Ian Marter and Richard Franklin as to who got the job. Franklin was eventually chosen, but Letts did not forget Marter and used him later on in one of the Pertwee stories he directed, *Carnival Of Monsters*, before casting him as Surgeon-Lieutenant Harry Sullivan – the new companion for the fourth Doctor - when Tom Baker took over in the role.

The final new character to be cast was an adversary for the Doctor - someone who was equal but opposite in every way. Letts and Dicks hit upon the idea of having a 'Moriarty' for the Doctor's 'Sherlock Holmes'. The character was the Master.

Roger Delgado:

"When it comes to casting a villain, or a fiend, and the producer is looking under categories of names, when he chances upon the heading 'vaguely Satanic', he will find my name. The qualifications speak for themselves; I have a beard around a menacing chin and eyes that can cut through the sturdiest of heroic men.

"*Doctor Who* had always eluded my grasp as an actor and my attempts to gain employment and do battle with both William Hartnell and Patrick Troughton had come to nothing. Destiny, however, held a trump card. Barry Letts remembered me from our days in the BBC Rep (Delgado was working on serials in the 1950s at the same time as Letts), and politely asked whether I would care to come and menace Mr Pertwee for a while. How could I refuse such an invitation?"

The Spray Of Death was commissioned from Robert Holmes as the first story of the season. Apart from having to bring all the new elements together, this story saw the return of the Autons.

Holmes:

"I didn't actually want to bring them back, but I had a couple of meetings with Terrance and agreed that there were still one or two more tricks to pull out of the bag with them. The second story with the Autons was meant to be far more sinister. The first just had a couple of shop window dummies coming to life. This time I wanted things like cuddly toys and armchairs that could become lethal Nestene weapons.

"Barry actually went for it and didn't hold back. I thought the idea of having a chair wrap around someone's head and squeeze the air out of him would have sent Terrance straight into a rewrite, but that wasn't the case at all. He stood by and supported some of the more outlandish ideas completely which, in view of the flack it caused afterwards, was quite brave of him."

Rehearsals began for the new season during the second week of September and one of the first sections of location filming was staged at the Robert Brothers Circus, which was rigged up in Edmonton. The four days of shooting started on 18 September with all the principal cast present and Delgado making his first appearance as the Master.

Delgado:

"The entire look of the Master was devised by the costume designer and the make-up team. I fancied the idea of being a bold

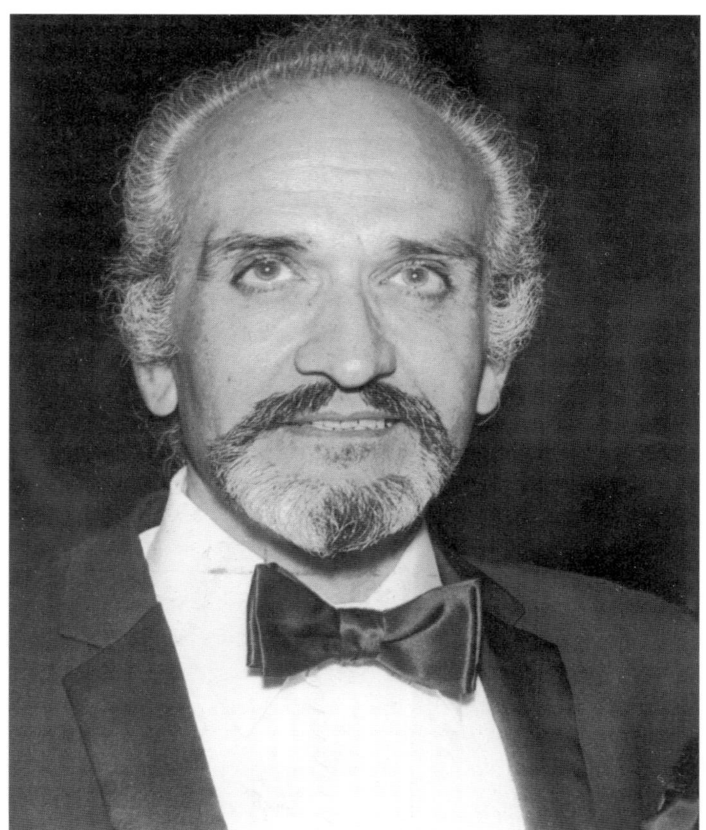

Roger Delgado.

Victorian, with flowing frock coat and cane, as the Master was, after all, a time travelling Moriaty.

"The finished product was what I can only describe as a malevolent Pandit Nehru outfit. It was inspired, and as soon as I put it on, I knew he would be the kind of man to wear black leather gloves. It seemed suitable and apt, and Barry Letts approved completely. I wanted a cigar or something to complement the attire but I was told this was 'too Blofeld' (a regular James Bond villain). For my final story, I may ask for a white cat for an accomplice!"

For Beacon Hill radar station, where the final battle with the Autons would be staged, the film unit moved to a Post Office complex near Dunstable. The set-ups took more time than anticipated and cut into the schedule quite badly.

Other locations included Hodgmore Woods in Buckinghamshire, where a nearby quarry was also used, and Black Park Cottage in Fulmer, in the same county, which doubled as the home of Farrel Senior. Closer to the production base back in west London, a milk depot was used as the rear of the Farrel compound and an afternoon was also spent in and around a shopping centre near Shepherd's Bush.

With several scenes still unshot, Letts had to plan out a way of completing them in studio. He opted for using CSO, which made the studio recording days more complicated as the additional material had to be shot around the sequences that were already scheduled.

From this story, retitled as Terror Of The Autons, onwards all of the studio sessions would be staged once every two weeks, the experiment tried out on *Inferno* having proved that Letts' system worked.

The Autons featured in the story were the same kind of drones that had been seen in *Spearhead From Space*, although the whole facsimile capability was left out of the second story. The blue boiler suit uniform was maintained but the masks were made far smoother and completely featureless. The vision and ventilation for the actor within was improved considerably as a result.

Timothy Combe was now back to direct the second story to go into production, *The Mind Of Evil*, which had been scripted by Don Houghton. Ray London was the designer. Houghton had

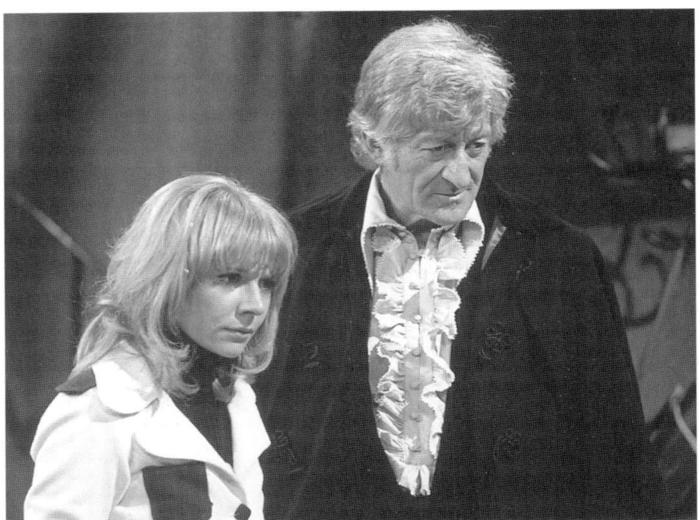

The Doctor and Jo during **The Sea Devils**.

completed the script rapidly as the eighth season had not been given permission to start production until transmission was well underway on season seven, with Pertwee proving to be very popular and ruling out any possibility of cancellation for the series.

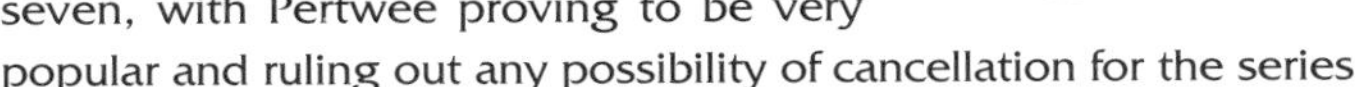

Houghton:

"I admired the kind of theories that Anthony Burgess had put into *A Clockwork Orange* (his controversial novel, which became an even more controversial film in 1971), and felt that the same principle of how far people can go to mentally alter the behaviour patterns of prisoners was an ideal topic to cover in *Doctor Who*.

"I pitched the idea at Terrance Dicks while we were working on *Inferno*, and he liked it. I think he realised that there hadn't been a story set in a prison before and that's where *The Pandora's Box* came from."

Houghton is referring to one of the working titles for the story, which was also known as *Doctor Who And The Pandora Machine* up until just before location filming began. His story involved a lot of action sequences, which could only be staged on location, and one thing was clear from the outset.

Timothy Combe:

"We knew at the beginning that it would be terribly expensive. It was fantasy mixed in with reality, and that costs. As was always the case with *Doctor Who*, there was never enough time on location. That's when you begin to go over budget without realising it, trying to get everything done at the same time. The money just seems to vanish in a puff of smoke!

"A lot of scenes were set around the grounds of a prison, so we thought we'd try to hold the shoot at a real one, but the Home Office said an emphatic 'No'. We looked at one or two castles that could be used as an alternative and Dover Castle seemed ideal."

A few days of location shooting in and around London came first, following straight on from *Terror Of The Autons*. Roger Delgado completed his scenes for the first two episodes during this time and would not be needed main studio session. The cameras moved from Kensington Gardens to Cornwall Gardens, with scenes set outside the International Peace Conference being staged at the Commonwealth Institute.

Delgado:

"The Master was first seen arriving in a horse box, which was hardly the most suitable vehicle to match with his sense of style. By the second story, when he was travelling around in a black limousine, I felt that the writers were beginning to understand his flair and panache.

"The Doctor had his little yellow car, I had my limousine. They say you can judge a man by the type of car he drives. Well, need I say more?"

By the beginning of November, the crew had moved on to Dover Castle where the main battle scenes between UNIT and the prisoners were staged over two days. The problem was that there were not enough extras and when Barry Letts saw the rushes, he told Combe to go back a few days later and get more close-up shots of both factions.

Combe:

"We had no money, no time and no actors, so we had to go for it ourselves. I even got a gun and some sunglasses myself and charged past the camera. We got everyone in; cameramen, sound

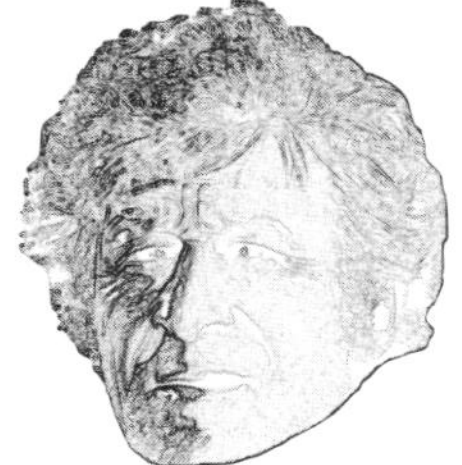

men, drivers, they were all either soldiers or prisoners. To be honest, they loved every minute of it."

The most complex sequence to be realised involved the hi-jacking of a missile. Letts had approached the RAF with a view to them helping out, and subtly dropped a mention into the conversation of how the Army had been so good to the programme with *The Invasion*. An unarmed missile was supplied with several willing uniformed extras who doubled up as both UNIT soldiers and mercenaries working for the Master.

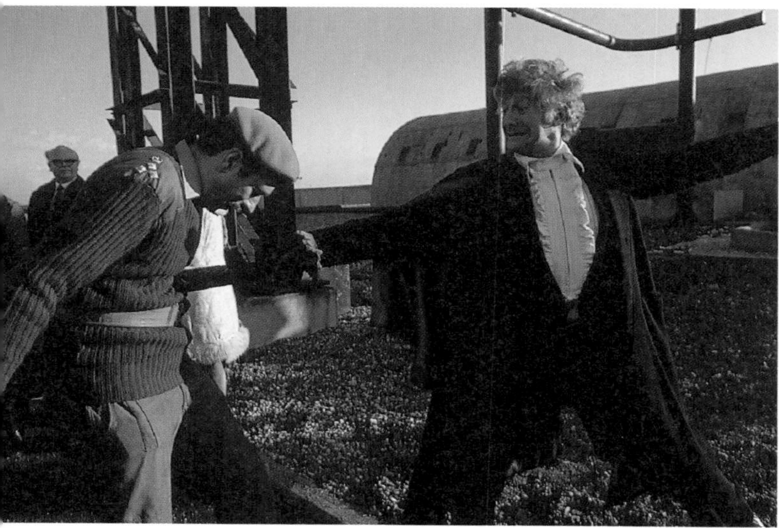

ABOVE: Larking around on location for **Claws of Axos**.
BELOW: Stephen Thorne as the **Last of the Daemons** – Azal.

Combe used an MOD airfield as a location and the main country roads leading to it as the sight for the confrontation. The BBC O.B. Helicopter was once again called into service, along with a couple of Land Rovers and a motorbike, which Richard Franklin managed to write off in an accident during filming. Combe kept the accident in the finished programme as Franklin was not hurt and the resulting footage looked spectacular.

The studio shots were recorded in London in TC3 at the beginning of December. One of the scenes involved a confrontation in the prison between the Master and the Doctor.

Delgado:

"We came to a point where the table standing between us was accidentally upturned. Far be it from me to play the wounded soldier, but I did fall and hurt my leg. In the heat of any theatrical moment such as this, you have to keep going, as money is lost on pointless moaning.

"To heighten the precarious nature of the scene, a jug of water fell on the table and smashed, turning the studio floor into what I can only described as an ice-rink. It was near impossible to keep any sense of balance, let alone stop yourself from laughing."

The story was completed on 18 and 19 December after which the cast broke up for their Christmas holiday. This was the last time both Combe and Houghton would work on the series.

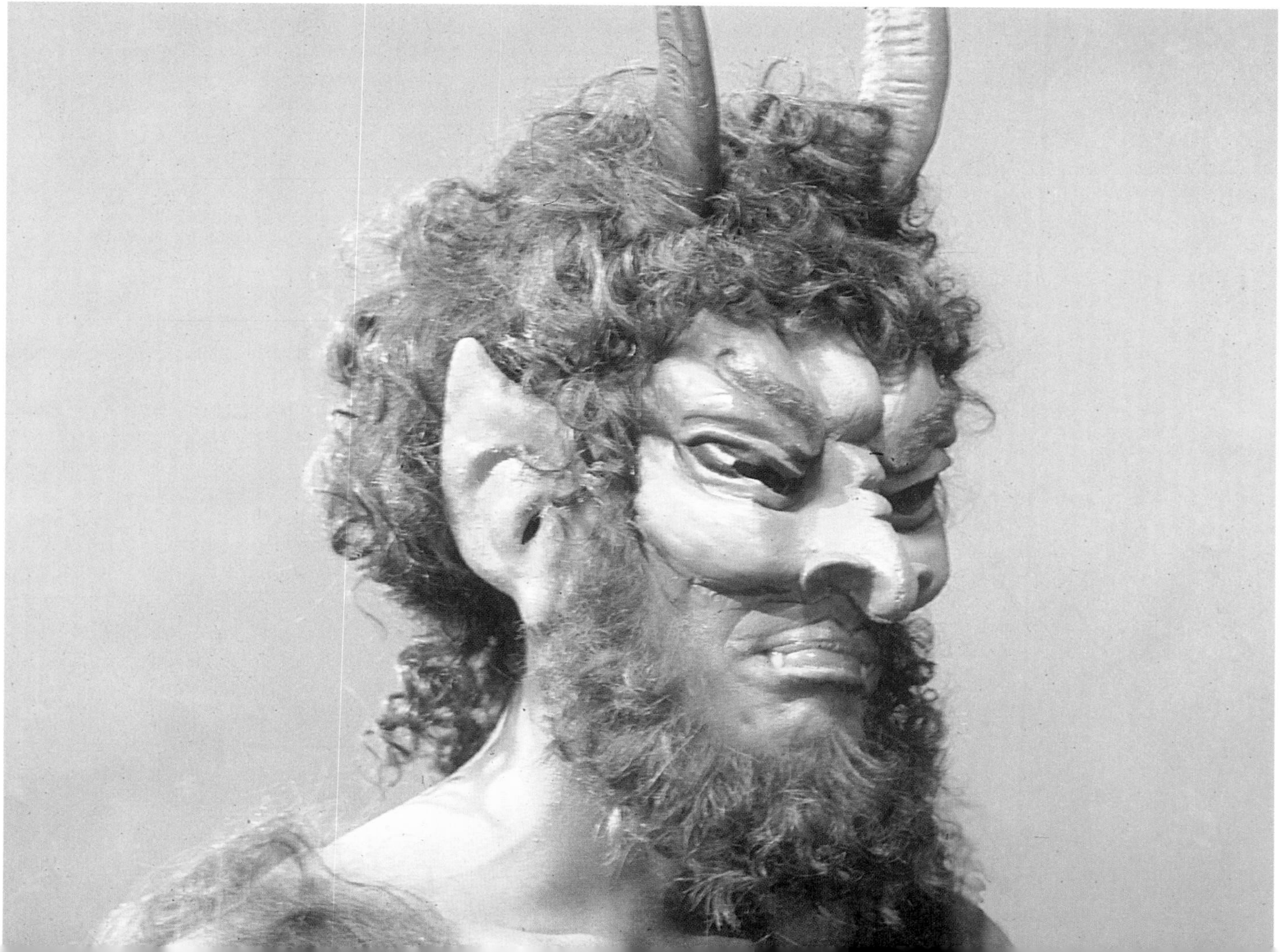

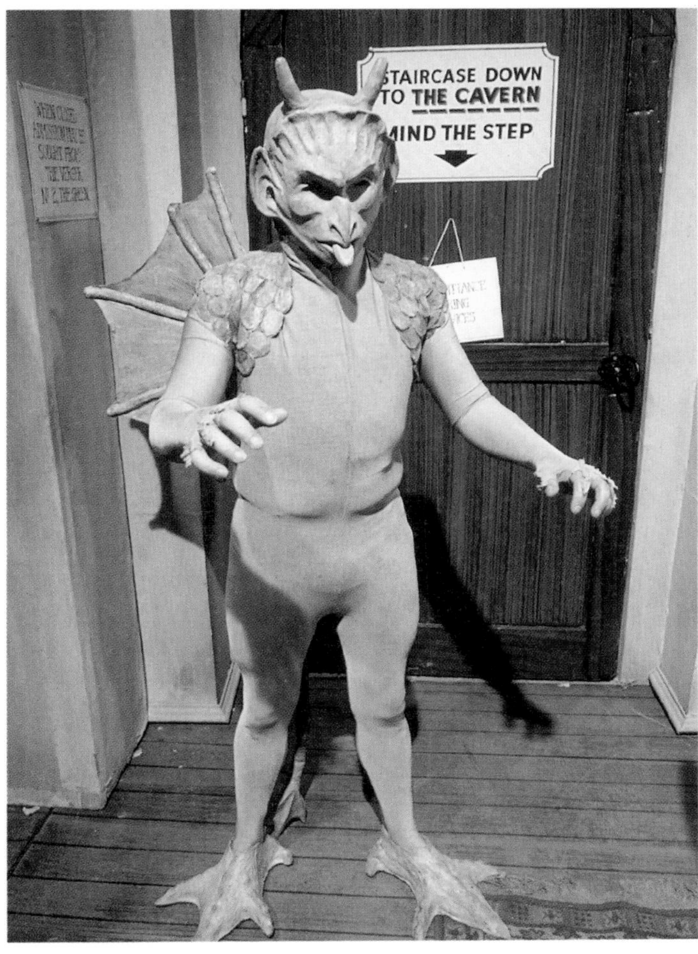

Stanley Mason as Bok during rehearsals.

The Bristol based writing team of Bob Baker and Dave Martin had been trying to get a commission to write for *Doctor Who* for some time. Dicks noted that there was potentially a good serial with *Vampires From Space*, which had been sent in as a potential seven-part serial. Heavily rewritten and cut down to four episodes, this became *The Claws Of Axos* and was scheduled as the third story of the season.

Following some brief rehearsals in the last week of December, the cast and crew left for a week's location filming as on 4 January 1971. Ferguson had found all the sites that the script required in and around Dungeness, the main scenes taking place at the vast power station and on the local beach along the Kent coastline.

The regular group of Land Rovers and cars were once again used to represent UNIT forces and the HAVOC team were brought in. This was the last time that they'd be used on the programme and they supervised an elaborate stunt sequence involving a trio of Axons attacking Yates and Benton in their Land Rover.

The Axons themselves came in two forms, one as a svelte race of golden skinned humanoids which were designed using a simple body stocking and gold face paint with specially moulded appliances to go over the eyes. The other was a walking mass of writhing tentacles. This involved a specially made suit that came in several pieces; gloves, boots, the body covering and a head mask. Painted with oranges, reds and yellows, the result was nearly impossible for the actor to see out of due to the surfeit of tentacles sprouting from the costume. The weather conditions during filming were totally unpredictable, with snow, rain and bright sunshine.

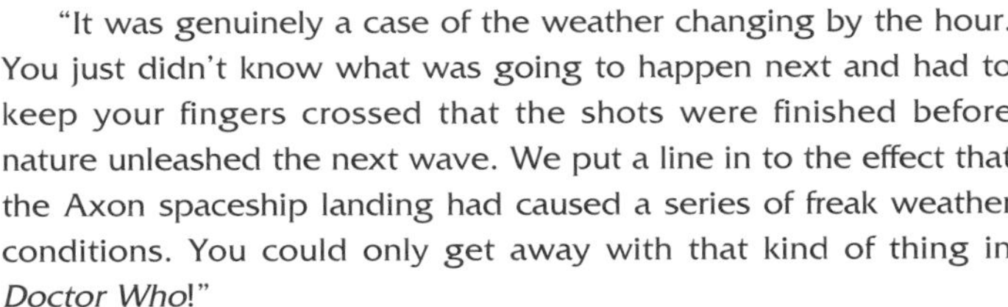

Letts:

"It was genuinely a case of the weather changing by the hour. You just didn't know what was going to happen next and had to keep your fingers crossed that the shots were finished before nature unleashed the next wave. We put a line in to the effect that the Axon spaceship landing had caused a series of freak weather conditions. You could only get away with that kind of thing in *Doctor Who*!"

Terror of The Autons had started transmission from 2 January, announcing the arrival of the Master to the programme with a front cover feature in the *Radio Times*.

Delgado:

"I was warned by Jon Pertwee about the effect of being associated with *Doctor Who* but I never saw it in person till after my first episode had been screened. Suddenly, it was no longer a case of being just another man walking down the street. After a while, I began to realise why children were staring at me.

"A knowing glance returned to their curious faces, saying, 'Yes, it's the Master, small child,' would send them diving for cover behind their mothers. The braver ones would stride up to me and ask for an autograph and advice on how to eradicate an unwanted teacher or baby brother."

The tentacled Axon costumes proved rather expensive to make and were retained in storage in case they could be reused. Eventually, a couple were redressed and used with a different colour scheme in the Tom Baker story, *The Seeds Of Doom*, the leather content in the composition of the costumes making them very durable.

Colony had been commissioned from Malcolme Hulke towards the end of summer 1970, following a favourable reaction to his last story, *Doctor Who And The Silurians* (this was the only time that the prefix of 'Doctor Who And...' was used in the broadcast episodes of the series. Originally, the story was called the less original *Doctor Who And The Monsters*).

Michael E. Briant was hired as the director on *Colony* having, like Combe, Camfield and numerous others before him, worked

The Doctor about to be grabbed by the Ogrons.

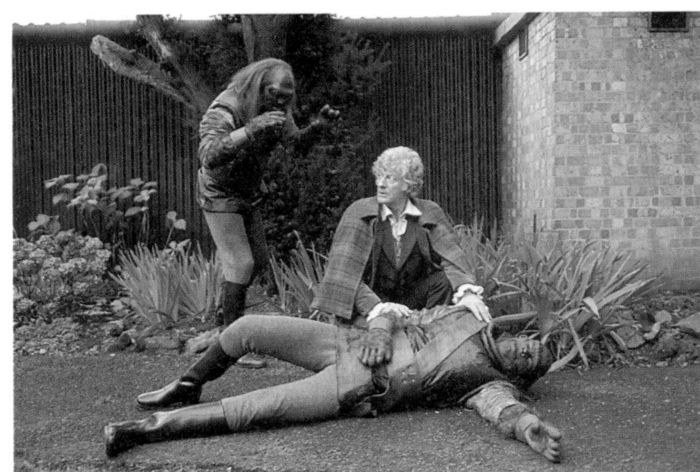

his way up through the ranks of the BBC, starting as a Floor Assistant on various shows, including *Doctor Who.*

Malcolm Hulke:

"I was fascinated with the history of colonialism and the repercussions it brings with it as the natural inhabitants of any given area become the servile species under such conditions. I spoke about the possibility of using that as a starting point for a *Doctor Who* story with Terrance, and he basically said, 'Have a go.'"

Briant scouted for various rocky landscapes, going to the usual quarries at Rickmansworth and Slough and eventually found the ideal setting in Cornwall at a Tin Mine in Saint Austell and a china clay quarry near Plymouth.

Several days of location filming were carried out between 14 and 21 February before the crew returned to London to begin studio rehearsals. Although Delgado was present in Cornwall, he would not be needed for some time as the Master did not return until the final third of the story. '*In Space*' had been added to the title as work began on the serial.

Colony In Space was the first story of the Pertwee era to send the Doctor beyond the confines of the Earth.

Hulke comments:

"There was a temptation to go straight back to the kind of formula they were using with Pat Troughton, but that would have been a very easy trap to fall into. *Colony In Space* was a one-off, just a reminder that the Tardis was still there, and that the Doctor could travel through time.

"Audiences tend to have a very short term memory and after nearly two years of UNIT on Earth, I thought a change with a space adventure would be something interesting."

One of the main special props for the story was the IMC Robot, a small tank-like creation with lengthy armatures.

Michael E. Briant:

"The robot was not exactly what you could call a success. The damn thing was huge and poor John Scott-Martin (the actor inside, who was used to such situations, having been a Dalek operator for several years) couldn't see a bloody thing. The dimensions were a bit out of sync with the set and every time it tried to get through the door, it smashed its head."

Season eight was proving to be a success with an average of between seven and a half to eight and a half million viewers each week. *The Mind Of Evil* episode one peaked at just over nine million.

Once twenty episodes were completed, the final story went into production. *The Daemons* was a five part story developed by Barry Letts and playwright Robert Sloman, who jointly penned the serial under the name of Guy Leopold.

Delgado:

"The whole idea of bringing the Devil himself, or what would appear to be that particular gentleman, into the series as a potential ally for the Master intrigued me greatly. The whole notion of him tapping into the pagan beliefs of mankind, and proving their origins to be alien, was inspired. It was the end of a perfect year for all of the cast. We had almost become a family."

Letts allocated two weeks of location filming for the story and Christopher Barry returned to the programme to direct with Roger Ford as his designer. The script had very specific location requirements – a pagan burial mound, a village pub and green (with enough space to land the UNIT Helicopter), and a rural church and graveyard.

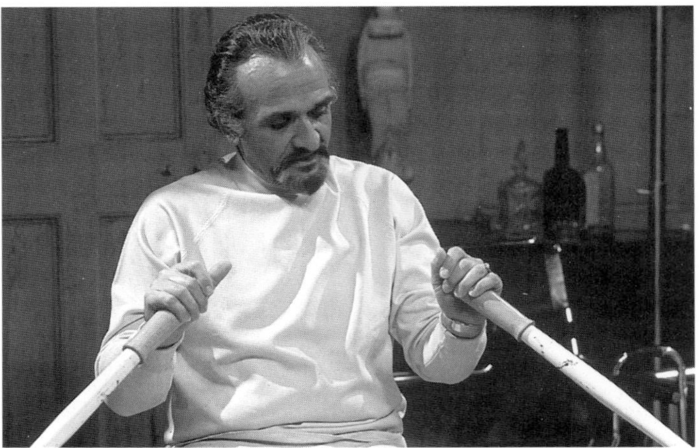

The Master.

The search for a suitable location ended in Aldbourne, in the heart of Wiltshire. With a burial site located to the north of the village and an old MOD airfield in nearby Membury, everything that Barry needed for filming was within easy driving distance.

After a week of rehearsals for all the exterior scenes, the crew set up base and started filming during the second week of April. All the heat barrier sequences were staged first, with an outside broadcast van doubling as a mobile UNIT headquarters and part of a hanger being used to act as the Doctor's garage. After a week of perfect conditions in bright sunshine, things turned a bit strange...

"It was the middle of April, and everything was fine for the first few days, then suddenly it started to snow," recalls Barry Letts. "There were panic stations at first, but it soon started to thaw and Chris Barry was able to get on with filming."

Moving into the centre of Aldbourne itself for the second week, the final few days' filming saw the first appearance of Bok, a small stone gargoyle brought to life by the power of Azal.

Delgado:

"We spent several delightful days in Wilstshire making my personal favourite, *The Daemons*. Little Stanley Mason was my pet gargoyle, Bok. He could throw balls of flame with the skill of an England fast bowler. Whenever he was with me, I would tell him to 'Sit', 'Stay', and all the things that a pet is meant to understand, but he didn't listen - perhaps this is the way of all gargoyles?

"I remember the final scenes for the sheer spontaneity of the crowd of villagers who were watching. They suddenly started to boo and hiss when I was driven away, as the prisoner of Jon and Nicholas Courtney. It only happened the once, and it was perfect and just for the occasion. I spoke to Jon about this later, and he said that was the kind of magic that *Doctor Who* could produce."

Bok was a simple character to create, the diminutive Mason wearing a grey bodystocking adorned with moulded wings, a set of claws for both feet and hands and, of course, a tail. His head was covered with a half-mask based on the classical tongue-pulling image of a gargoyle.

Back in the studios at the beginning of May,Stephen Thorne played the character of Azal, the last of the Daemons:

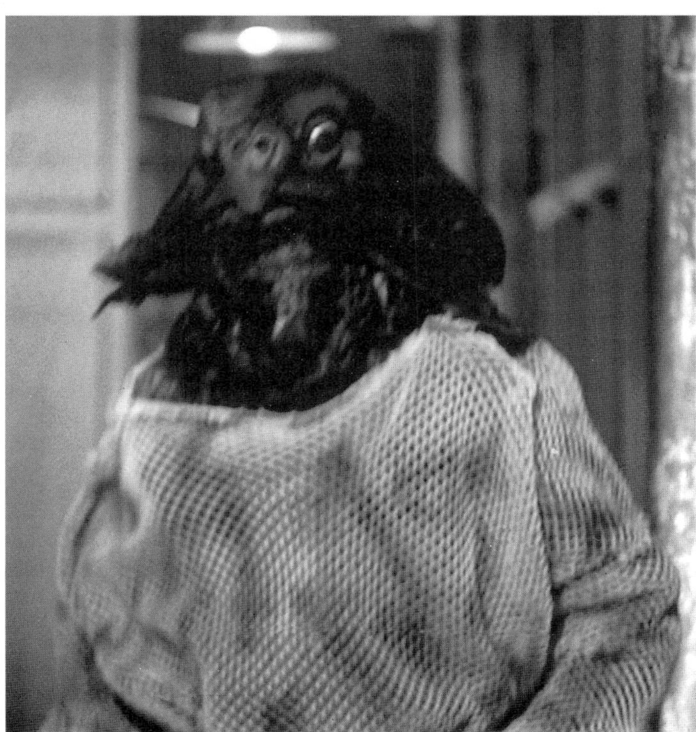

A scantily clad Sea Devil.

"I looked a bit like Pan, but without the pipes. I was all fur-lined legs and hooves, with a curly chest wig that matched the beard and hair they put on me (the costume was completed with a face-mask which left the mouth clear for a pair of specially made elongated fangs). I just had to stand in front of a blue screen and be menacing on cue!"

The Daemons achieved the highest ratings of the twenty five week run. As the cast broke up for the summer, plans were already well underway for the start of the ninth season, with Dicks commissioning scripts for a September start date. Every year needed a good 'opening night', as the head of the department termed it. The first story had to have the vital element that would attract the casual viewer's interest.

Season seven had the fact that *Spearhead From Space* would see the debut of a new Doctor, while *Terror Of The Autons* introduced the Master for the following year. Season nine would celebrate the return of an old adversary as Letts finally gave way to the continual requests he was receiving.

"People did keep asking, 'When are you going to bring the Daleks back, then?' It was about five years or so since they'd last been seen, so they were dusted down again."

Louis Marks, who had last written for the series on *Planet Of The Giants*, had submitted a storyline called *The Time Warriors* which dealt with terrorists travelling back through time to assassinate a government minister who would corrupt the future of the planet. It became a case of 'What if the Daleks ruled this 'Future Earth'?' and so the scripts were suitably altered. There was a problem with the actual execution of this plan, however, as the BBC had very few working Dalek costumes left. In fact, there were three and, although their new paint scheme made them look impressive, when it came to the location filming in the second week of September, there was no way that director Paul Bernard could make them look anything like an invasion force.

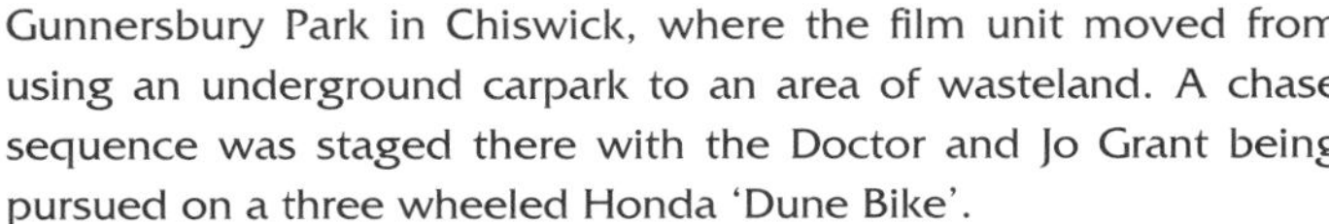

Retitled as *The Day Of The Daleks*, several days were spent around Gunnersbury Park in Chiswick, where the film unit moved from using an underground carpark to an area of wasteland. A chase sequence was staged there with the Doctor and Jo Grant being pursued on a three wheeled Honda 'Dune Bike'.

Michael E. Briant comments:

"Barry (Letts) always liked to get some form of 'new' vehicle in for Jon to use - something that was new on the market and wouldn't become a common sight for some time. It gave a futuristic look to the programme without a great deal of expense. So we had moon-buggies (*Colony In Space*), three-wheeled motor bikes and jet-skis (*The Sea Devils*) way before anyone watching would actually know what they were."

The Day Of The Daleks film crew then moved to the Brentford canal, using a tunnel by the canal itself for several battle scenes between Daleks and UNIT troops, while a nearby stately home was used as Auderly House in the story.

To publicise the story, a trailer was shot announcing the return of the Daleks, restaging scenes of them moving around famous London landmarks. It was screened on BBC1 several times around Christmas 1971, a couple of weeks prior to the start of season nine on Saturday 1 January, 1972.

The Day Of The Daleks was one of only two stories to feature UNIT during the new series and Delgado was now no longer the recurring villain in all the stories. Fearing overkill with the character, Letts and Dicks had opted to give him only selective appearances from now on.

Delgado:

"I have to admit that there was some cause for concern on my part about appearing in *Doctor Who*. Much as I enjoyed it and looked forward to returning to each story where the Master appeared, I found that it had a restrictive effect on my career. The industry as a whole regards the programme as being continuously in production, and due to my 'presence' throughout my first year, they tended to think that I was shooting all the time, which was not the case at all.

"With only the odd battle here and there with the Doctor, I think producers and directors tended to think I was unavailable for other things, as *Doctor Who* took up all my time. As a consequence, I found myself twiddling my thumbs for longer periods than I would care to, and that's why I felt it was time for me to move on. But the Master had to go in style!"

Work continued on *The Day Of The Daleks* with a new breed of monsters introduced for the serial. The Ogrons were towering creatures imbued with incredible strength but little brain power. They were the creation of John Friedlander, who was now regularly sculpting the masks for the various alien races appearing in the programme.

By using latex appliances, and keeping certain parts of the actor's face free - the mouth and eyes - he was able to bring a more realistic quality to them. The masks were also durable, whereas before there was always a danger of damage (as with the Krotons, for example), the production team knew these would last and, like the Axons, survive to be used the following year. They were eventually seen again in *Frontier In Space*.

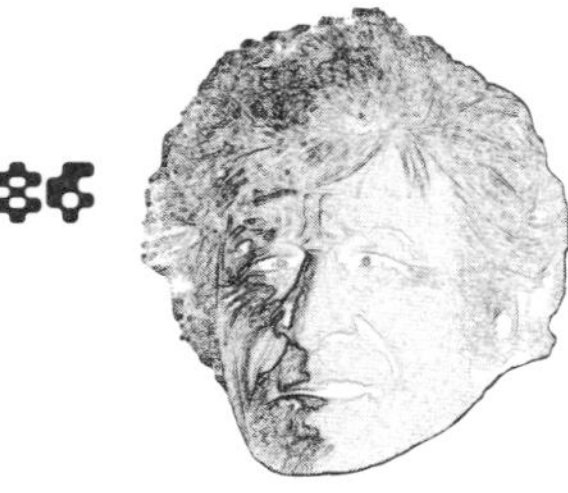

Friedlander was again called in to help create Malcolm Hulke's new reptilian race, *The Sea Devils* which, although broadcast third in the season, went into production as the second story, in order to take advantage of the weather before the onset of winter to complete the extensive marine location filming that was required.

Roger Delgado returned to resume his role as the Master, now held in prison after his capture at the end of *The Daemons*, and Michael E. Briant took on his second directing assignment for the programme, with Tony Snoaden as his designer.

Hulke's script had started out as *The Sea Monsters*:

"I thought a great deal about trying to do a sort of sequel to *The Silurians*, which I thought had worked really well, especially in the execution of the monsters. The problem was that we'd blown them to kingdom come at the end and you could hardly do something as contrived as saying they didn't actually get hurt because they were in a different cave when the explosives went off. So, I thought it wouldn't be unreasonable to suppose that there were other similar races inhabiting the planet at the same time."

With the history of both the Army and the RAF helping out on the programme already, Barry Letts approached the Navy to sound them out on the possibility of participating. The reply came back that they would make available whatever hardware and facilities were needed, as long as the service was portrayed in a good light.

With this in mind, the cast and film crew left for six days of location filming on 23 October aboard *HMS Frazer* and *HMS Reclaim*, where the diving bell sequences were staged. The main naval base seen throughout the story was the *HMS Frazer* gunnery school, where all the main cast and the Sea Devils themselves were needed for battle scenes. Six Sea Devil costumes were made, but did not meet up with Briant's expectations when he saw the finished product on location.

Briant:

"They looked obscene! I didn't want to have naked monsters wandering around, so we got some rope netting and put sections of that on them. It looked rather like string vests. I liked to think that it was bits of old fishermen's nets that they'd found at the bottom of the sea.

"The other problem was the heads. The costumes were a kind of overall which was fine, and the masks were worn like hats so that the actors (several members of the old HAVOC team) could see out of the creatures' necks. Whenever they actually ducked under the water, an air bubble got trapped in the top of the mask, and it sent them flying off like bullets. It was hysterical! These things suddenly shot out of the water, and then you'd see Terry (Walsh) and Pat (Gorman) get up and start wading around trying to find their heads!"

For the remainder of the shoot, the crew moved to the Isle of White, where all the sequences involving the special prison holding the Master were filmed. Norris Castle and its surrounding grounds were used, while some time was also spent working around the beaches of Whitecliff Bay. As in *Fury From The Deep* in season five, the script called for an oil rig and the production team found themselves in the same frustrating situation.

Briant:

"We couldn't get onto a rig at all, so I had a bit of a brainwave and remembered that there was an old sea fort, like the one we used in *Fury*, near the Isle Of White. We used that instead.

"We wanted Roger to go out on a sea scooter we had, but he took me to one side and admitted that the mere thought of water terrified him, so we used a stunt man. When it came to the Doctor and the Master escaping in some survival suits, and having to

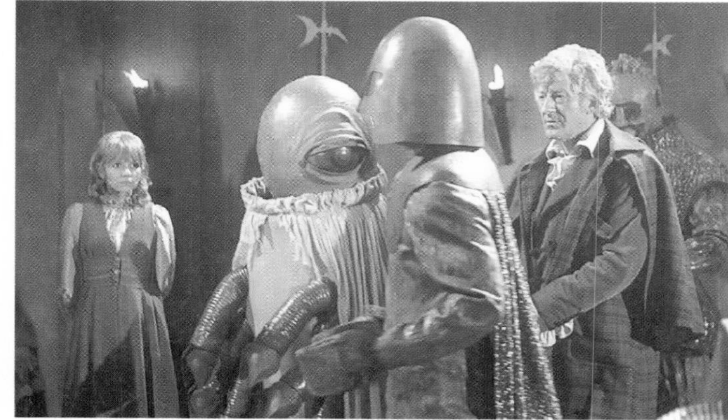

ABOVE: The giant green Alpha Centuri and an Ice Lord during rehearsals for **The Curse Of Peladon**.
LEFT: During rehearsals Brigadier Lethbridge-Stewart often appeared without his military moustache.

float in the middle of the sea wearing them, Roger agreed to do one take, which was incredibly brave of him. He got through it somehow and he was quite ill afterwards, but everyone admired him for doing it."

By 8 November, the cast were back on dry land rehearsing for the first studio sessions.

Delgado:

"I have to admit that one of my favourite moments came in the story *The Sea Devils*, where I was held in prison. One scene had the Master watching a children's puppet series (*The Clangers*) on a vast television screen and he was convinced that these things were some advanced alien civilisation. He was deeply disappointed when he was told the truth. I think it would have been rather fun to have him join forces with them!"

The story was completed with the recording of episodes five and six on 13 and 14 December after which the cast broke up for Christmas. Letts made the decision to bring production of the next serial forward, so transmission would begin at the end of January a week after *The Day Of The Daleks* had completed its run. The schedule suddenly became very tight for Director Lennie Mayne and his designer Gloria Clayton. They had just over a month of production time to get all four episodes of *The Curse Of Peladon* ready for broadcast.

Brian Hayles had written the four part script which had been developed from a submission he sent to Terrance Dicks called *Doctor Who And The Brain Dead*.

Hayles:

"I followed the new UNIT set-up when Pertwee came into the programme and thought it would be an idea to have the Ice Warriors invade earth. The idea I sent in had them using a device that could turn the human brain to ice and make men into zombie-like slaves who obeyed their every command. Terrance was not keen."

Dicks and Letts wanted to explore the possibilities of presenting detailed alien cultures within the framework of the programme. To this end, Hayles formulated a plot that would present a much more intimate adventure.

"I said, 'Why not try the *Ten Little Indians* plot device (an Agatha Christie book, where a group of people are gathered together and as they're murdered one by one, it becomes clear that the killer is one of them), and have the Ice Warriors as the immediate suspects, when in actual fact they're totally innocent?' That's where *The Curse Of Peladon* came from.

"The director was a loud, colourful Australian called Lennie Mayne, who took one look at the working title, which was then *The Curse Of The Peladons* (originally, it was just *The Curse*) and said, 'No way! That sounds like a case of the clap!' It was suitably changed."

Due to the fact that they were made of thick latex and fibreglass, the Ice Warrior costumes had survived intact during storage and Sonny Caldinez, who had appeared as one of the creatures in both *The Ice Warriors* and *The Seeds Of Death*, effectively got his

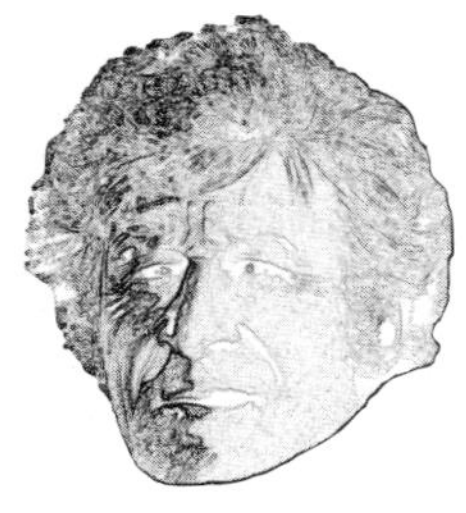

old costume back for his role as Ssorg. One warrior was needed alongside the Ice Lord, Izlyr, and again an old costume had survived well enough to be adapted and augmented with the addition of a cloak and chest plate. Alan Bennion returned to the programme, having previously played the Ice Lord Slaar in *The Seeds Of Death*.

Hayles script called for several other creatures to be created. There was Aggedor, the Royal Beast of Peladon, which was played by stunt man Nick Hobbs. This was a dark fur-covered body-suit, with claws, a moulded snout and eyes, and a horn on top of its head.

Arcturus, one of the Galactic Federation delegates, was operated by veteran Dalek actor, Murphy Grumbar. He had to sit inside the creature's box-like life support system which had glowing tubes of liquid on its sides, powered by a car battery. Arcturus itself was housed inside a glass dome on the top of the structure. The whole thing's movements were limited to turning left or right, and little else.

Alpha Centuri, another delegate, was by far the most elaborate costume of the story. With the main body built around layered hoops, which were supported across stunt man Stuart Fell's shoulders inside, the front featured six arms that could all be moved. They were connected to Fell's arms which worked the upper pair. When he moved his arms, the other limbs mirrored his gestures.

The huge spherical head was made of fibre-glass, with a vast single eye, which was made like a double-mirror so Fell could easily see out of it. The eye-lid could also be operated, so that it blinked occasionally. Neither of the two stunt men provided the voices for the characters, though they had to learn the lines to fit the cues of Ysanne Churchman's and Terry Bale's vocalisations for them off camera.

Hayles:

"Alpha Centuri caused a bit of a problem when it got into the rehearsal rooms as Lennie took one look at it and said words to the effect of, 'What the hell's that meant to be? A giant green dick?' The costume people quickly dressed it up with a large yellow cape, but it did little to lessen the effect. After that, it was known as 'The green dick in the cloak'."

The cast returned from their holiday during the first week of January, and went straight into filming several sequences at Ealing including the Doctor and Jo's arrival on the mountainside of Peladon's castle and the fight between the King's champion, Grun, and the Doctor, which was done in the empty water tank at the studios. This heightened the effect of the two men effectively being in an arena.

Hayles:

"It was strange to see David Troughton in the series (he played King Peladon). Having last worked on *Doctor Who* during his father's time with the programme, I could see one or two hereditary mannerisms, but he was a good actor in his own right, and I thought he brought a unique quality to the part."

The Peladon scenario worked well and Hayles began to consider writing a sequel:

"The whole structure of the society, struggling to overcome the barbarism of its past and meet new technology head-on, was intriguing. I thought about continuing the story, taking up practically where it left off, but that would have been too easy. It was talking to Terrance that sparked the notion off going further down the line, taking off a few decades into their future rather than a few weeks, so I started playing around with a few ideas."

Episode one saw the programme reach a new high in the ratings for the colour era of the programme, with just over ten million viewers. Episode two reached eleven million, the highest figure since *Galaxy Four* way back in September 1965.

While Mayne was editing *The Curse Of Peladon*, the cast and crew left to start the location filming for the next story, *The Mutants*. Christopher Barry returned once again as the director, with Jeremy Bear as his designer. The scripts were written by the team of Bob Baker and Dave Martin, or 'The Bristol Boys', as they became known.

The plotline was inspired by a synopsis that Barry Letts had submitted for consideration when Gerry Davis was still the script editor in the mid-1960s. Baker and Martin expanded on it greatly, taking in themes of colonisation and pollution.

Christopher Barry selected Chiselhurst Caves in the heart of Kent for the main location work, with the nearby Finsbury Caves also being used. The rest of the sequences on the surface of the planet Solos were staged at a local chalk quarry.

Six elaborate 'Mutt' costumes were needed for the main scenes, with the actors playing them being cast for their size as the Mutts were meant to be quite small. Their shells were made from a wire frame with fabric pulled over them to act as their skin. Production assistant Chris D'Oyly John remembers one of the more unpleasant aspects of the job for the actors involved.

"The Mutts had heads like insects, with mandibles on their jaws that twitched. The only way to do this was to attach them in some way to the actor's face and it was literally a case of clipping them to their cheeks with clothes pegs. They were in agony and you had to take the masks off as quickly as possible between scenes. There were so many bruises at the end that they looked as though they'd been in a fight."

Jon Pertwee commented in 1973:

"There is a constant source of pleasure in seeing the inventiveness of the costume designers and coming face to face with their efforts. Some are utterly believable. We had a race of insects scuttling around some caves in Kent last year and they looked wonderful. The rule is to never test exactly how 'real' they are though, because one poke to what you think is a hard shell could easily rip some delicate fabric and leave a damn great hole in the monster's side!"

For the finale of the season, Robert Sloman completed his first solo script for the series with *The Time Monster*. It called upon the myth of what happened to the lost city of Atlantis, which had already been covered to some extent with the Troughton story, *The Underwater Menace*.

The director assigned to the story was Paul Bernard and his designer was Tim Gleeson. *The Time Monster* was only the second story to feature UNIT that year and it also saw the penultimate appearance by Roger Delgado.

"It was a fascinating idea to mix the modern science of *Doctor Who* and the mythology of Atlantis. The Master was, for I think the only time so far, at his most romantically charming. The most evil men in history have always had the ability to seduce with their power, and the Queen (Ingrid Pitt) was totally entranced by his skilled manipulation of her gullible emotions. I relished the

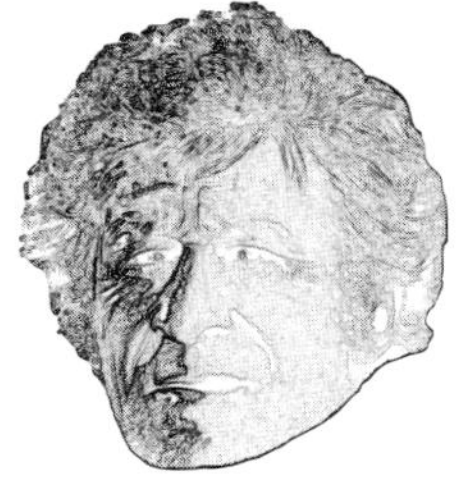

opportunity to play on this because I am convinced it is something the Doctor could never do."

Rehearsals for the location filming began in the first week of April, followed by five days in and around Reading. Some time was also spent at Gunnersbury Park, in Chiswick, where Bernard had taken the film unit previously for *Day Of The Daleks*.

The final two instalments moved to Atlantis itself, with Hammer horror star Ingrid Pitt now joining the cast.

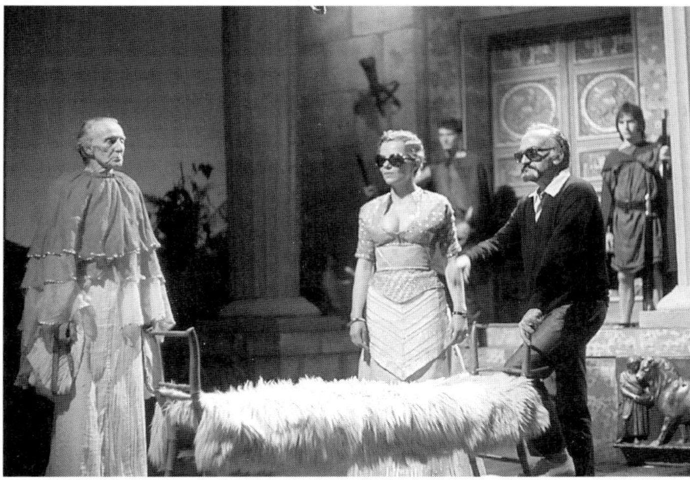

The Master in casual attire rehearsing for **The Time Monster**.

Delgado recalls:

"It occurred to me that the Master could quite easily have stayed and ruled Atlantis with the Queen, as I liked to think that he was quite taken with her. But I realised that this was not the kind of ending he deserved. The Master would need to face a threat of his own creation, which turns on him and forces him to destroy it, thus killing himself in the process – but it would not be as an act of redemption. It would be as an act of self-preservation that went horribly wrong.

"I broached the scenario with Barry Letts and he jokingly said, 'Why, you're not thinking of leaving us, are you?' to which I solemnly had to confess that I was. I did not want to fade out quietly, cryptically left so that I might return one day. It had to be a final, undoubted demise that would in some way effect the Doctor's very soul.That's how I wanted to go."

The story was completed in TC3 on 23 and 24 May, winding up the season. The first episode of *The Time Monster* was broadcast on the previous Saturday. With the tenth season confirmed, and a departure story for the Master the obvious way to end it, plans got underway through the summer for other ways to celebrate the tenth anniversary year. It was clear that something special had to be done.

Barry Letts:

"Over the years, people used to say again and again, in the pub or whatever, 'I've got a marvellous idea. Why don't you have all three Doctors together?' I resisted this for a long time because it seemed to go right against the idea of having the Doctor regenerate. To have them all together seemed to make nonsense of the whole continuity of the character."

Every year, the production team tried to come up with a 'First night' episode to kick off the new season that would be an automatic draw for the viewers and win the vital *Radio Times* cover article to herald the programme's return. The casting of the Master had worked, as had the return of the Daleks for season nine. The idea suddenly became appealing as a way to kick off a tenth anniversary run.

Letts:

"We suddenly thought, 'Well, why not have the three of them together? Surely we can come up with a plausible reason, and work out how it can be done, in terms of the Time Lords and their technology'. To a certain extent, I think we succeeded but, of course, we did run into the problem of dear old Bill Hartnell not being able to play a full part in the proceedings."

Patrick Troughton:

"Barry Letts approached me, and sounded me out about whether or not I'd be willing to go back. I'd only been gone for two or three years and I wondered whether it might be a bit too soon to go back, but the fact that I'd had so much fun before overcame any real doubts. Besides, as my sons pointed out, I hadn't been seen in colour before, so I could hardly miss out on an opportunity like that, could I? It did come as quite a shock when I heard about Billy. Nobody knew he was so ill."

Barry Letts:

"I'd spoken to Bill on the phone and he'd said he'd love to do it. We were quite happily, going ahead with the scripting and making plans for the first Doctor to play a full-sized part.

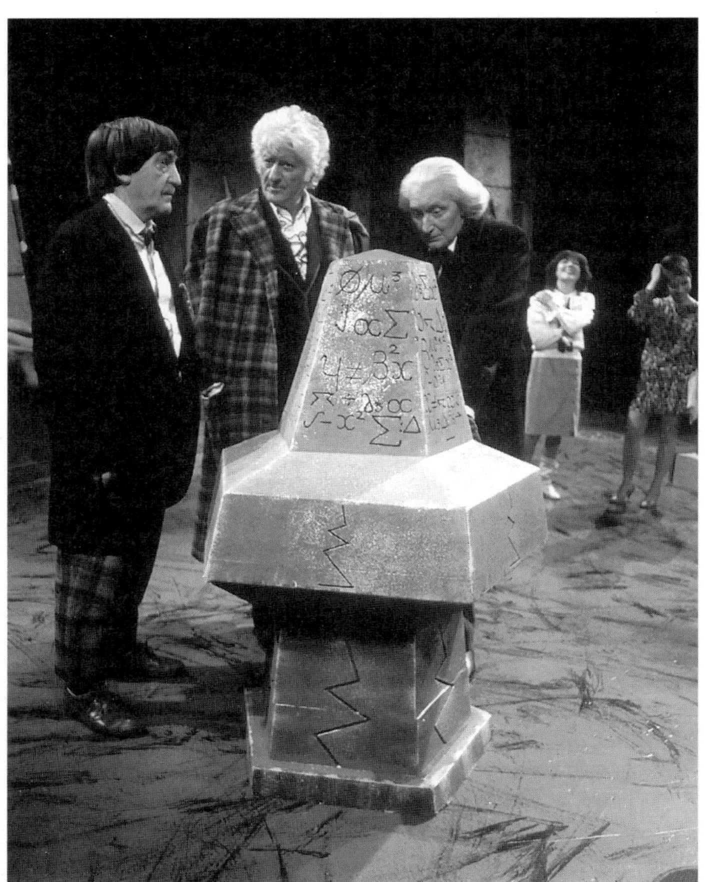

The Three Doctors.

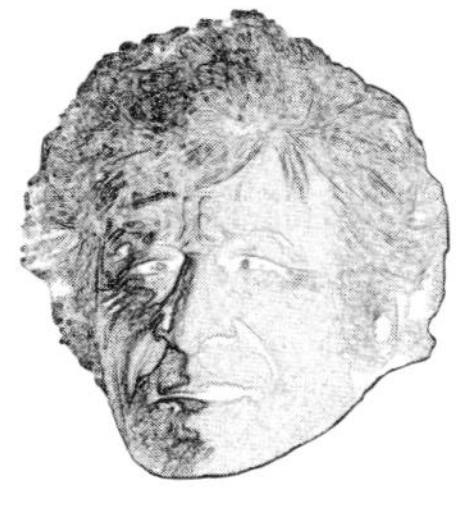

"We were well into that process when his wife rang me up and said, 'Bill says that you've asked him to be *Doctor Who* again'. I said yes and explained what we were doing, and she said, 'I'm sorry, but I knew nothing about it. I should have warned you. He just can't do it, he's just not well enough to do it. He's got atherosclerosis of the arteries of the brain. You happened to get him on a good day. On a bad day, he can hardly remember who he is, let alone lines in a script.'

"By that time, we were committed to it, and the whole thing had been announced. It was panic stations, and Terrance and I had to sit down and figure out how on earth we could do it."

Patrick Troughton's schedule made it difficult to make the story any earlier than November, so there was time for rewrites while two other stories for the tenth season were made.

Robert Holmes:

"I'd always found the thought of freak shows and how man could have the fascination to stand and stare at the malformed and mutated quite disturbing. I came up with the notion of having a Barnum-type showman who had a peepshow machine in which he kept all the monsters of the galaxy in miniaturised versions of their natural environments. It wasn't a circus, it was all computerised and as big as a stool, and you had to peer through the top of it to see the Dalek or the Cybermen, or whatever...

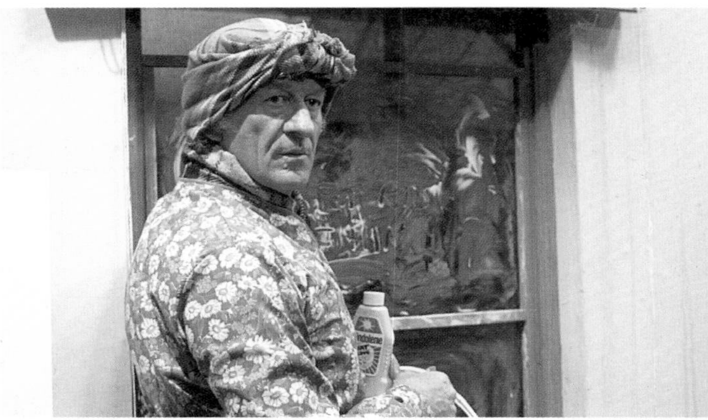

ABOVE: An unusual outfit for The Doctor in **The Green Death**.
BELOW: The Doctor, Jo and the Professor working on a new superglue for the Brigadier's moustache.

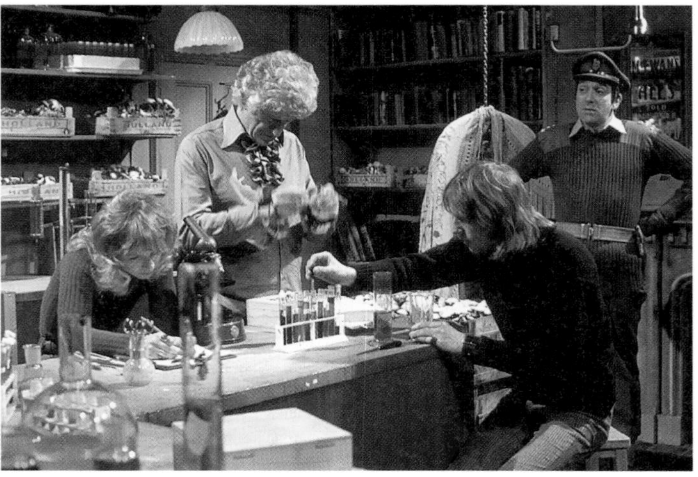

"The idea was to have the Doctor and Jo land in one of these environments and only begin to realise that something's wrong when the find they're on a ship in the 1920s and it's attacked by a prehistoric monster! I tried to write it with two basic settings, as Barry wanted a cheap story to direct at the end of the year, but it apparently ended up costing quite a bit!"

Peepshow became *Carnival Of Monsters* and was shot as the last story of the ninth season's recording block. Letts was directing and Roger Limiton worked as his designer.

The location shooting for the 1920s ship was carried out on the SS Bernice, off the River Medway, in the first week of June. For the Doctor and Jo's encounter with the Drashigs, gigantic reptilian monsters inhabiting a swamp - in reality, glove puppets that were shot later on. Holmes: "If you rework the word Drashig, you'll find it's an anagram of Dishrag..." - a day was spent with Pertwee and Katy Manning filming at Burnham on Crouch Marshes, in Essex.

The story saw the first appearance in the series by Ian Marter, as Captain Andrews, Letts having remembered the actor from his audition for the role of Captain Yates. In just under two years, he would be working as one of the regular cast members of the programme.

The final two days work on *Carnival* were spent in the studio on 3 and 4 July. After that point, Pertwee and Manning departed for their summer break, with work due to resume on season ten at the beginning of September. One decision that had been made by Letts and Dicks was that a tenth anniversary series would not be complete without a certain race of aliens.

Malcolm Hulke:

"Terrance and Barry had hatched a plan to do a mammoth Dalek story. Not a four parter, or even a six, this was going to be twelve weeks long. I knew this had already been done, and I think they spoke to one or two people who said it wasn't such a good idea.

"They decided to split it in two, with a build up that would reveal the main villains to be the Daleks at the end of the first half, while the second half involved them *en masse*. Terrance asked whether I'd handle the first chunk, which had the Master in it. I knew and liked Roger Delgado a great deal and I enjoyed writing for his character (Hulke had already done so twice before, with *Colony In Space* and *The Sea Devils*). That, I'm afraid, was a far greater incentive than writing for the Daleks, whom I always thought were a bit one-dimensional and flat. Terrance got the only man who knew how to do anything with them in for the latter six episodes, and that was Terry Nation."

The working title of *Frontier* became *Frontier In Space* as production grew closer. Hulke's other instruction for the plot of his serial was to bring back the Ogrons, who had proved to be very popular after *Day Of The Daleks*. Terry Nation, meanwhile, started drafting out *Destination Daleks*, as the second half of the story.

Just over three months after completing *The Time Monster*, Paul Bernard was back with the programme to handle the directing on Hulke's story with Cynthia Kljuco as his designer. The Ogron masks were still intact and usable from *Day* and John Friedlander was brought in to handle a new race of monsters, the Draconians. Based on a design by Bernard, the creatures overall look drew heavily on the stylised images of Japanese Shogun Warriors.

Jon Pertwee said in 1973:

"I admired the Draconians tremendously as they were the first time that I felt totally convinced that this was an alien race I was

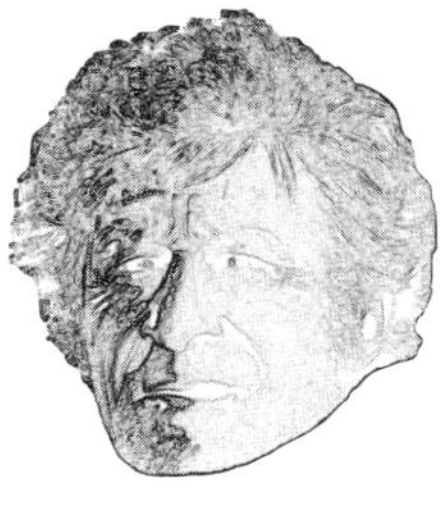

The Whomobile made its debut in **Invasion Of The Dinosaurs**.

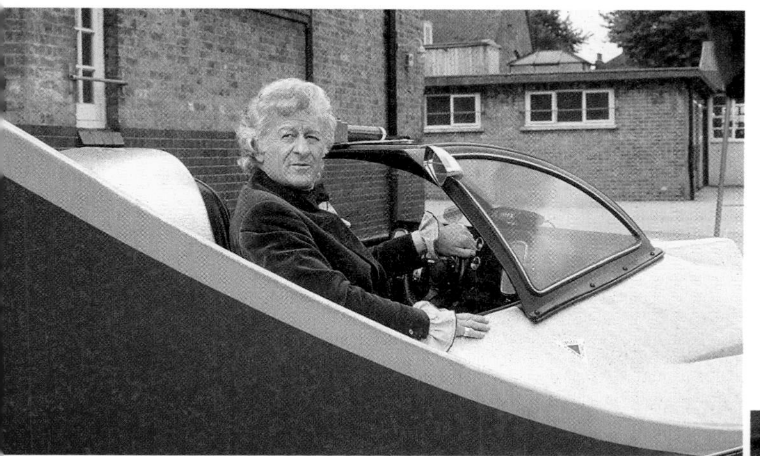

"I'm keen to go out in a blaze of glory, as I firmly believe that the great villains should have their own equivalent of a heroic end. I have been well served by the writers so far, who have given me wonderful dialogue, and the directors, the cast, the crew... it has been a truly happy working experience."

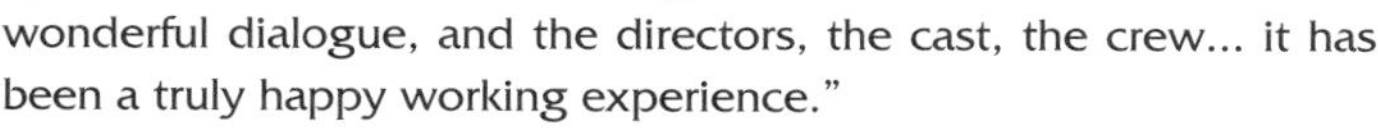

Patrick Troughton returned to the series to start rehearsals for *The Three Doctors* at the end of that week, with the title having been changed from *The Black Hole* to a more obvious alternative. By now, Letts had managed to overcome the situation with William Hartnell.

"I spoke to Heather Hartnell at length and managed to establish that Bill would be able to sit and read lines to camera, and

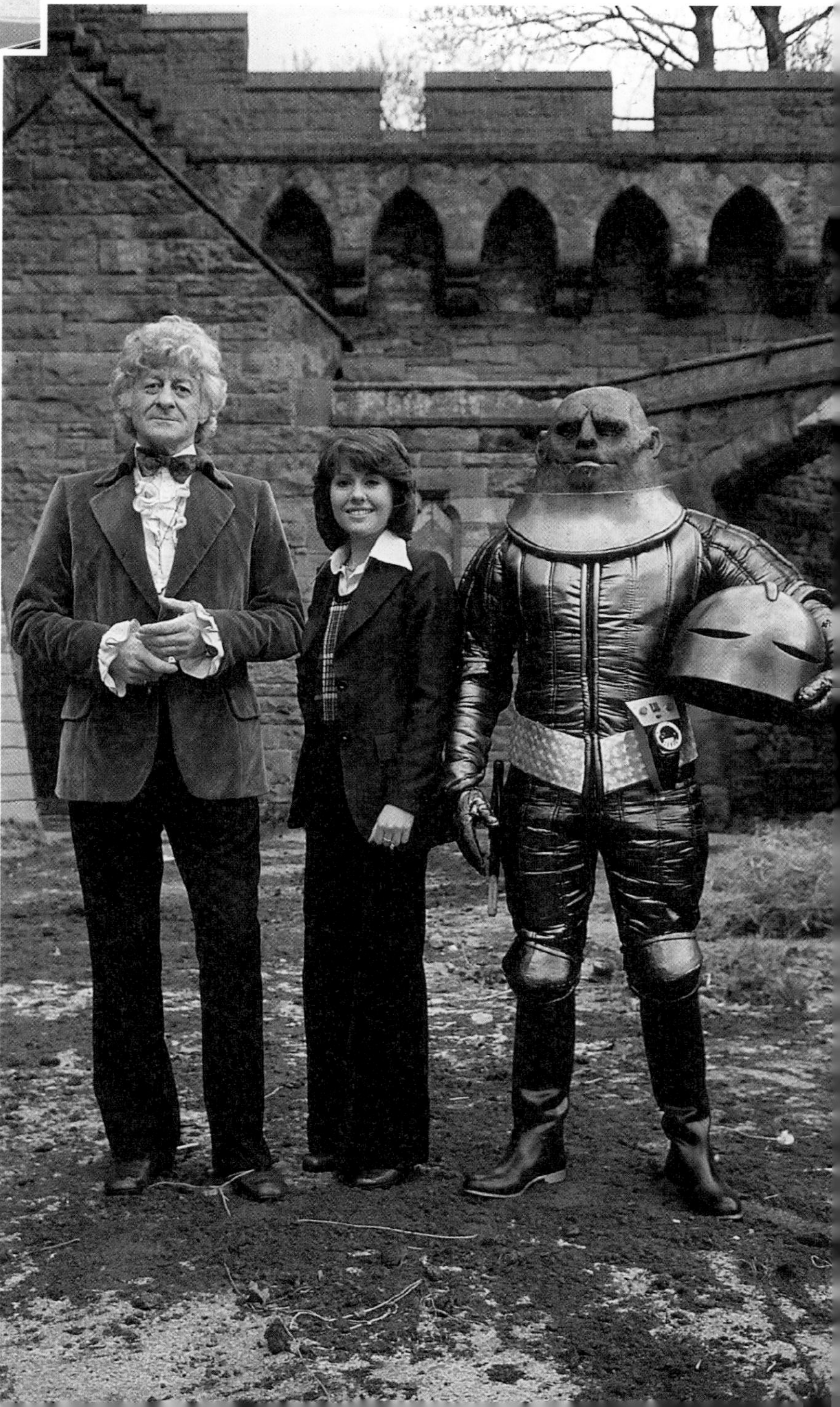

meeting. I remember sitting talking to one of the actors in one of the quarries where we were filming and forgetting totally that he was really as human as I was. The make-up was that convincing."

Roger Delgado:

"Jon Pertwee came up to me and told me how wonderful these new reptilian monsters were and that he couldn't understand how the make-up technicians had made them so convincing. I simply said, 'That's the magic of *Doctor Who*', and Jon said, 'Yes, I suppose it is, isn't it.' He wandered off, totally forgetting that that was what he said to me when we were in Wiltshire (on *The Daemons*)."

The masks had intricate scales across the high-domed head and face with the actor's chin and eyes left free, although the chin was concealed behind a delicate beard and all flesh tones were painted to match the mask colouring. The actors wearing them made their first appearance in front of the camera along with the Ogrons on the first location shoot for the story.

Following several days rehearsal, work began around the exterior of the Royal Festival Hall on London's South Bank on Sunday, 10 September. Following this, the grounds of a private house in Highgate Hill were used for a day, before the cast and crew moved to the Fuller's Earth Works quarry in Reigate, Surrey, where Delgado arrived to complete his first few scenes on the story.

Several days work at Ealing followed, with Pertwee completing specially staged scenes of him making a spacewalk around the exterior of a spaceship. All the extensive model shots for the story were completed using a variety of cannibalised models that had been purchased by the special effects department from Gerry Anderson's company, Century 21. The ships seen in *Frontier In Space* comprised of bits that came from series ranging from Thunderbirds to *UFO*.

Delgado was keen to get his teeth into the final story for the Master, as he said only a few days after completing his first recording block on *Frontier*:

Liz Sladen joined the Doctor as reporter Sarah Jane Smith in 1973.

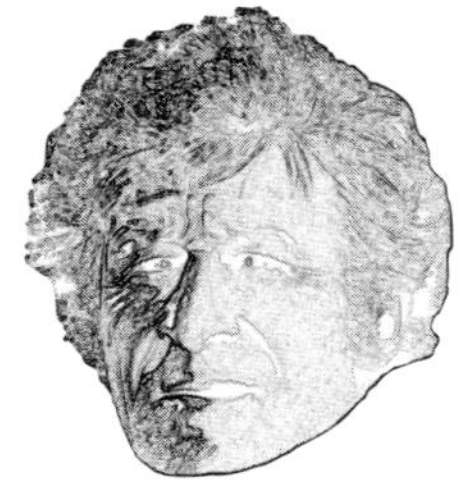

that he'd be fully aware of what was going on. It wasn't that he'd gone completely do-lally, or anything remotely like that, it was just that he would never have been able to cope with learning a script and then having to act the part.

"We got him down to Ealing and shot all his stuff in one day's filming. He sat in his chair and did it all from cue cards. He knew exactly what he was doing and was able to give a very good performance. It was a treat to watch him work, actually."

The only other material of Hartnell that was used in the story was a brief shot of the first Doctor wandering around a garden, seen on a screen by the Time Lords when they attempt to take his incarnation out of its time stream. This was filmed in an afternoon at William Hartnell's cottage in Hayfield, Kent, where a series of photographs were taken of him together with Pertwee and Troughton. The *Radio Times* also mounted a studio bound photo session, with Hartnell present, to get a shot for a front cover on the magazine.

Scenes outside UNIT's Headquarters were filmed at Haylings House in Denham, while the rest of the location filming was spent working around Rickmansworth Quarry. Director Lennie Mayne was working from a script by Bob Baker and Dave Martin, and Roger Limiton had returned as designer. As with *The Curse Of Peladon*, Mayne was racing against time to get the serial ready for transmission, which was due to start on 30 December. A large set for the UNIT HQ interior, with corridors running outside the Doctor's laboratory, was erected in TCI for the first studio day on 28 November.

Troughton enjoyed being back:

"It was an added bonus to have Nick there as well (Courtney, who had worked with Troughton on *The Web Of Fear* and *The Invasion*). It felt a bit odd suddenly being back on the Tardis set again and I was a bit worried about whether I'd be able to pull it off after the gap, but it was no problem at all, really."

The second studio block ran from 11 to 12 December with the large sets of rogue Time Lord Omega's palace in TC8. Stephen Thorne returned to the programme to play Omega:

"Lennie Mayne could make his feelings felt on certain matters in, shall we say, a slightly florid way. He didn't mince words. Omega had these guards that were meant to be anti-matter blobs, or something like that, and the costumes were hysterical. They looked like melted lumps of jelly!

"Lennie took another view and when he saw them in rehearsal, he took one look and said they looked like swollen parts of the male anatomy! I also remember him being terribly upset about the sets for the throne room. He wanted some grandiose palace like the Taj Mahal and all he got was a few painted flats. There just wasn't the money to do anything else."

With the immense publicity surrounding the story, the tenth season got off to a spectacular start at the end of the month. Episode four actually had the highest ratings figure for any of the Jon Pertwee stories. Just under twelve million viewers tuned in.

After the regular Christmas break, work resumed in the last week of December, as David Maloney returned to Direct Terry Nation's half of the Dalek epic, now titled *Planet Of The Daleks*. Letts was now talking with Robert Sloman about ideas for a 'final' Master story for Roger Delgado, who had told him about the problems he was facing getting work beyond *Doctor Who*.

Letts:

"I told Roger I was very sorry to hear that he wanted to go, from the point of view of the programme, but that I completely understood his situation as an ex-actor myself. I said, 'Well, you tell me. Do you want to go out in a blaze of glory, with a big bang? Or, do you want to just quietly finish? And he said, 'Oh, I'd much rather go out with a bloody great bang!'

"Bob Sloman and I were talking over an idea to kill him off, and Terrance was in on it as well. We'd always played around with the idea that the Doctor and the Master were bound together in some way, that maybe they'd been friends at college, or something like that. There was the question of why didn't the Master kill the Doctor when he had him in his power? It always seemed to go wrong.

"We thought we'd capitalise on this, and have the story left ambiguous at the end, with an enormous great cosmic explosion happening... maybe even creating a black hole... as a direct consequence of the death of the Master. No one would never know whether he allowed it to happen because he couldn't face the fact that if he didn't do it, it would mean killing the Doctor, or whether it was accidental, or whether you ultimately had to put it down to the fact that the Doctor had killed the Master. We were going to leave it completely in the air and let everybody make their own interpretation."

Four new Daleks were made for *Planet Of The Daleks* , which brought the number of working casings up to seven, counting the three that already existed from as far back as the original Dalek story.

After close to three years working on the programme, Katy Manning asked Barry Letts about leaving at the end of the tenth season. The final six-part story, which was being written by Malcolm Hulke, was accordingly structured to send Jo Grant out on a high.

Planet Of The Daleks was completed with two final days in TV Centre, on 19 and 20 February. The finished story would be transmitted as the fourth of the series, and episode one achieved the highest rating for the year, next to *The Three Doctors'* record, with eleven million viewers drawn to watch by the return of the Daleks.

Michael E. Briant was now back with the production team to helm *The Green Death*, with John Borrowes as his designer. Hulke's script was addressing serious issues of environmental pollution, which Letts was keen to see the programme tackling.

Hulke:

"*Doomwatch* was able to hit the viewers with far more graphic scenes of realistic problems with ecology and the damage industry was causing, but I realised that only *Doctor Who* could get away with actually having the waste in question create genetic mutations.

"Wherever there is rubbish, you're bound to find an infestation of flies buzzing around and I couldn't honestly think of a more horrific insect to enlarge than a fly and its maggots. A spider is a spider and they're pretty innocuous, but a fly can spread germs and decay in an instant. I find them far more repulsive."

The story started with chemical waste being poured down empty mine shafts and Hulke consequently chose a Welsh setting.

"I had the whole thing taking place in a tiny mining village, where there was a typical industrial take-over, with the 'men-in-suits' brigade destroying the land and heritage without a care for the local population.

"Another element we included, that *Doomwatch* couldn't quite get away with and remain in the boundaries of science fact, was to have a 'thinking' computer. Originally it was just a harsh metallic voice, like a Dalek or a Cyberman, but Michael Briant came up with a brainwave and cast John Dearth, whom he'd known since he was a child actor, as BOSS's (the computer) voice. He gave it a whole personality that I hadn't considered possible. He was never seen, and gave a wonderful performance."

While casting was underway to find the new girl for the series, the cast and crew of *The Green Death* left for Wales to start the location filming from 5 March. All of the main sites that Briant needed had been found in and around Deri, in Mid-Glamorgan, where the crew were based for two weeks.

A Scotch Tape Factory doubled up for the exterior and grounds of the Global Chemicals plant seen in the story and a disused National Coal Board Mine and its nearby quarry were also used for several days. In the quarry, Briant had to shoot a scene with thousands of the 'giant' maggots being bombed by the RAF. He takes up the story:

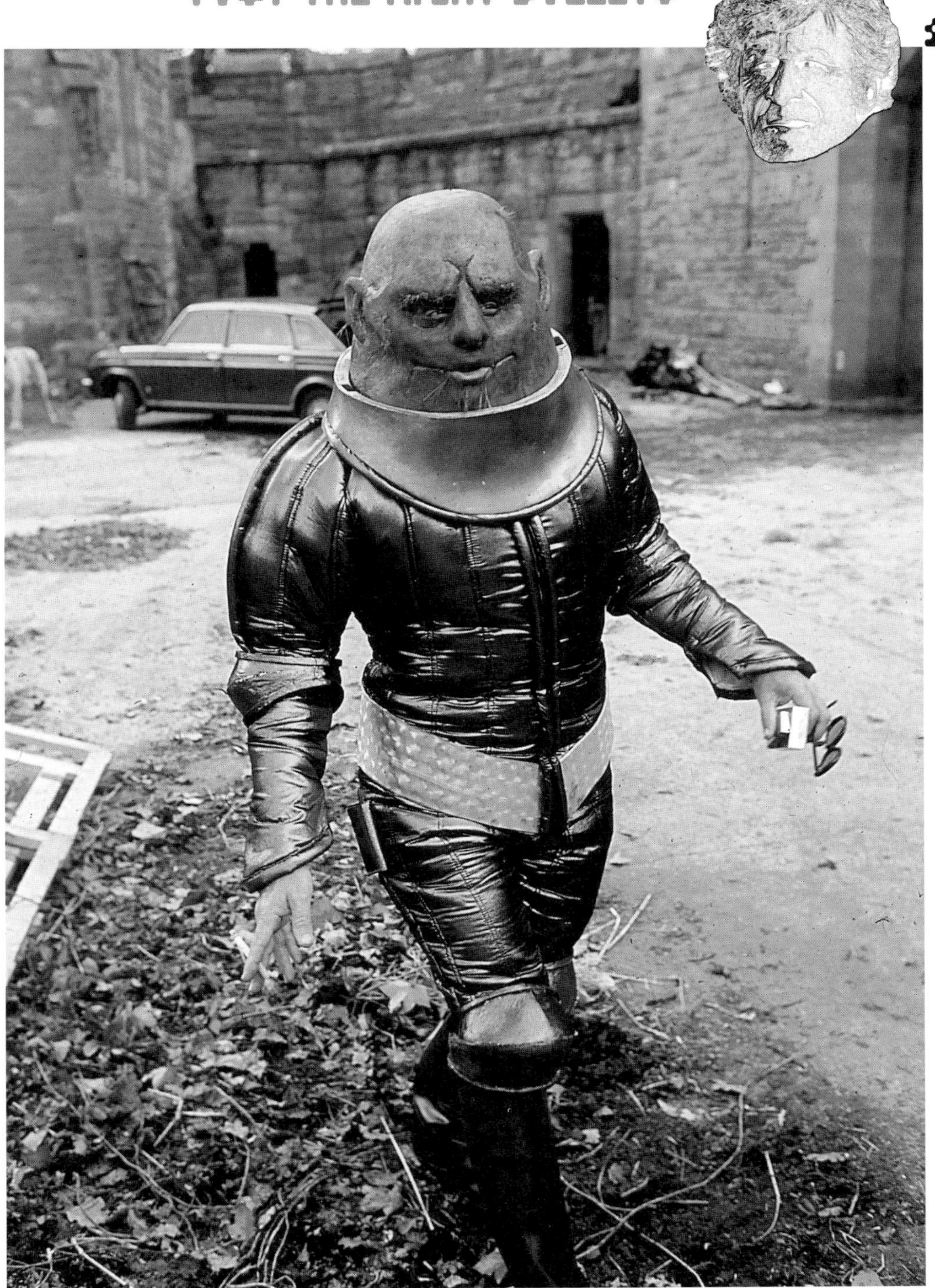

Linx taking a Sontavan fag break in **The Time Warrior**.

"We couldn't get hold of some real jets, so we had to use an old helicopter that the BBC had in Wales. It looked as though it could barely get off the ground. The bombs themselves were basically toilet ballcocks loaded with explosives – all we could find that looked vaguely bomblike. So, apart from having a battered 'copter dropping firebomb ballcocks, we had to create an army of maggots...

"These were inflated condoms, strategically placed around the slag heaps. After a while, the winds got up and they began to take off like balloons. The condoms had to be tied down because the slipstream off the helicopter also caused chaos with them. That was the scenario we had to work in, imagine how many straight faces were kept...

"The special effects people had spent so much time making puppet maggots with snapping teeth for the close up shots, that they had barely any money or time to make the giant fly we needed at the end. It wasn't exactly what you'd call convincing, and poor Jon had to drive through the freezing cold wind in the condom-infested quarry with this flapping bit of latex squirting green ink at his windscreen!"

Back in London for the last week of March to start rehearsals, the new companion was confirmed as being Elisabeth Sladen. Robert Holmes was working on the script to introduce the new character of Sarah-Jane Smith. This episode would go straight into production after *The Green Death*, and be held over as the first story for the eleventh season.

The first studio block for Manning's final story went into TC3 on 2 and 3 April. There was a certain 'tense' atmosphere through-

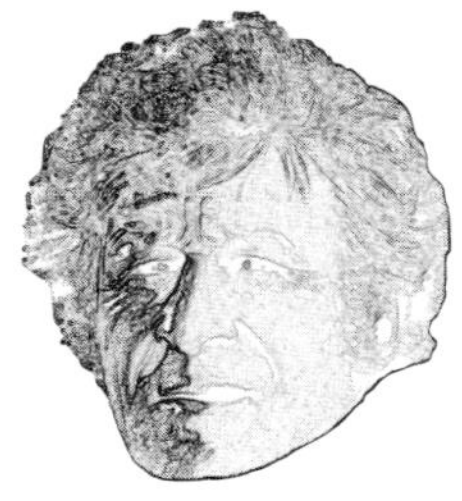

out the story due to the presence of Stewart Bevan. He had been cast as Professor Cliff Jones, who wins the heart of Jo Grant. Bevan was Manning's real-life boyfriend and there was a feeling from the other members of the regular cast that he was taking part of their 'family' away from them. Briant recalls the rehearsal rooms getting a bit 'edgy' at times.

Holmes had submitted a storyline to Terrance Dicks earlier in the year, with his tongue rooted firmly in cheek, about a battle report from a Sontaran Officer called Holmes, to his commander, Terran Cedicks. The production team had asked for a historically based story, which would be the first since *The Highlanders*, and Holmes put a twist on it by having a war-mongering alien land in mediaeval England. He won a commission and, working with Dicks, added the journalist-companion role for Sladen to the four part story which went from *The Time Soldier* to *The Warrior Of Time*, to the far more simple *The Time Warrior*.

Veteran director Alan Bromly, who had produced the anthology series *Out Of The Unknown* for its final two seasons, was hired to direct the story, with Keith Cheetham working as his designer. The main problem to begin with was to find a suitably battle-worn castle for the main bulk of the location filming. Work began with several days filming at Peckforton Castle, near Tarporley, in Cheshire.

Kevin Lindsay had been cast as Linx, the Sontaran warrior stranded on Earth. He had to cope with wearing a thick latex mask that totally encased his head, making breathing and vision difficult, especially when the character had to wear his helmet as well. His costume was heavily padded to give the look of the squat muscular build of the race, and as Lindsay was already suffering from a heart condition, the filming proved to be a considerable strain for the actor.

Robert Holmes:

"I wanted Linx to be incredibly pompous, a sort of a typical Colonel Blimp character, but totally alien at the same time. The Sontarans lived and breathed for war, spending every hour thinking about it, and every minute trying to instigate it.

"The twist was that he ended up in a society that was probably more blood-thirsty than his own and saw the chance to hone their fighting skills, and cheat a little as well, by giving them guns and weapons that were centuries ahead of their time. I toyed with the idea of having him occasionally filing reports into his computer, commenting on what he was doing. That could have been very funny with his observations on mankind, but it would have jarred the narrative continually, making it stop and start, so I never bothered with that."

As *The Green Death* was drawing towards the end of its run on television in mid-June, the cast and crew broke up for the summer. They were due to start work on the eleventh season's remaining stories from the beginning of September. Letts and Sloman were now planning to actually sit down and write the Master's final story, but a tragedy intervened within a week of finishing work on *The Time Warrior*.

Roger Delgado had been offered the type of comedy role that he longed for in a French-financed film to be shot that summer, called *Bell Of Tibet*. Delighted by the opportunity to change his villainous image, he left for the location work in Nevshir in Turkey, on 18 June. His plane was late arriving there and the driver who picked both Delgado and a pair of technicians up tried to make up lost time by speeding to the film set.

Travelling too fast, the car spun off a bend and plunged into a ravine. Delgado and one of the technicians were killed. He was fifty three years old. In the interview that was conducted with him during the making of *Frontier In Space*, he was asked to sum up the character of the Master as he saw it. His answer was simple, quoting a line from *Don Quixote*.

"He is the Master of everything, and the owner of nothing..."

Delgado's death traumatised the entire production team and cast on *Doctor Who*, and was partially behind Jon Pertwee's decision to leave the programme. With Katy Manning gone, Delgado's tragic death and with the UNIT stories he was so fond of becoming less and less frequent, Pertwee decided that it was time to move on. He asked Letts if he could leave at the end of season eleven.

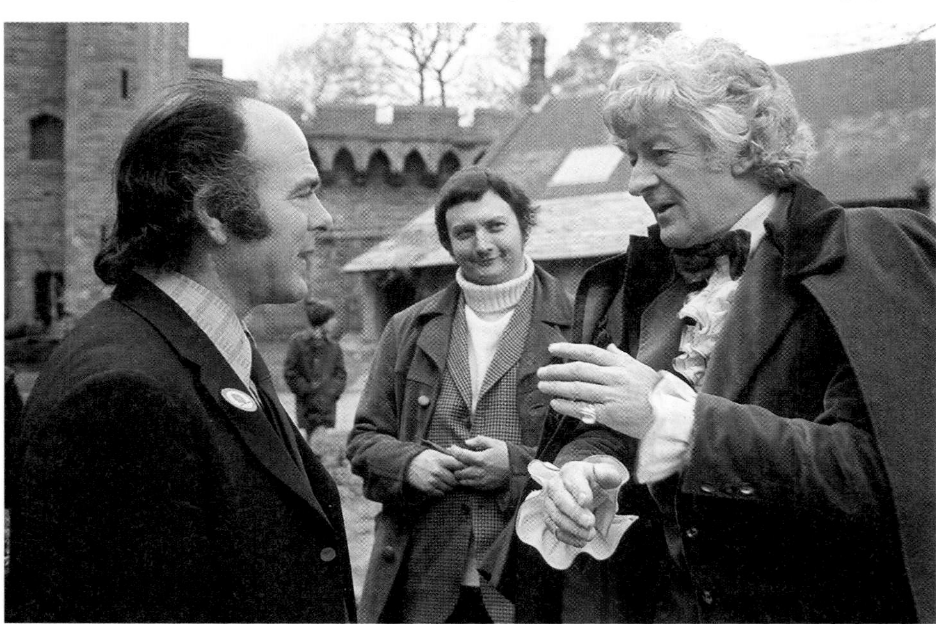

John Pertwee, Terrance Dicks (Script Editor) and Barry Letts (Producer) on location with **The Time Warrior**.

The timing was not good, as the amount of work this would entail (such as casting the new Doctor) would need to be planned out throughout the Summer break and both Letts and Dicks were committed to another series for that period. Both men had wanted to leave after their third year with *Doctor Who*, but were persuaded to stay by their head of department. Anxious to explore a more realistic avenue of science fiction, they put forward a proposal for a series called *Moonbase Three*, which was accepted and the six episodes were to be shot before work started on *Doctor Who* again at the end of August.

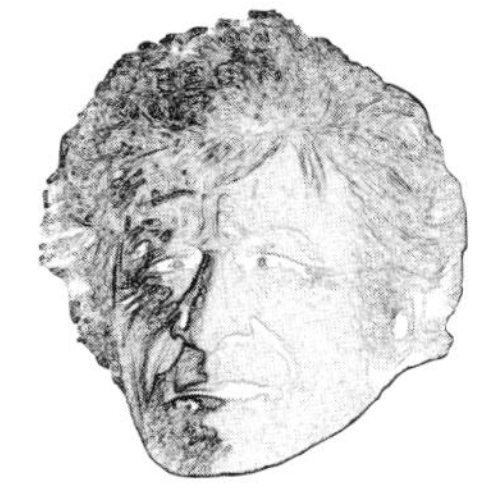

Many *Who* regulars were drafted in to help with the workload that summer, including Dudley Simpson to handle the music, Roger Liminton as the designer and Christopher Barry as one of the two directors. John Lucarotti, who had not worked on *Doctor Who* since the Hartnell era, wrote two episodes and in doing so, re-established a working relationship with the production team. This lead him to submitting a storyline for the twelfth season.

For the final four stories that were needed to complete season eleven, Dicks had commissioned writers whom he knew he could rely on to get on with the work while *Moonbase Three* went before the cameras; Terry Nation had a Dalek story, *The Exxilons*, and Brian Hayles was drafting a sequel to *The Curse Of Peladon* (which he remembered as having a working title of *The Betrayal*). Robert Sloman was hired to work on the finale for the season, which would be the last adventure for the third Doctor.

While The *Time Warrior* was still recording, *Operation Golden Age*, by Malcolm Hulke, was being completed and Letts approached a director who had not been on the programme since William Hartnell's days.

Letts:

"I went to Paddy Russell to ask her if she would like to come and do a *Doctor Who*, and she said, 'As long as I don't have to Direct any tin cans!!'"

She was given Hulke's script, now called *Invasion Of The Dinosaurs*, with a promise that there were no Daleks in sight.

Hulke:

"Barry wanted to do a dinosaur story, as the model stuff on a show he'd done (*Carnival Of Monsters*) had convinced him it was possible. It was actually Terrance Dicks who came up with the idea of putting them in the streets of modern London and that triggered off the idea of having a group of scientists trying to alter the course of mankind's development."

To accomplish the extensive location work that Hulke's scripts called for, Russell had to plan out her shooting schedule like a military campaign. Some of the first shots to be done were actually carried out while *The Time Warrior* was still in production with the director and a cameraman completing several establishing shots of the deserted city for the first episode in mid-June.

The next batch of shots were filmed on 2 September, still some time before the main bulk of location work would be executed. The crew moved from Whitehall to Billingsgate, Trafalgar Square and Westminster Bridge. This was when 'The Alien', or the 'Whomobile' as it was later named, made its first appearance before the cameras.

A suggestion was made for the Doctor to have some form of futuristic vehicle that could be used in the earth-based stories as an alternative to Bessie, which had been in use since season seven. Letts was reluctant to carve any money from his production budget for this, so Pertwee himself invested in having such a car built. The result looked like a futuristic hovercraft and was designed within the restrictions imposed on the dimensions of cars on the road, so that it could be driven through the streets legally. The prop was not quite finished in time for the filming but for its second and final appearance, in *Planet Of The Spiders*, it had been completed.

Seven further days of filming came three weeks later. The exteriors of UNIT's makeshift headquarters were shot around the base of the Central Electricity Board in Ealing. Other sites included Smithfield Market, Southall Gas Works, Covent Garden, Kingston Meat Market, a Pickford's Warehouse in Ealing again, Wimbledon Common and the entrance to Moorgate Underground Station. The crew faced the same problem there that Douglas Camfield had done on *The Web Of Fear*, with costs proving too high to actually be able to film inside. Designer Richard Morris had to recreate the platform of the station in studio.

Between the location filming and studio work, the model work that was needed to bring the Dinosaurs to life was shot. Hulke had included five main types in the script; a T-Rex, a brontosaurus, a tricerotops (for the Underground sequence), a stegosaurus and a pterodactyl, which was the only one used on location, as a rod and glove puppet.

Barry Letts:

"*Invasion Of The Dinosaurs* should have been the *Jurassic Park* of its day and it could have been a lot better. It was going to be done the same way as we'd done the Drashigs, with CSO, model work, the whole business... "

There were two main problems. Firstly, it hadn't been taken into consideration how difficult it would be to match the location shots with the model work in studio to and the finished scenes looked as though the Dinosaurs were 'floating' against the backgrounds. The other problem was that none of the main BBC visual effects designers were available, including John Horton, whom Letts had specifically asked for because of his work on the Drashigs, so the job had to be farmed out to an independent company.

Letts:

"What they did was to make the creatures with a very limited movement range. They were just built around bent wires. It looked very primitive and very bad. I was very angry about it."

Hulke:

"After *Dinosaurs*, I remember someone asked me how I could tell my *Who* stories apart as I'd done so many of them, and after a moment's thought, I said, 'You can colour code them by the shades of Jon Pertwee's jackets. Black for the early stuff, green for the middle, and a definitive purple at the end'."

An Axon is helped into his costume.

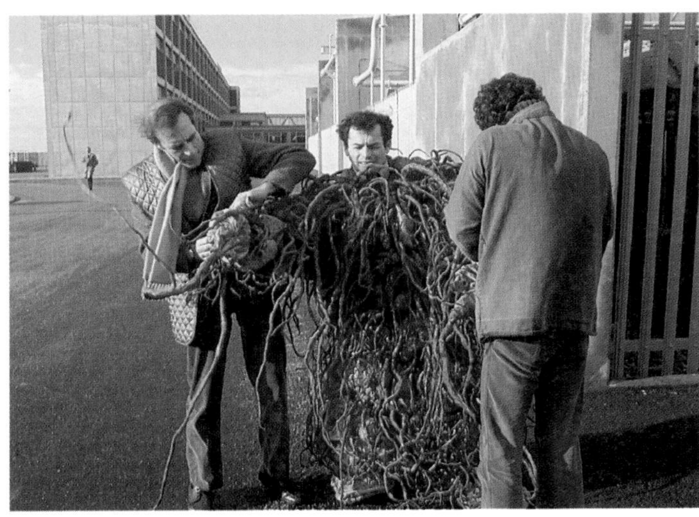

Pertwee's costume did change quite frequently. He had originally started out with a sombre black outfit and cape for the seventh season, and thereafter developed a taste for a variety of velvet smoking jackets. They became his Doctor's trade mark, along with the sonic screwdriver, a device that was suggested as an idea by Michael E Briant's idea when *Fury From The Deep* was being made.

Briant:

"I think the greatest disservice I ever did to *Doctor Who* was to come up with that screwdriver. Hugh David went for it when I suggested it to him and by the time I was actually directing episodes, every time I came back there was some point in the story where the Doctor got out of deadly peril by playing around with his sonic screwdriver. I felt it was a bit of an easy way out."

Briant was now back with the production team, scouting for locations for *The Exxilons*, which was retitled as *Death To The Daleks*. With the pressure now on to get material 'in the can' before the Christmas break, production began to overlap.

Invasion Of The Dinosaurs was completed in studio on 12 and 13 November with episodes five and six in TC3, while location work had already started on *Death To The Daleks*. Briant, working with Colin Green as his designer, had started to film sequences on the 13th at a quarry near Gallows Hill in Dorset, using the guest cast members for sequences that did not require Pertwee or Sladen.

The Daleks were now in quite a poor state and Briant used a mixture of the survivors from the 1960s and the ones that were built for *Planet of The Daleks*. He was not keen on the colour scheme and asked for them to be repainted using the silver markings he remembered from working on *Power Of The Daleks* and The Daleks' Master Plan in the mid-60s.

John Friedlander was brought in to create masks for the Exxilons, using a general sculpted one for the extras and a more detailed version, which involved taking head-casts of the actors, for the ones with dialogue, such as Bellal.

Briant:

"I wanted the Exxilons to have a strange, eerie pulsating glow on their skin, so we covered the costumes with strips of scotchlite tape. This was being used for roadmarkings at the time, and when you used certain types of lighting, although you couldn't see it with the naked eye, on screen it looked rather good."

One of the problems that Briant had to overcome on location, was how to get the Daleks to move successfully across the sand in the quarry.

Briant:

"There was this stuff called 'Elmac Track' that the cameras ran across to get a smooth image. Unfortunately, nobody realised how fast the Daleks would be able to go once they were mounted on it. We had a shot where they were meant to be coming down a slope, and once they were given a shove, the effect was lethal. They must have gone at nearly one hundred miles an hour, and all you could hear was the little voices inside going, 'Help! Help me!' We nearly died laughing."

After final studio sessions on 17 and 18 December, Pertwee and Sladen took their Christmas break. Brian Hayles' scripts for the new six-part Peladon story, now called *The Monster Of Peladon*, were ready for their return at the end of December when extensive work at Ealing was carried out for many of the scenes set in the mines of the planet.

Hayles:

"It was at the time of the great strikes and I wanted to draw attention to the way the Miners were being treated by the authorities. That's why there's a subplot in the second Peladon story."

To maintain a sense of continuity on screen as well as off, many of the same cast and crew from the first story were rehired; Lennie Mayne as the director, Gloria Clayton as his designer, Nick Hobbs donned the Aggedor costume again and Stuart Fell and Ysanne Churchman joined forces to bring Alpha Centuri back to life, complete with a new darker green colour scheme for the head.

The Ice Warriors were out in force four being needed in total, including an Ice Lord. Both Alan Bennion and Sonny Caldinez reprised their roles in rank, but as different characters, while the other two warriors were put together from the costumes that were still intact from *The Ice Warriors* in 1967. One of the heads is noticeably a different size from the others, denoting that it was Varga's, as worn by Bernard Bresslaw in the first story.

As studio rehearsals began, Letts was busy seeking out a new actor for the title role in the series, while Dicks was working closely with Robert Sloman on the final rewrites of *Planet Of The Spiders*, which Letts had chosen to direct to bring both the season, and the Pertwee era to a close. One final story would be made by the producer/script editor team before they left the programme as well, with production overlapping on *Planet Of The Spiders* for the first story to feature the fourth Doctor.

As *The Monster Of Peladon* went into TC8 for episode one on 28 January, *Invasion Of The Dinosaurs* was well underway on television, enjoying some of the highest viewing figures for the past few years. Both episode one and three were seen by eleven million viewers.

Hayles:

"I noticed that quite a bit had been done to try and make Alpha Centuri look, shall we say, less suggestive. I think the cloak was a bit fuller, because whenever it swept down a corridor with burning flambards along the walls, it looked as though aliens had invaded a Jane Austen novel."

Episodes three and four were completed in TC6, on 11 and 12 February. Hayles never wrote for the series again, although he did novelise some of his own scripts. Things were about to change radically with the presentation of *Doctor Who*, as a new producer, Philip Hinchcliffe, was waiting in the wings and Robert Holmes was now trailing Dicks to take over as the script editor.

Hayles:

"I had one or two ideas to do a third and final Peladon story, as the idea of introducing an entire civilisation and following it through several centuries of development fascinated me. The idea behind it would have rounded the whole thing off as a trilogy and the Ice Warriors would have been there again with Alpha Centuri.

"The idea was to have a threat to the planet in the shape of an unseen invasion force and the various alien factions of the Galactic Federation would have been trying to win the approval of the King, Queen, or whoever, to defend it on their behalf. The Doctor would have arrived and realised that the threat was probably within the group trying to defend it Perhaps someone, someday will take up the story where I left it, and finish it off properly."

The main bulk of the location work for *Planet Of The Spiders* was carried out in the second week of March. Letts wanted something spectacular that would call on all the main stuntmen who had worked on the Pertwee stories, and give them their own small scenes as a kind of 'thank you' to them. So, sequences were staged for Stuart Fell as a tramp, whom the Doctor drives over in a hovercraft, Terry Walsh was seen mooring a boat and everyone had their fifteen seconds of fame.

The unit moved from Hopton Army Barracks in Wiltshire, where the UNIT Headquarters scenes were filmed, to Membury Airfield where a one-seater alto-gyro (a miniature helicopter) was used. It was pursued by the 'Whomobile', which was seen to take off thanks to CSO matting. Bessie was also present on location, so both of the third Doctor's cars were used together for the first and only time.

A boat chase was shot around the River Severn and the meditation centre exteriors were filmed in Staines, in Surrey. Letts returned to take his cast into rehearsal at the end of March. All of the scenes that required the UNIT regulars, such as Nicholas Courtney and John Levene were done over this block, to allow them to start rehearsing for the debut of the fourth Doctor. This would start its location work while the final scenes of *Planet Of The Spiders* were still in studio. Terrance Dicks had completed the script for the next story and Christopher Barry was waiting to start work with the actors. As the episodes being shot out of sequence, the regeneration scene between the third and fourth Doctors was staged over these first two days.

The second studio block dealt with all the meditation centre scenes for the story, and saw the last work on the show as a regular character by Richard Franklin, who was also moving on after the end of the season. All the scenes on Metabilis Three came next, which was itself a bit on an in-joke. Whenever the Doctor tried to take one of his companions on holiday in the Tardis, it would be to see the wonders of Metabilis Three, but the journey always deviated in some way. He eventually got there only to find that it had turned into an incredibly hostile environment (*The Green Death*) and now it was to lead him to his death confronting the giant spiders that ruled the planet.

One commentator in the press mourned the passing of the third Doctor as the final episode of *Planet Of The Spiders* was transmitted on 8 June.

"With Jon Pertwee's departure from *Doctor Who*, we have lost the third Time Lord in a row of what has become a national institution and treasure. William Hartnell was popular, as was Patrick Troughton, but I feel that Pertwee has surely secured its future, presenting a character that can be accepted by both young and old alike.

"It is a hard act to follow, and although Tom Baker looked secure enough when he was presented to the press a few months ago as the fourth actor to take on the part, it must surely be an intimidating track record he has to overcome. Pertwee has always expressed a concern that *Doctor Who* should never be seen using a gun, or threatening anybody with one. If that was the case, his Doctor still held just the right bullets to win through."

Not only was the longest serving actor to play the part about to make his debut, he would also see the programme soar to the highest ratings peak in its history. He would appear in stories that were far darker in tone than anything that had been shown before. Tom Baker formally took over as *Doctor Who* on 16 February, 1974, when he faced the press for the first of many occasions.

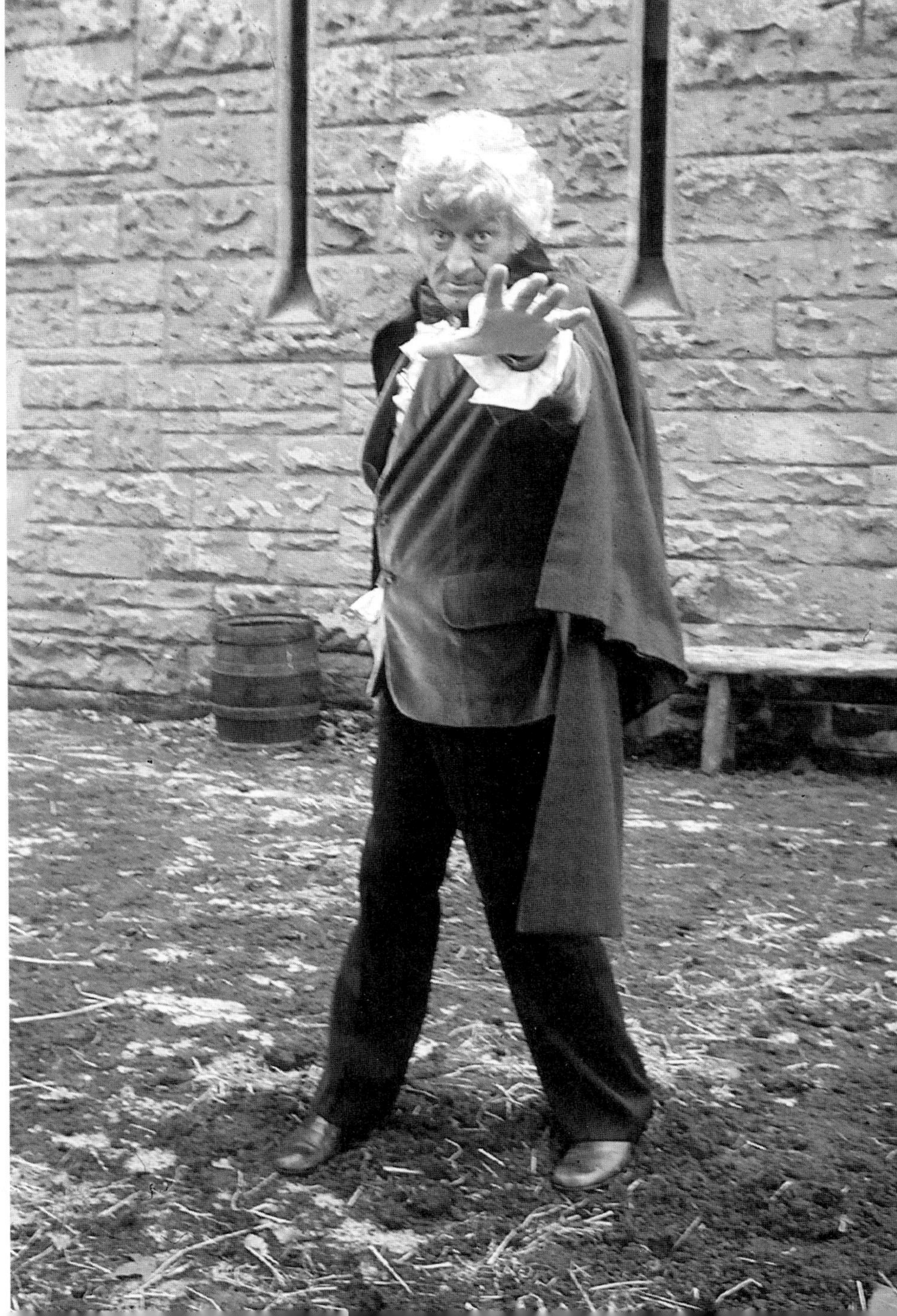

Chapter

The Vortex of Immensity

THE VORTEX OF IMMENSITY

THE VORTEX OF IMMENSITY

"I met Tom in the BBC canteen just before I took over, but I couldn't hear a word he said to me. *Top Of The Pops* was being recorded while we were trying to talk! It was really a bit daunting, I mean, there was a whole generation out there who had grown up with him as 'their' Doctor..."

PETER DAVISON Unpublished interview – November 1982

"Tom was like a blast of wildly eccentric energy when you first met him. Pat Troughton always used to say that an actor playing *Doctor Who* had to be more eccentric than an eccentric, and Tom certainly managed to fit that bill with honours. I couldn't quite believe it when somebody told me he used to be a Monk," recalled Robert Holmes. "I cornered him and said, 'Why did you leave the order then, Tom?' and he gave me one of those boggle-eyed stares of his and said, 'I was in a continual state of priapic euphoria and if I didn't get out when I did, I would have spent the rest of my life with a considerable stoop!' Then he stalked off. You had to take Tom on a day to day basis."

The quest to find the fourth Doctor had taken a long time and in the process, Barry Letts had seen a wide range of very well known faces.

Letts:

"I was getting in touch with people and not saying, 'Would you like to be *Doctor Who*?' but, 'Would you like to come and discuss the possibility of being *Doctor Who*?'

"Graham Crowden, for example, came along and said, 'I love the idea of being *Doctor Who*, but I don't think I could commit myself to three years at it (I felt they ought to do it for at least that length of time) because at the end of the first year, if I was offered a wonderful part at the National Theatre, I'd want to go and play it. I wouldn't want to stay.'

"Michael Bentine felt that he wanted to be involved with the scripts. He said, 'I've never done anything where I wasn't involved in that area!' We had to say to him, 'Look, in the first place, we wouldn't want to give up our control of the scripts, and secondly, you just would not have the time."

Richard Hearne was also approached. He'd enjoyed huge popularity in the 1950s and 1960s with his character, Mr Pastry, and children adored him.

Letts:

"Richard was terribly sweet but I just hadn't realised how old he'd got (he was 65), and he really couldn't understand what I was saying. I told him I wanted to discuss the possibility of him playing the Doctor and he said, 'Well, I'm very flattered that you should ask as I've always liked the programme but I don't really think that Pastry is right for the Doctor.' And I said, 'It's not him we're asking for as the Doctor, it's you.' He said, 'Yes, yes. I understand that, but Pastry's always been a comic character,' and he could not get it out of his head that what we were asking him to do was repeat his Pastry performance as the Doctor."

The popular *Carry On* star, Jim Dale, was also under consideration by Letts along with Fulton McKay, when another name was added to the list by the head of Letts' department, Bill Slater.

Letts:

"While all this was going on, Bill said to me at one of our everyday meetings, 'How are you getting on?' And I told him, and he said, 'Have you ever thought of Tom Baker?' I said I'd never even heard of him.

"Bill said, 'He played the doctor for me, in *The Millionairess*, when I directed it for *Play Of The Month* for BBC2. He gave a marvellous performance, he really is an excellent actor. He was the chap who played Rasputin in *Nicholas And Alexandra* (made in 1971).'

"I'd never seen that, so Bill asked whether I'd like to meet him. We got on like a house on fire and I thought he was ideal for it. He was very much a personality and a great eccentric in his own right. I told him I thought he would make a marvellous Doctor Who, but I didn't even know if he could act, because I'd never seen him in anything.

"Tom said, 'Well, as it happens, I'm appearing at this very moment at a Cinema in Victoria in *The Golden Voyage Of Sinbad*, playing the villain.' I thought right, we'll go and see this, and I went back to the office and said, 'Come on, Terrance. Drop whatever you're doing, we're going to the pictures!' We went and saw it and when it was over I went straight back to the office and rang Tom and said, 'Would you like to be the Doctor, because I think you're just right for the part?'"

Tom Baker was put under contract and faced the press for the first time on 16 February, accompanied by Elisabeth Sladen and long-standing *Doctor Who*-extra Pat Gorman who donned an *Invasion* Cyberman costume for the occasion.

Robert Holmes:

"One or two of the reporters thought that we'd hired Harpo Marx because Tom had this manic grin and a mop of brown curly hair. There were one or two ideas to make him up with a white shock wig like Albert Einstein, or give him a

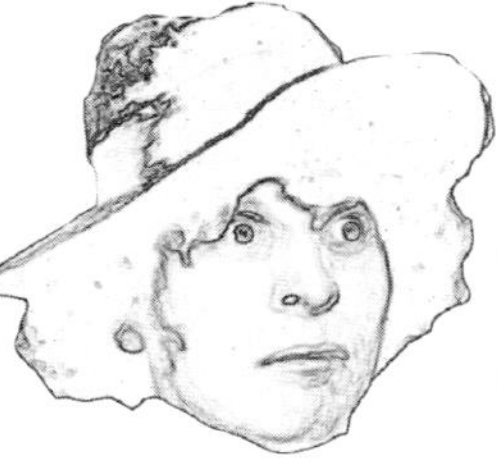

deer-stalker and turn him into Sherlock Holmes (which Holmes would actually do much later on in *The Talons Of Weng Chiang*), but I think it was Barry who said, 'No. Just leave him as he is.'

"I think Tom had an idea about making him look like one of those bohemian artists that worked in Paris in the 1920s who spent their evenings sketching at the Moulin Rouge. Jim Acheson (the costume designer who took care of the 'look' for the fourth Doctor), must have latched on to that line of thought because that was the kind of image that was eventually achieved."

To complement the wide-brimmed brown felt hat and red corduroy jacket, the outfit was completed with a scarf. Tom Baker takes up the story:

"Jim Acheson wanted a colourful scarf and purchased a sufficient quantity of different shades of wool to bring one to life. The problem was that the task of actually making it fell to one Begoria Pope, who was over the moon to be working on *Doctor Who* and just got on with it without asking a single question. Jim had bought far too much wool and she used every last thread of it because he'd failed to say what kind of length he wanted. When it came and I tried it on, I nearly drowned in the wool! It was hysterical; it seemed to go on for miles! We decided to keep it because it was so funny."

Letts had introduced a new character to act as a second companion for the Doctor. It was uncertain how 'strong' a character or what age the Doctor would be before Baker was cast, so a younger, stronger man was brought in as back-up. Surgeon Lieutenant Harry Sullivan was played by Ian Marter, whom Letts had remembered auditioning for the part of Captain Yates in 1970 and from his work in *Carnival Of Monsters*. The name of the character was mentioned as being the UNIT medical Officer in *Planet Of The Spiders* and his first appearance came in *Robot*. Terrance Dicks had completed writing the story, with Robert Holmes now script editing, by April 1974.

Holmes:

"I wanted a strong visual element for the first story. We couldn't use the Daleks or Cybermen because stories had already been commissioned featuring them later on in the run. We came up with the idea of a sort of *King Kong* story, where Sarah Jane would develop an empathy with a giant robot. The problem was that if you want a giant robot, you have to make a giant robot. That's easy enough, but then you had to get it to move."

Having already had experience seeing in a 'new' Doctor with Patrick Troughton's debut, Christopher Barry was brought in as *Robot's* director to see Tom Baker through his first adventure. Philip Hinchcliffe was now trailing Letts for his final story as producer and the main production team included Ian Rawnsley as Barry's designer.

The cast and crew departed for location recording for five days from 28 April to 1 May. All exterior sequences were now being shot on video to make it easier to integrate video effects with the footage. The vast majority of the five days was spent in and around the BBC Training Centre at Wood Norton which was also the site of the first scenes to be shot for Jon Pertwee's debut in *Spearhead From Space*.

The KI Robot costume was built by an independent firm of contractors and Michael Kilgarriff was hired to play the creature due to his height (6ft 7"). Kilgarriff had already played monsters in previous stories including the Cyber Controller in *Tomb Of The Cybermen* and an Ogron in *Frontier In Space*, but working as the Robot proved to be a nightmare.

Kilgarriff:

"My costume was so incredibly heavy and claustrophobic, I could hardly move. I kept keeling over or just falling to my knees when we were on location. It was horrific. I was waking up in the middle of the night with the most horrific nightmares about getting trapped in that damned suit. I went to Christopher Barry and told him that I couldn't go on like that and wear it through all the rehearsals in the studio. He came up with a lightweight version, which was just the head and shoulders, the feet and the claws, and I only had to put the full whack on at the last minute. I don't know how I got through it."

Following two weeks of rehearsals, the initial recording block was hit by a BBC strike in progress at TV Centre on 21 May 21st. The scene shifters were refusing to dismantle the sets and an episode of the children's magazine programme *Blue Peter*, which was then being presented by ex-companion Peter Purves, had to use TC3 with a *Doctor Who* laboratory set still left up from that day.

The studio material was remounted across 1 and 2 June 1st when all the UNIT lab scenes were completed using the same basic set as in *Planet Of The Spiders*. The completion of ROBOT marked the end of the year's recording. Terrance Dicks had now moved on and Barry Letts stayed for a few months in an advisory capacity. During the summer break, Tom Baker made the first of many publicity appearances, some accompanied by Marter and Sladen, to heighten public awareness of the fact that a new Doctor would be in residence on the programme's return. *Robot* was scheduled to start transmission from 28 December that year.

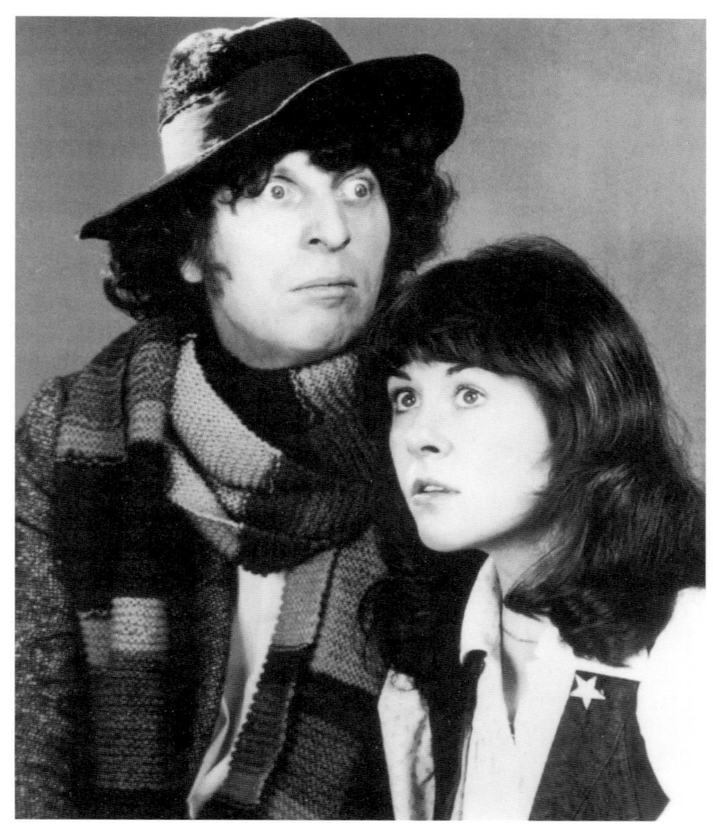

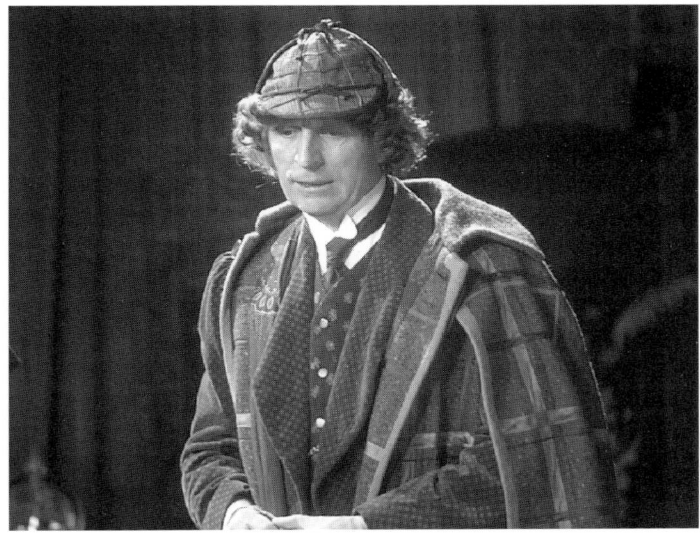

Holmes:

"With *Robot*, Tom had effectively lined up a series of fireworks showing us what he could do and it was just a case of figuring out which blue touchpaper to light for each story. You never knew what he would do with a script as he was a great believer in adding his own ideas... which five times out of ten you actually used... but it always seemed to come together in rehearsals, and nearly always at the last minute. There was this wild energy about him and he used to go off like a rocket in the studio. Some directors actually found the thought of working on the series quite intimidating because they were used to actors saying, 'Yes, certainly, Mr Director. I'll do it like that. All too happy to oblige.' Tom just wasn't like that at all."

Tom Baker:

"One always gets asked about the methods and the train of thought that lies behind a performance but I honestly didn't know how I was going to play it when I first started on *Doctor Who*. I just tried to anticipate how he would react as we went along and I suppose you could say it was a happy accident when we found out it was working!"

For the Pertwee era, the main bulk of the story output had consisted of six-part stories, which was a format on which Holmes was not particularly keen as he felt they always tended to 'sag' in the middle episodes. He and Hinchcliffe decided to try a cost cutting experiment for the rest of season twelve.

The plan was to keep the same director and crew for the normal period it would take to make a six-parter which would entail a week of location work followed by the studio sessions. By using the location week to make a two-part story needing no studio material, the time that would normally have been spent in TV Centre could be used to make an entirely separate four-parter. There would effectively be two stories for the price of one.

To cut back on costs, a decision was made to reuse the sets of the four-parter in some way and it was Holmes who came up with the idea of using a space station in the first story which would reappear in the second, suitably redressed, at a distant point in its future. Holmes drafted out a plan as follows:

"We planned it so that the studio-bound four parter on the space station would come first, followed by the two-parter entirely on location with the Doctor and his companions being sent off from the station to do something. As they try to get back there, they get diverted into another six-parter, before finally getting back for another four-parter which would reuse the space station sets."

The three stories Dicks had commissioned were worked into this scenario; John Lucarotti was drafting up *The Ark In Space*, Terry Nation had a six part Dalek story called *The Genesis Of Terror* and Gerry Davis had started work on *The Return Of The Cybermen*. There were, however, problems with the first of these stories.

Holmes:

"John's scripts were proving to be very '1960s' as they started to come in (Lucarotti was still living in Majorca) and they were a bit strange, with slightly archaic dialogue that just wasn't Tom. He had these headless creatures (the Gelf) playing golf with their limbs and using their heads as the golf balls! The special effects team would have had a field day on that one but it was dangerous ground. It was one of those scripts that could have turned out to be hysterical if the visuals weren't convincing."

Holmes also claimed that the original version of the script was meant to be six episodes long and that the location filming would have required forests and stretches of wilderness for the interior jungles of the Ark. Whatever the case, he set about totally rewriting Lucarotti's scripts (keeping the setting of the Ark), and approached Bob Baker and Dave Martin to handle the two-part story, as he had no time to write it himself.

As rewrites on *The Ark In Space* finished, with Holmes taking the on-screen credit as writer, he turned his attention to *The Return Of The Cybermen*, which would be shot back to back with *The Ark In Space*, using the space station sets.

Holmes:

"Gerry was writing a Cyberman story as they'd always been done. It was as though there was a formula that he knew worked well and he couldn't bring himself to break it. I started to tinker with it as soon as I'd finished on *The Ark In Space*, and I heard later on that Gerry thought I'd made the Cybermen slightly farcical

The Doctor meets Harry Sullivan and the Brigadier in **Robot**.

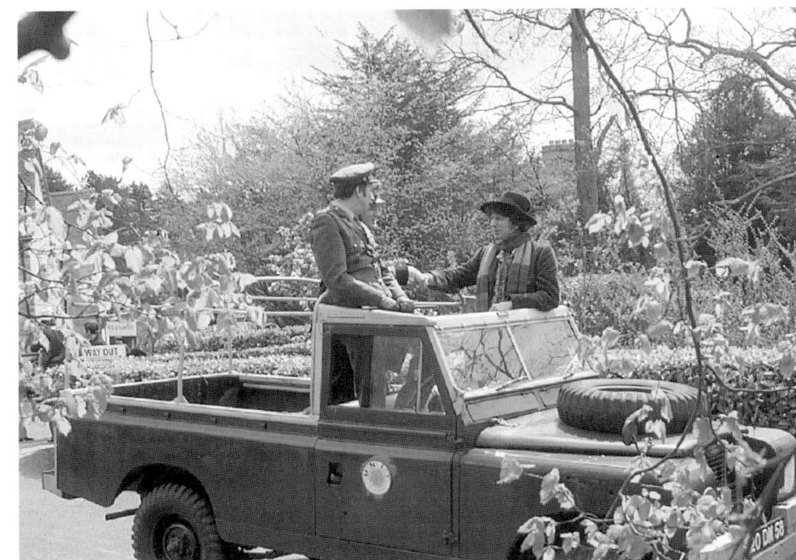

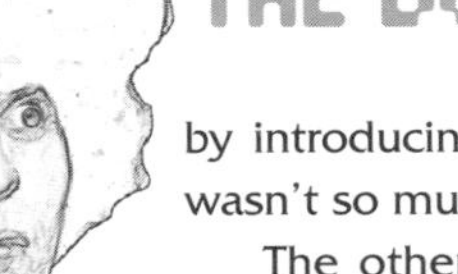

by introducing their gold dust allergy. It wasn't so much farcical, as fallible."

The other story, which would come between *The Destructors* and *The Return Of The Cybermen*, was Nation's Dalek saga. This was shot as the fourth story in production order in January 1975, so Holmes would not have to start editing work on it until December.

Harry and the Doctor wondering how to deal with a dead Wirrn in **The Ark In Space**.

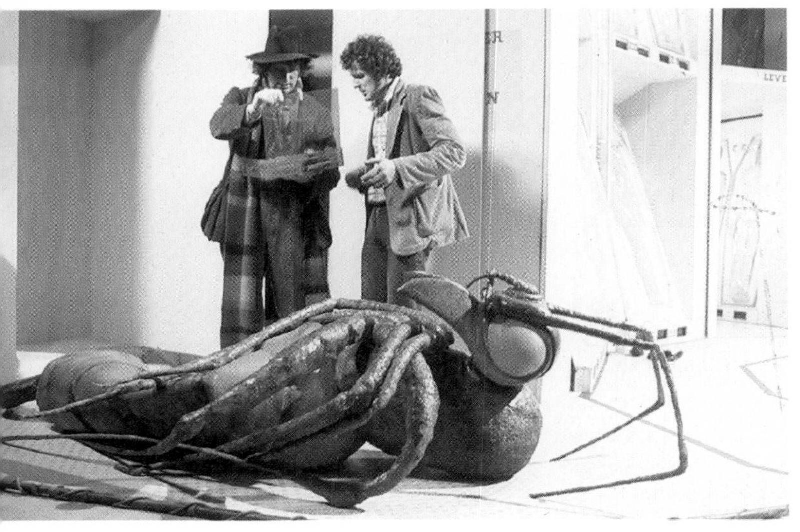

Hinchcliffe hired Rodney Bennett to direct the block of six episodes that would encompass *Ark* and Baker and Martin's script, which was now called *The Sontaran Experiment*. The two-parter called for a location that could represent the solar-flare decimated Earth landscape and Bennett opted for the heather-strewn wilderness of Dartmoor. Developments in video technology now meant that outside broadcast equipment could be easily used in such places, whereas before only film cameras could be.

When it came to casting the Sontaran, having viewed *The Time Warrior*, Bennett brought back Kevin Lindsay to play the role. John Friedlander redesigned the mask slightly so that the problems Lindsay had experienced on the first story would not happen again. The make-up did not enclose the head so much and the mouth was wider, which made breathing easier. The heavy mask had been worn for much of the time in the first story but was only used for one brief scene this time, and the bifurcated three fingered gloves were replaced by gloves with five digits.

Filming went smoothly enough for the first three days but on 29 September, working on scenes where Sladen was held in a force-field dungeon surrounded by rocks, Tom Baker slipped and fell, breaking his collar bone.

Tom Baker:

"It was all wonderfully dramatic and I was carried across the moors on a stretcher. Terribly heroic, I thought, but I was deflated slightly on my arrival at the hospital when I was told that broken collar bones were as common muck when a rugby team was playing in town. When I arrived back at the hotel, I think you could have knocked Barry Letts and Philip Hinchcliffe over with a feather. They were sitting very quietly and solemnly at the bar, probably wondering about the future of the programme without their lead actor, when suddenly there he was, right by their side, offering to buy them a drink!"

Baker completed the filming for the final three days with his arm strapped up in a sling. Because he was unable to move very well, Terry Walsh doubled for him in all the subsequent shots where the Doctor was seen clambering across the rocks. Stuart Fell doubled for Lindsay for the fight between the Doctor and the Sontaran, Field-Major Styre, at the conclusion of the second episode.

The cast and crew returned to London and began rehearsing for *The Ark In Space* after 8 October.

Holmes:

"I went over to the natural sciences unit and asked what the nastiest type of insect was and they rattled off a list of spiders that could kill with a single bite, but I wanted something a bit more unnerving. One of the girls there mentioned this wasp from the middle east, which laid its eggs inside the body of a caterpillar so that its young had something to eat when they hatched.

"That's where the idea for the Wirrn came from, because I simply turned the whole notion around, and thought, 'What if there was a giant wasp, that could do the same type of thing to a human?' It was obvious that the human would have to be at its most helpless and that would be when they were asleep, or in cryogenic suspension. Story conferences on *Doctor Who* used to get a bit stomach churning at times."

The Ark In Space featured sets designed by Murray-Leach. The Nerva Beacon space station consisted of vast curved walls with viewing panels set in front of a backdrop which could had a space cyclorama across it.

Tom Baker:

"I remember the sets were beautifully designed so that there was a real feeling of outer space about them. Walking inside the chamber where the sleeping humans were being stored was like walking into a miniature cathedral; it was breathtaking."

Two types of the insect-like Wirrn were needed for the story and John Friedlander worked on both of them. The grubs were made out of a cocoon of blister pack sprayed with green paint and latex, while the fully-grown creatures were hooped tubes of material with a head mask and mandibles at the front which could be operated by the actor inside.

Michael E. Briant was brought back to direct the next story and David Spode worked on Murray-Leach's sets to make suitable alterations suggesting that time had elapsed on the space station since *The Ark In Space*. The title of Gerry Davis's script had been altered to *Revenge Of The Cybermen*, with extensive rewrites being carried out on the text by Holmes, who explains:

"I didn't exactly find the Cybermen to be convincing villains. They were expressionless tin soldiers, and there's not a lot you can do with a concept like that. So I brought in the whole subplot about them trying to destroy Voga (the planet of gold – the one substance that can kill them), and made them the very last batch of Cybermen still alive, travelling around in the last of their battered battleships.

"The other reason behind the whole Vogan subplot was that we had more money available for the story than we thought, and location shooting was suddenly a possibility. I drummed up some fight scenes in a cave and Mike Briant went down to Wookey Hole to shoot it."

The filming at Wookey Hole Caves, in Somerset, started in the third week of November, following a rehearsal period that began as *The Ark In Space* studio sessions finished. The location itself was reputed to be haunted and, as Briant explains, things were far from easy down there.

"Well, to start with, we had small boats on the river there, and they ran right into the rocks. Liz (Sladen) fell into the water and started to get dragged underneath, because there were incredibly strong currents there. Terry Walsh who was there for the stunt work, leapt in and saved her but was terribly ill for a while afterwards.

"One of the cameramen fell off a rock and broke his leg. It was terrible, and it was all because of the Witch of Wookey Hole. There's a rock formation there that looks rather like a witch's hat and we were warned not to make fun of it. All this happened about five minutes after a couple of the technicians had dressed it up with a broom and a cape! We'd obviously brought the curse to life..."

Apart from the Cybermen, which had new costumes built by an outside contractor, the Cybermats were also brought back. Briant used the same kind of puppetry technique with CSO that he'd employed on *The Green Death* to bring the giant maggots to life. The Vogans were created using head masks, once again designed by Friedlander, which left the chin and lips free to give the actors unrestricted mouth movement. The two studio recording sessions took place in TC3 back at TV Centre, where the corridors of the Nerva Beacon were once again erected for 2 and 3 December and the main studio cave interiors were used on 16 and 17 December. One line that should have been edited out by Robert Holmes before recording slipped through the net, as he explains:

"There was one howler in the Cyberman story, where Tom and Liz Sladen are tied up in the space station which the Cybermen had aimed to crash into a planet. They had to face each other and say something about heading for the biggest bang in history! God knows how they got through it."

The cast broke up for Christmas, while work began on Terry Nation's scripts, dealing with the creation of the Daleks. David Maloney was brought in to direct, having already worked with the problematical props on *Planet of The Daleks*, while Roger Murray-Leach stayed with the production team for one further story to handle the design work.

Holmes:

"Terry had come up with the notion that the whole regime behind the creation of the Daleks would be like Nazi Germany, which was picked up by the costume designer who came up with the Gestapo-like motif."

The creator of the Daleks was brought into this story as a crippled genetic scientist called Davros, who was given the wonderful design twist of having his wheelchair, or life support unit, look exactly like the lower half of a Dalek casing. Actor Michael Wisher had a head-cast taken by John Friedlander, who sculpted the intricate latex mask he would have to wear in front of the cameras. To get used to this during rehearsals, Wisher took an unusual step, as Tom Baker recalls:

"It was painfully funny during rehearsals with Mike Wisher, because he took to wearing a kilt and a paper bag over his head to get into the character. I'm afraid it reduced me to tears on several occasions."

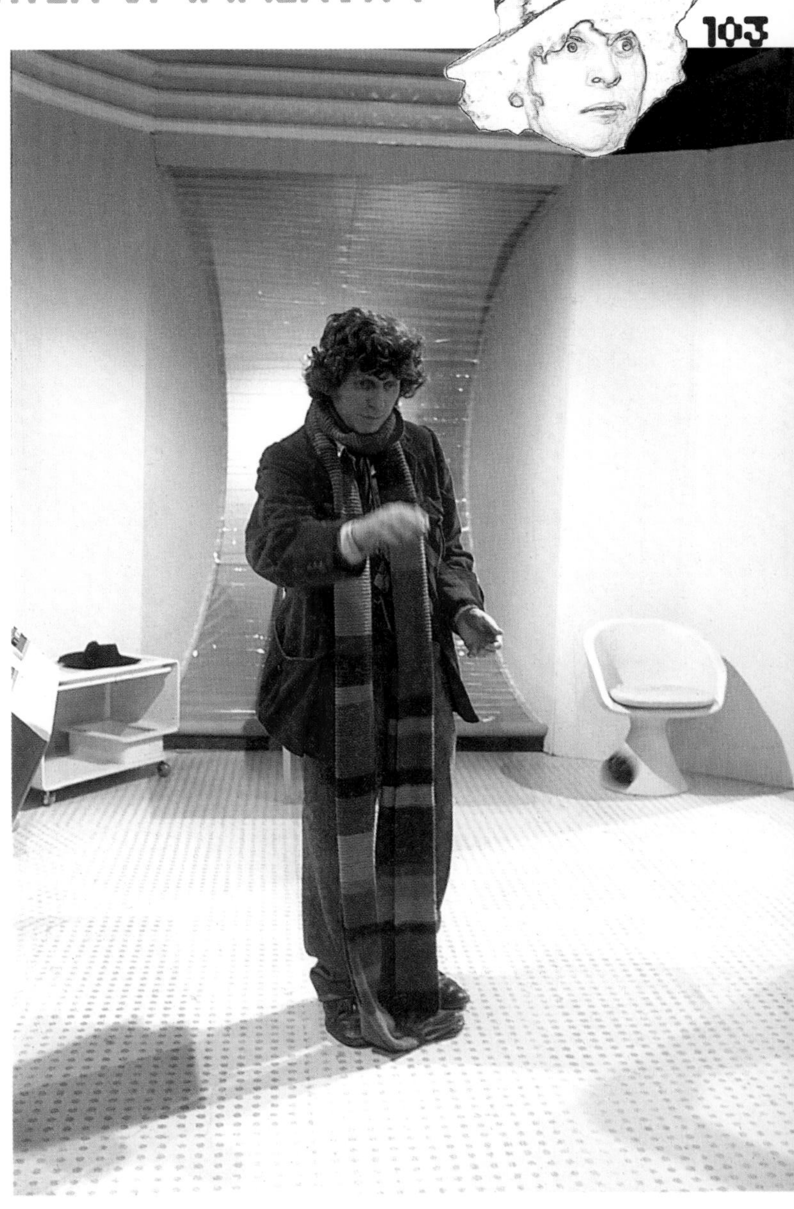

The Doctor demonstrates his prowess with a yo-yo aboard **The Ark In Space**.

The cast were brought back together as January started, to work on the scenes that were due to be shot on location. Remembering the quarry he'd used in *Planet Of The Daleks*, David Maloney elected to use it again and several days were spent at Fuller's Earth Works in Surrey.

Robot had started broadcasting and over ten million viewers tuned in for each of the first three episodes. The current story in production was now called *Genesis Of The Daleks* and studio work began with the bunker scenes where Davros's laboratory was concealed.

Holmes:

"There was a tried and trusted trick that had been used in the past, where the Doctor played a mental game with the villain of the piece, just to remove any doubts that the guy in question might have an ounce of sanity left. We tried to take this to an extreme between Davros and the Doctor, with Tom pushing to see if Davros would use genocide to become all powerful.

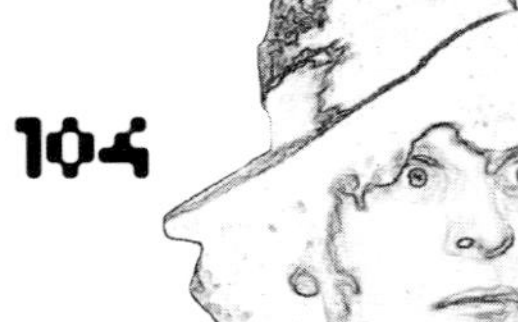

"On paper it worked fine and read well, but when Tom and Mike Wisher got hold of it and David Maloney staged it with nothing but tight close-ups, it became quite extraordinary. There was a real buzz on the set while we were making that one. It was almost as though people knew they were making something that was above average, which was odd for me as I'd fought quite strongly against doing it at all."

Since Jon Pertwee had made his debut, the series had traditionally kicked off as a major part of the New Year season on BBCI, the first story starting off in the last week of December or the first week of January. Now the programme planners wanted to move it to a September start date, which meant that the production team would have to continue beyond the planned six stories in the recording block of season twelve, to meet the demand for material that there would be at the end of the year.

One move that would give them a bit of headway would be to curtail the run of stories currently being broadcast, so the planned finale, which Robert Banks Stewart was working on under the title of *The Lock Ness Monster*, was pulled from following on from *Revenge Of The Cybermen* so that it could be used to start season thirteen come September. season twelve finished broadcasting with only twenty episodes having been screened.

Stewart's script entered production in February 1975. Douglas Camfield returned to the series as the story's director, with Nigel Curzon as his designer. The original plan had been for the serial to run for six episodes, but as it was being used to start the next run, Holmes cut it down to a four-part adventure instead.

Holmes:

"Dougie Camfield was a brilliant judge of scripts and he used to come in and work with me on the final edits on the story before they were dished out to the actors. I think that, with the exception of Michael Briant and David Maloney, he was the only Director we had who did that sort of thing."

The budget would not stretch to the cast and crew actually going up to Scotland to film around the real Loch Ness, so Camfield found an alternative in the shape of Bognor Regis and a small village near Chichester called Chorlton. Location work started in the third week of March and covered five days. The final day was spent at a quarry in Littlehampton where all the scenes involving the Zygon spaceship being destroyed were shot.

The Zygons themselves were the joint effort of John Friedlander and costume designer James Acheson. The basic notion was to make their shape similar to that of a human fetus, covered in symmetrical patterns of nodules based on the suction cups on an octopus's tentacle. The costumes came in two halves, the lower torso worn as trousers supported by heavy braces while the chest and head came in one piece that had to be pulled over the actor like a jumper.

Three such suits were made but only the lead creature, Broton (played by John Woodnutt) required a microphone to be hidden in the heavily padded costume as the dialogue of the other two creatures was prerecorded by the actors.

Several days were spent at Ealing filming the extensive model work of oil rigs being destroyed and the Loch Ness monster itself, the Skarasen, which was brought to life with the rare use of stop-motion animation.

Douglas Camfield:

"We had hellish problems with the Loch Ness monster because we'd run out of money, and there was still this last shot to do of it rising out of the Thames. There was only one way to do it in the time we had and that was as a glove puppet... which is exactly what it looked like on screen.

"One moment it was a carefully animated model, then it was something like Sooty, so it was a mixed show as far as the monsters are concerned, although the Zygons were marvellous."

As with any season, several scripts that were initially commissioned fell through during the development period, but one that is of interest from that year saw the brief return to the show of Dennis Spooner, who was working from his plotline called *Nightmare Planet*.

Spooner:

"I had this notion of a world where the masses were kept under control with a continuous supply of drugs in the food and water, which they didn't know about. Whenever somebody does something wrong, the drug is stopped and they see these awful monsters and horrific images all around them, and die of fright. Bob (Holmes) got a bit worried by the implications of the drug taking. The idea went pear-shaped and fell through."

Holmes was having to commission scripts rapidly as the shooting period on the programme was now going to continue until the end of the year, with only a few weeks off in September for the cast. Technically, the separate production blocks of season twelve and thirteen had been merged together. Terry Nation's second Dalek plotline for the year had been turned on its head when Holmes told him to redraft the basic concept and create a new set of monsters for it. *The Kraals* was the result. Terrance Dicks was brought in to work on *The Brain Of Morbius*, which was another one of Holmes affectionate homages to the old horror films of the 1930s, 40s and 50s.

Holmes:

"Terrance had done *King Kong* with *Robot*, so I gave him *Frankenstein* to play around with on *Morbius*. It was always so much easier for the audience if they were watching and could say, 'Ah, it's like *The Curse Of The Mummy's Tomb*', rather than, 'Oh, it's the ugwats killing the zagwits', because if it was a more familiar story, they could relate to it far easier.

"I'd given a nod to the Quatermass stories with the two Auton adventures and I gave Lewis Grieffer the Mummy legends, and Bob (Robert) Banks Stewart *The Thing From Another World* (*The Seeds Of Doom*). I always liked to leave a thread of recognition there, and if people guessed what I was borrowing from, that was just fine by me."

Grieffer's Mummy story was next into production, under the title of *The Pyramids of Mars*, but it was subjected to a major rewrite before the director, Paddy Russell, started work on it.

Holmes:

"I knew Lewis from way back when and he'd done a fair bit of science fiction work for ITV in the past, so I thought that there was a fair chance he'd come up with a good *Doctor Who* script. I can't remember why, exactly, but Lewis had to go off to Tel Aviv for some reason and wasn't available for the rewrites that were needed, and there were plenty.

"I dug up a few books on Egyptian mythology because Horus and Sutekh were the kind of things I wanted to use - these almighty, all-powerful 'Old Gods' - and I redrafted the entire thing, using a pseudonym on the credits. It was only when I rewrote something one hundred per cent that I used my own name on screen (as with *The Ark In Space*), so we used Stephen Harris on that one."

Location scouting was carried out towards the end of March and the beginning of April. The story's requirements were for an old manor house, with a courtyard large enough to accommodate designer Christine Ruscoe's vast pyramid for the story's finale, and a cottage in its surrounding woodlands. Stargroves near Newbury in Berkshire, which was owned by Mick Jagger at that time, was ideal and the cast and crew set off for four days filming from Tuesday 29 April. The house and the surrounding woodlands were used, and with no cottage in the vicinity, a substitute was found by using the exterior of the estate's stable block.

The Mummy costumes made their first on-screen appearance during the location work, with the actors inside barely able to see out of the thick 'bandaged' masks. The costumes worked on the same principal as the Ice Warrior designs. Leggings were held up by braces, with straps across them holding up the arm coverings. The chest and the head area were part of a wire supported shell which had to be lowered over the head and shoulders of the actor from above.

During one afternoon, Tom Baker had to don a full Mummy costume for the sequences where the Doctor disguises himself as one of the robots. Rather than have a double in his place, Russell insisted that Baker go through the motions himself.

Baker:

"She was sure that people would be able to tell it wasn't me if there was a double, because there was a certain way that I walked that could not be imitated. I thought this was nonsense, but unfortunately actors have to listen to the directors and do as they're told, even if it does mean near suffocating in the process."

Transmission of *Revenge Of The Cybermen* was complete by the third week in May, with Baker's debut season having proved to be a huge success. An all-time ratings high for the series up to that point was reached with episode two of *The Ark In Space*. Over thirteen and a half million people tuned in. The rest of the season never dipped below the eight million mark.

The Pyramids Of Mars also marked the first appearance of the Tardis console room for the Tom Baker era, using the same basic prop that had been introduced during season eight. The original console, which was actually painted a light shade of green, was last seen in Inferno before being taken out of service for good.

For the next story into production, Holmes once again used horror movies as a reference when he briefed the writer. Like Lewis Grieffer, Holmes had known Louis Marks since the mid-60s, when they were both jobbing writers submitting storylines to the numerous serials that were being made by the independent companies at that time.

Holmes:

"I gave Louis Marks *Doctor Jekyll And Mister Hyde* as a starting point, with the Id Monster from *Forbidden Planet* (made in 1956) thrown in for good measure. That in itself was a 'rip-off' from a Shakespeare play (*The Tempest*), so in a roundabout way, you could say *Planet Of Evil* was influenced by the Bard himself!"

Following on from his success with *Genesis Of The Daleks*, Hinchcliffe asked David Maloney to return to direct the story. He joined the production team barely three months after completing the Dalek story and began pre-production in May. Roger Murray-Leach returned as the designer with a brief that he had to build an alien jungle.

The resulting set was erected at Ealing, where filming began at the end of the second week of June. Murray-Leach had even managed to accommodate a small river into his design, with endless trees and vines that had all been carefully positioned, following consultation with Maloney, to allow for clearings where the cameras could be positioned.

The Id monster anti-matter creature idea that was 'borrowed' for the story from *The Forbidden Planet* was intended only to be seen as a vague outline, just as it had been in the original movie, but the BBC could not afford to use cell by cell animation techniques for this production. An extra wore a heavily padded silver costume, with huge eyes and draped in dozens of tentacles. When harshly lit against a blue background, its resulting outline was transferred onto the main image by CSO. This meant that the creature could appear from nowhere, attack and vanish again quite effectively.

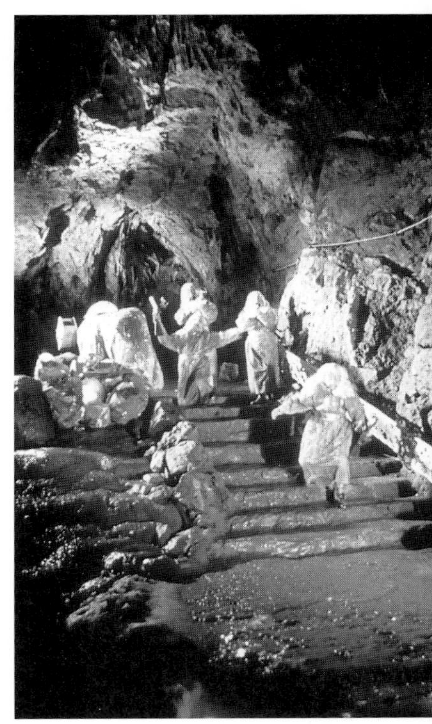

On location at Wokey Hole Caves in Somerset for **Revenge of the Cybermen**.

For the next story, Baker and Sladen's old boss returned. Barry Letts directed Terry Nation's new four-part story, which had been retitled as *The Android Invasion*. Letts' plans to work on a series based on the life of Marie Curie had fallen foul of BBC politics and been delayed by a year, so directing a *Doctor Who* was an ideal way of taking up some of the 'spare time' he now had. Philip Lindley took on the task of designing the sets for the story.

The cast departed for four days' location work on Monday 21 July, filming at the newly constructed Harwell Atomic Power Station in Berkshire. The crew completed their scenes before the facility had been formally opened. Material that had to be shot in woodlands came next, with the unit working around Bagley Woods in nearby Radley. The village scenes were staged in East Hagbourne, where much of Baker's free time was spent signing autographs for eager onlookers as the local school had broken up for its summer holidays while they were there!

The story was the last to feature any actors from the original line-up of UNIT until season twenty, when the Brigadier would be brought back for *Mawdryn Undead*. For this story, only Benton (now promoted to RSM) was present while Ian Marter returned for one final appearance as Harry Sullivan. Both Holmes and Hinchcliffe felt that UNIT stories had run their course and that there was no place for them in the current format of the programme.

Holmes:

"We had nothing against the performers at all, it was just that there were only so many times that the Brigadier could blow things up, and there were only so many times that aliens could invade earth and remain unnoticed by the general public. It was stretching credibility, and we just wanted to move on, so that's what we did."

Letts remembers Tom Baker collecting various plant seeds from Bagley Woods and pocketing them, intent on planting them in all the cracks in the pavements around Notting Hill Gate, where he was living at that time, in the hope that he could bring some colour to the streets when they bloomed.

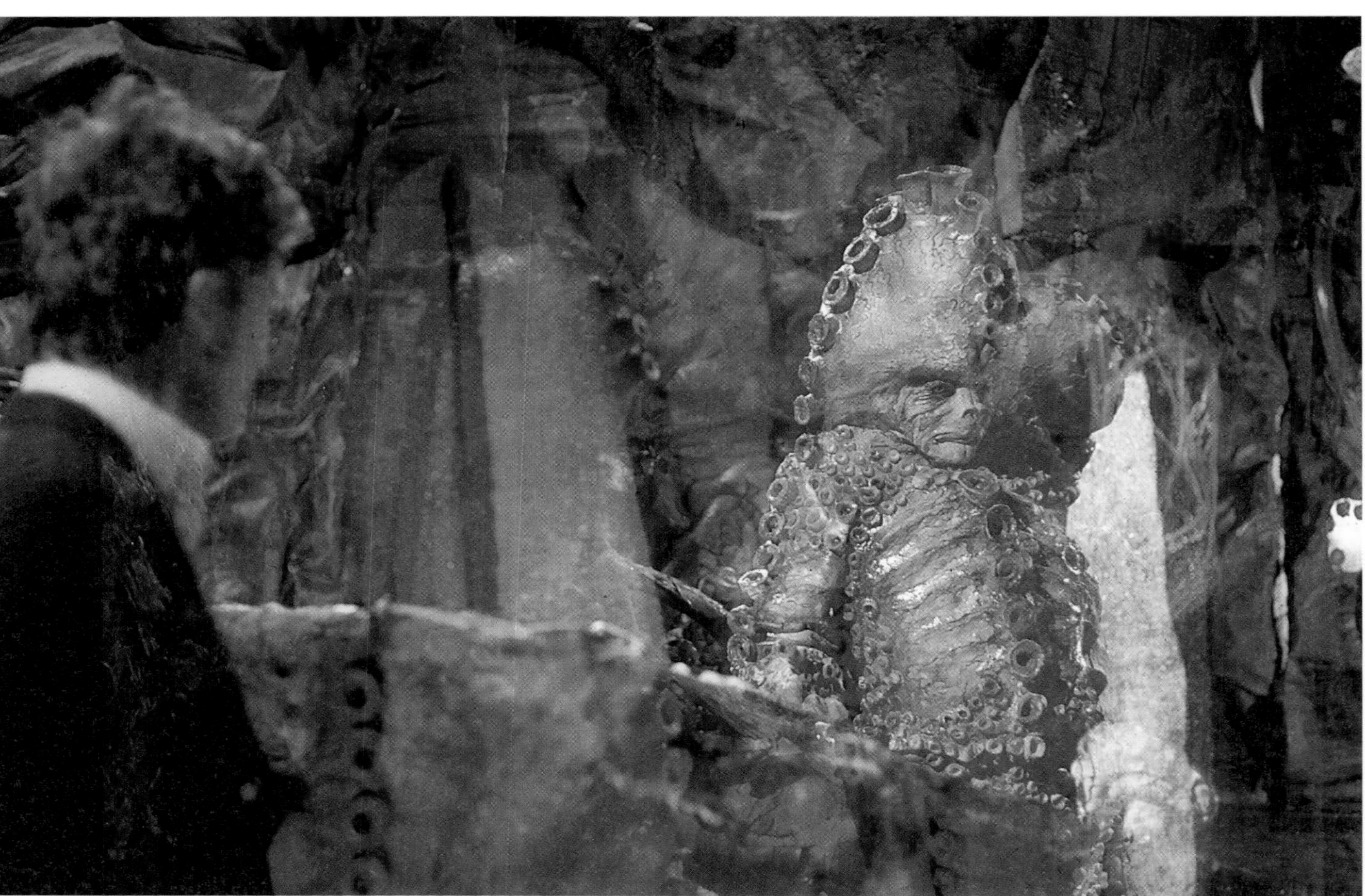

Terror of the Zygons was originally called The Loch Ness Monster.

As Shaun Sutton commented:

"Tom was wonderfully eccentric. There were always tales filtering through of what he'd got up to, or something that had gone on while they were filming. I remember someone saying that there never seemed to be much acting involved - perhaps he really was Doctor Who."

The first two studio days, completing a mix of scenes from all the episodes, ran across 11 and 12 August. The Kraals made their first appearance in studio on the second day, with their leader, Stygron, having already been used in East Hagbourne.

Three heavily padded costumes were made for the actors playing the creatures, with the heavy face masks having been made by John Friedlander, who gave them thick Rhino-like skin, and made them rather bulky, ungainly figures. Nation's scripts actually described them as elegant insect-like lifeforms, but this was changed by Hinchcliffe and Letts in pre-production.

The second studio session moved to TC8, and work on the story was completed on August 25th and 26th. Up until very late in the day, just prior to rehearsals, it had been assumed that Nicholas Courtney would appear as the Brigadier in the story, but he was away on a theatre tour so the part had to be slightly rewritten and changed to Colonel Faraday, played by the veteran *Avengers* actor, Patrick Newell.

Having worked continuously for close to eleven months, Baker and Sladen were given a couple of weeks off before the final two stories for the thirteenth season were recorded. *Terror Of The Zygons* started transmission on the Saturday following the last studio day of *The Android Invasion*, with the season's 26 week run due to go through until March 1976. With Holmes and Hinchcliffe now free of the last vestiges of material commissioned by Dicks and Letts, they were guiding the show in a much darker direction than ever before.

Tom Baker:

"There was undoubtedly a dark, gothic edge of horror while I was with the programme, but then again, children love to be terrorised in that particular way. There may be the most foul smelling fiend imaginable confronting me, about to try and inflict unspeakable harm, but all they have to do is turn and look on either side of them, and they'll see their family sitting alongside. I've said it before, but *Doctor Who* is a family event.

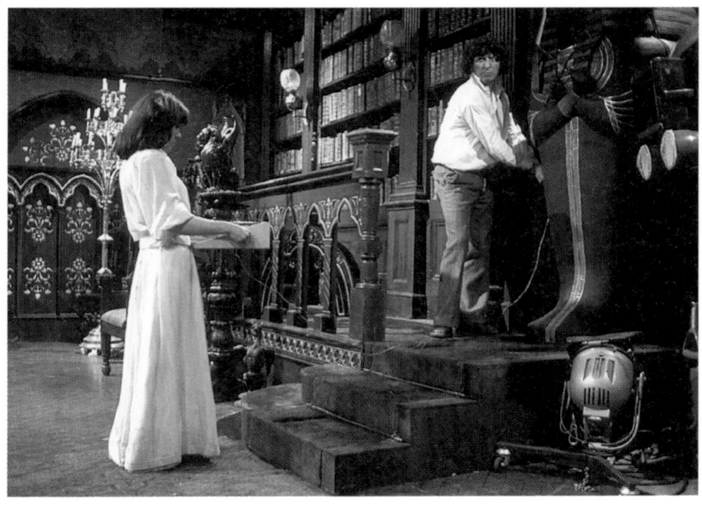

On set for **Pyramids of Mars**.

"I've spoken to countless children over the years, and now adults who were children at the time, and none of them ever thought for one moment that it was real. They all knew that my Doctor was totally infallible, and besides, all they'd have to do is look in the *Radio Times* for the following week and see that I would still be there, but being able to suspend belief for half an hour each week is incredibly healthy for the mind. I should know, I have enough trouble coping with reality."

Robert Holmes always went through the scripts prior to production with a pencil, and as he explains:

"I used to underline a paragraph or two where the plot got a bit heavy, and I thought it would raise the hackles on Mrs. Whitehouse's neck (Mary Whitehouse, then head of the TV watchdog team, the National Listeners and Viewers Association). There was never any intentional grimness, I think it was more a case of trying not to patronise the viewers. If a monster killed someone, we showed it, because there's nothing worse than having someone sitting at home, and saying, 'Oh, they didn't have the guts to show it.' We only ever did that when it was vital to the plot, and necessary to expand the narrative. We were accused of being ghoulish, but then again, those people never saw what I had to cut out!"

By the beginning of the fourth week of September, Tom Baker and Elisabeth Sladen were back rehearsing the next story, which saw two veterans of the show return once more, with Christopher Barry Directing and Barry Newbery Designing *The Brain Of Morbius*, which had the false name on the scripts of Robin Bland.

Holmes:

"Terrance (Dicks) handed in these scripts where the whole centre of the story revolved around this elaborate robot trying to put a body together for his master, Morbius, whose head was the only bit to survive intact from a space crash. Well, Philip decided that we couldn't actually afford to make the kind of Robot costume that was needed, and as it was there was a lot of cost cutting going on, which led to that story being studio bound.

"Terrance was away, and I had no choice other than to redraft the thing myself, which is when the story swapped the robot for the scientist, Solon, and the severed head became a brain which needed a new home, and the old scientist eyes up the Doctor's as being an ideal cranium. Anyway, when Terrance got back, he was far from happy, and wanted his name taken off it, saying I should use something bland in its place. So that's exactly what I did with Robin Bland."

The first two recording days were spent in TCI on 6 and 7 October with the desolate landscape of Karn being created with a vast set that had to be erected in one of the larger studios at TV Centre. The body that has been put together from various space crash victims to house Morbius's brain was described in the script as a 'potpourri', a mix of bits and pieces of different creatures, and to this end a suit was created for stuntman Stuart Fell to wear, with the only recognisable human feature being a left arm. The effect was achieved by building the muscles of the body around a cotton jump-suit, which was then given dark skin tones and a vast claw for the right arm. A clear plastic helmet with metal eye-stalks was later attached to the neck of the creature, with the brain being housed within.

Tom Baker:

"Philip Madoc (Solon) was killingly funny during the rehearsals, and there was one scene which will always be imprinted on my mind, where the jar containing the brain was knocked to the ground, and Philip just looked down and said, 'Sorry, Morbius.' I was in pain for quite some time following that."

Holmes had commissioned a four-part script from Robert Banks-Stewart shortly after *Terror Of The Zygons* had been completed, with the working title of *The Krynoid Invasion*.

Holmes:

"We ended up with a gap of two episodes and nothing to fill the space, so I asked Bob (Banks-Stewart) to fill out his story for an extra two weeks. I wasn't that keen on the six-part format, and the only way I could get it to work was to bring in a sudden twist that would change its direction totally in the middle of its run. You had to effectively interweave a pair of stories to get anything that was any good.

The Doctor indulges in a little swordplay in **The Masque of Mandragora**.

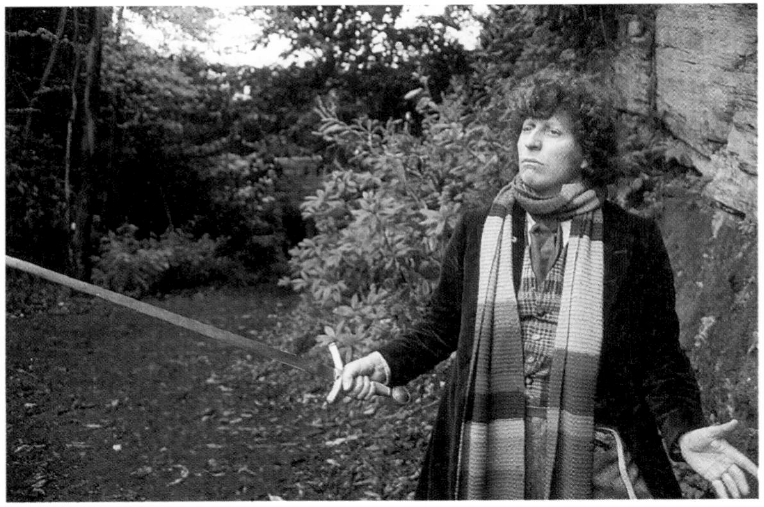

RIGHT: **The Brain of Morbius**.
BELOW: Antarctic peril for the Doctor in **Seeds of Doom**.

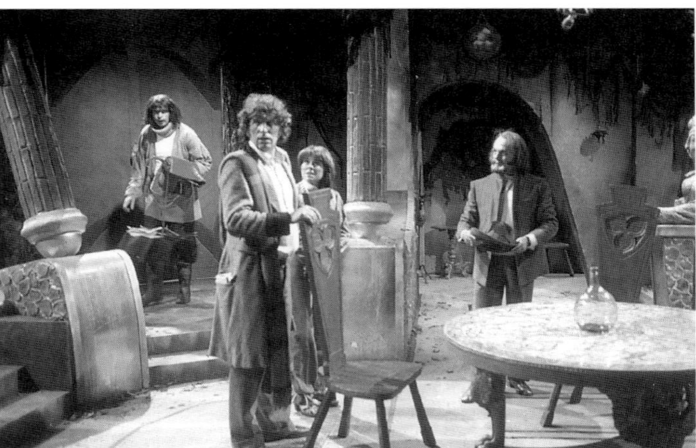

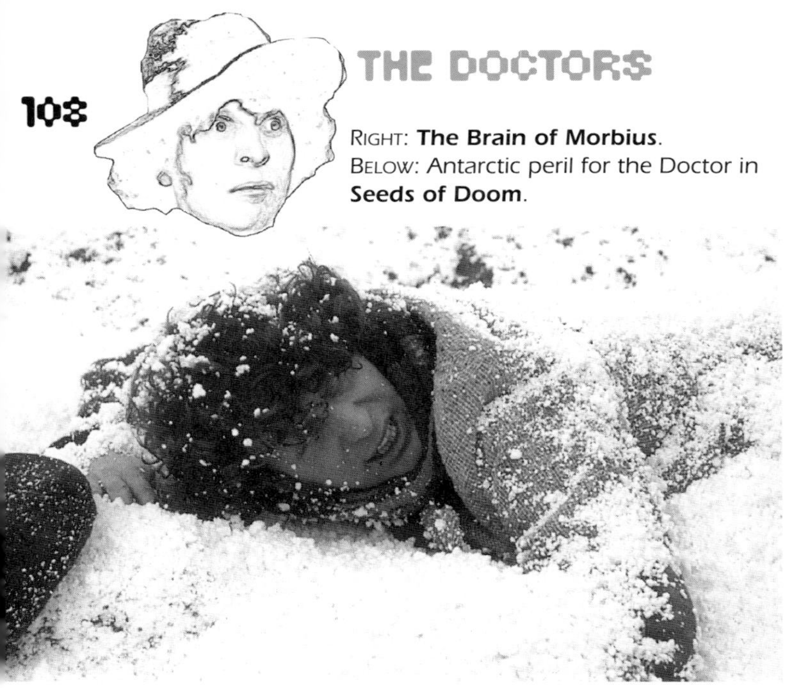

"I think Bob was working on other things, and didn't exactly have much time to come up with any more material, so I sat down with Dougie (Douglas Camfield, returning to the show as the story's director), and we tried to turn it into a rip-off of *The Thing From Another World* (1951), because the main consideration was to try an make the extra two parts as economically as possible."

Roger Murray-Leach returned as designer on the story, and with more work now being added to his load, another designer was brought in to help with the first two 'sub-plot' episodes, with Jeremy Bear joining the team, having last worked on the programme as the sole designer on *The Mutants*. He would handle the antarctic requirements for episode one and two, while Murray-Leach concentrated on the manor house and other settings for episodes three to six.

Five days of location work were needed in total, and the ideal setting for the villain Harrison Chase's mansion was found in Athelhampton House near Dorchester. All of the arctic sequences were shot in a heavily snow-machined area of Dorking Quarry, where some portacabins were erected to represent the snow-bound base where scientists have excavated the alien Krynoid pods.

Once infected by the spores, humans mutated into the vast vegetable based, multi-tendrilled shapeless creatures which Holmes admits were an affectionate nod of appreciation to the first *Quatermass* serial, where the climax featured a similar beast in Westminster Abbey. While the final creature was seen on screen destroying Chase's mansion as stop-motion animated effects, the degeneration stages from the initial infection of the human were done in several ways.

Simple green make-up for the 'sting' became layers of latex as the skin started to mutate and tendrils began to grow, while the still humanoid Krynoid saw the old Axon costumes brought out of storage, with the original mass of tentacles being pruned down slightly and the orange colouring being changed to a suitable shade of green. The next stage, before the animated version took over, was effectively worn like a tent, supported by a framework inside, which had enough room for the operator to manipulate some of the tendrils.

Before studio rehearsals began, a final few shots were taken outside TV Centre itself, with the entrance to the main reception area doubling as the exterior of the World Ecology Bureau. The first two day studio session took place in TC4 during 17 and 18 November.

Holmes:

"I took a joint decision with Philip quite early on to not use any of the old regular characters for the UNIT scenes. They were genuinely only seen for the last couple of episodes, and there really wasn't enough material to justify bringing Nicholas Courtney or John Levene back. I think to give them a call, and say, 'OK, chaps. Time to put the battle fatigues on again', and then only give them four or five scenes would have been slightly insulting. It also helped to distance Tom's Doctor from that tradition of earth-bound stories, so I told Bob to draft in some new characters (Major Beresford and Sergeant Harrison) to take their place for that one story."

The Seeds Of Doom would be the last formal appearance of UNIT, until they were revived for one story (*Battlefield*) in 1989. Philip Hinchcliffe intervened during production and insisted that some of the more graphic Human-to-Krynoid transformations be toned down.

Camfield:

"One of the characters was tied to a bed, with Tony Beckley (Harrison Chase) and his men eager to see his mutate. Well, I had these shots where you saw a close-up off his face as it turned green with tentacles sprouting out of the skin. Philip thought this would be taking things a bit too far. I disagreed, but you have to concede sometimes because the producer is ultimately responsible for what goes out, and if there's trouble, he's the one who gets his knuckles rapped."

The Seeds Of Doom was completed with the last studio work being done in TC8, on 15 and 16 December. Both Baker and Sladen were now released to enjoy a lengthy break, with work due to start on season fourteen in April. On screen, both *Planet Of Evil* and *The Android Invasion* were scoring high ratings, with episodes regularly getting over eleven million viewers. *The Seeds Of Doom* would bring the televised season to a close on 6 March, with *Doctor Who* due to start again in September, in its now regular Autumn slot.

Having completed three seasons with the series, Elisabeth Sladen told Hinchcliffe that she wanted to move on and leave the show but, rather than bow out as a last minute rewrite at the end of *The Seeds Of Doom*, she was persuaded to stay on for the first couple of stories for the next season so that Holmes could commission a suitable finale for her.

Holmes:

"Liz was very insistant that she just went, with no fuss, but she'd been around for quite some time, and it would have been unfair just to have her vanish. So, we made her very central to *The Hand Of Fear*, having her possessed and that sort of thing, making it a show piece for her."

Bob Baker and Dave Martin started work on the scripts, which were originally called *The Hand Of Time*, as work on *The Seeds Of Doom* was completed. Her penultimate appearance in the programme would be in the new season's opening adventure, which Holmes had commissioned Louis Marks to write as *The Catacombs Of Death*.

Holmes:

"I think Philip was taking a page out of my handbook, by asking writers to base their work on old films, because I think he told Louis Marks to do a historical story like *The Masque Of The Red Death*, which was one of those lurid Poe adaptions with Vincent Price. I was actually loathe to try and do stories set in the past, but Louis had a fascination with astrology in the Renaissance period and came up with a wonderful idea of the Doctor accidentally transporting this malevolent energy (The Mandragora Helix) to Italy, where it took over the leader of a satanic coven.

Hinchcliffe was keen to use some extensive location work, and with director Rodney Bennett, they decided to use Portmeirion in North Wales. A village of mixed architectural styles built by Sir William Clough-Ellis, it was famous for being used as the main location of Patrick MacGoohan's classic thriller series of the late 1960s, *The Prisoner*. The actual look of the place could easily be augmented to give it the right period feel, and this task fell to Barry Newbery, once again taking on the job of designer.

Another part of Newbery's brief for the story was to redesign the Tardis console room, as Hinchcliffe felt that the regular one had been seen often enough. He thought it was time for a change. Newbery created a wood-panelled set, which was almost Victorian in style.

Newbery:

"I thought of the old Jules Verne novels, and tried to come up with something along similar lines to the control rooms he had for Captain Nemo (in *20,000 Leagues Under The Sea)*†and his other characters. The console itself was meant to look like an old writing desk and it actually had a flap that came down, with paper and a quill pen inside. The walls' 'wood' look was actually achieved using wallpaper with a wood pattern on it."

Baker and Sladen arrived back to start rehearsals for the location work at the beginning of April 1976. Baker was now fully aware of the kind of responsibility the actors playing *Doctor Who* had to their audience.

Baker:

"There is one part of the audience out there you must never let down and disappoint, and that's the children. The adults can look and say, 'Oh, there's Tom Baker walking along the pavement over there', but to the children, it's *Doctor Who*. I could and would never be seen smoking or drinking in public, because it would cause great disillusionment, and there's nothing worse than breaking a child's belief in one of their heroes."

Baker and Martin's scripts had undergone a title change to *The Hand Of Death*, before settling on *The Hand Of Fear*. Lennie Mayne returned as the director for the story, having last worked on the programme on *The Monster Of Peladon* during Pertwee's final year, and Christine Ruscoe came back as well, having completed design work on *The Pyramids Of Mars* during the previous year.

Holmes:

"I threw *The Hands Of Orlac* (made in 1960) at Bob and Dave as a reference point for their script, but they took it one step further by bringing *The Beast With Five Fingers* into the plot as well, by having a severed hand moving around on its own. They'd come up with an idea of having Tom avert some nuclear disaster for one story, so by combining all these elements, they came up with *The Hand Of Fear*."

For research into nuclear power stations, the writers were given access to the Central Electricity Generating Board nuclear power station at Oldbery, near Avon. The CEGB were all to happy to help and made it clear that the story itself could be filmed there, so with Mayne approving it as a location, that's exactly what happened, with three days of location work being carried out there during the second week of June.

Two more days on location followed at the nearby ARC Quarry in Thornbury, where a miscalculation during the filming of an explosion resulted in one of the three cameras shooting the scene being destroyed under the resulting rubble. The final scene for Elisabeth Sladen, as Sarah departs from the Tardis for the last time, was shot in a street in a nearby village on one of the last days of filming.

The first of two studio sessions began on 5 July in TC8 at TV Centre, and ran until 8 July. On the second day, all of the Tardis scenes were recorded, and so the farewell scene between the Doctor and Sarah-Jane was staged, with Baker and Sladen apparently reworking a lot of the dialogue themselves, with Holmes' complete approval.

Holmes:

"Tom and Liz had developed a hell of a rapport over the years which would have been criminal to ignore when it came to that last scene. To be honest, it was a favourite pastime of Tom's to try and rewrite most of the scripts anyway, but in that instance, he really worked hard with Liz to get it just right.

"Because they didn't know exactly what we wanted to do with Sarah-Jane, Bob and Dave had left the final couple of scenes unwritten. I handled the stuff that was done on location, but when it came to the studio recording, it was one of the last things to be done on that particular set, and it became an effort shared between the three of us."

The second studio session, running for only two days, but again staged in TC8, ran from 19 to 20 July. Sladen departed after that point, leaving the Doctor on his own in the Tardis to go on to the next story alone, for the first and only time in the programme's history.

Holmes:

"Philip wanted to explore the mythology and the actual structure of the Time Lord society, which was something that had never really been touched on in depth before. I liked to think of them as a slightly classical race of scholars, with an incredible

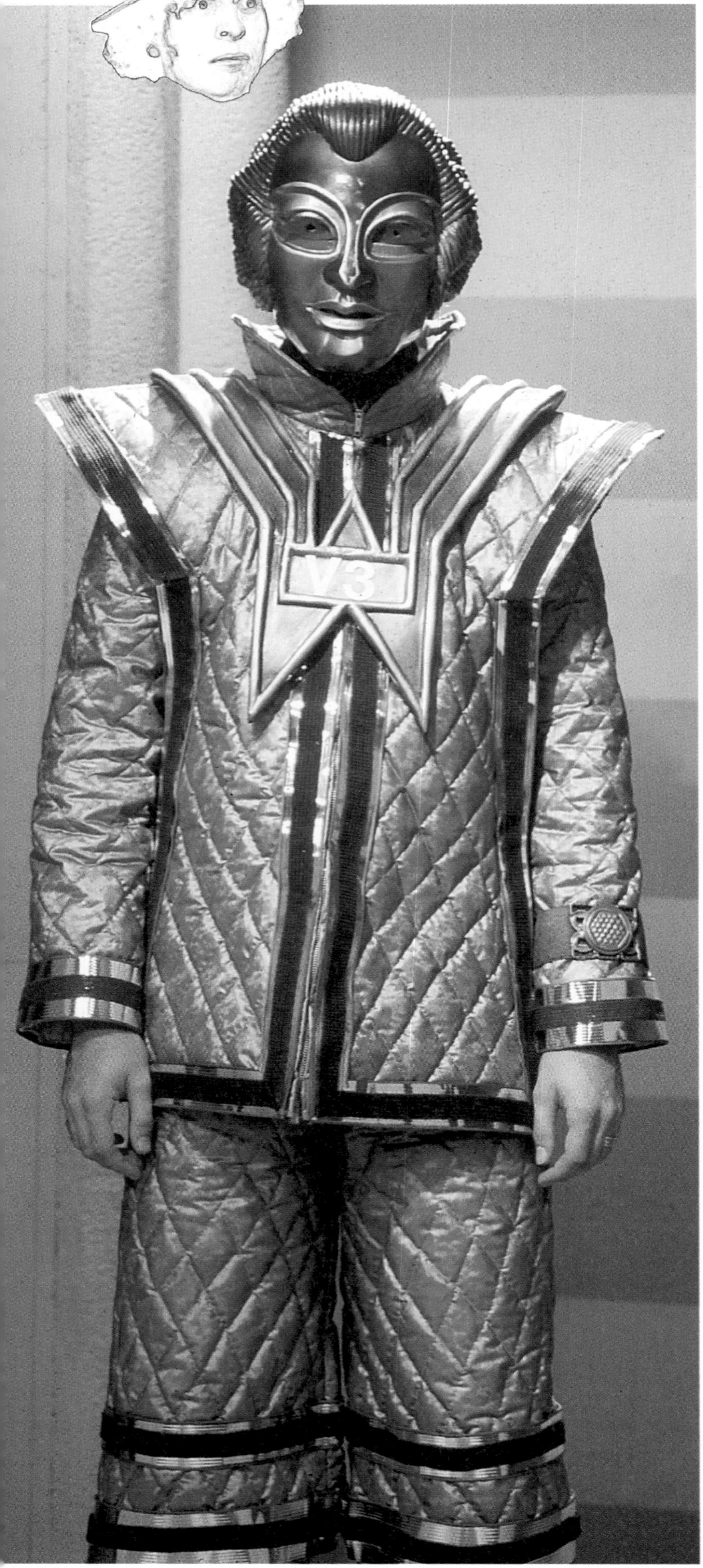

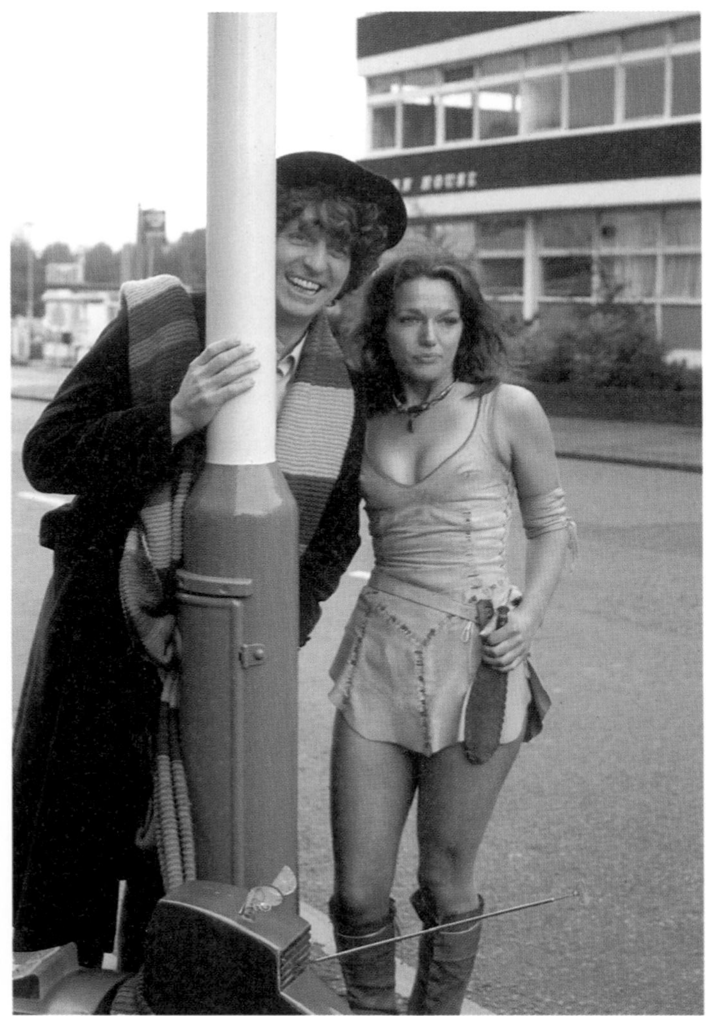

Above: *Leela became the Doctor's new companion in* **The Face Of Evil**.
Left: *An Art Decco robot from* **Robots of Death** *– minus its gloves!*.

sense of discipline and order amongst their ranks - but, as with anything like that, if you scratch at the surface, you'll find something pretty rotten underneath."

Holmes started work on the idea as *The Dangerous Assassin*, and again, called on a favourite film for his inspiration.

Holmes:

"I brought in elements of the paranoia of the main character being manipulated, and being unable to do anything about it, from *The Manchurian Candidate* (1962), and had the Doctor go through the same kind of crisis. That led to the idea of having the Doctor being framed for the assassination of the President of the High Council on his home planet. Both Philip and I agreed that the ideal manipulator would be the Master."

With Roger Delgado having died in 1973, a way to recast the role had to be figured out, so Holmes came up with the idea of having the character at the end of his final regeneration, with his body in a state of rapid decay. Both script editor and producer were planning to move on at the end of the season, so they could leave the ending open ended so that the Master could be brought back as a different actor by the new production team, if they so wished. Peter Pratt was cast for *The Deadly Assassin,* and had to work wearing a heavy latex mask, which made visibility very difficult.

David Maloney was hired as the Director, having won the admiration of the production team for his work on both *Genesis Of The Daleks* and *Planet Of Evil*, and he was once again teamed with his *Planet* designer, Roger Murray-Leach. It was clear that the story would require extensive location work due to the sequences which ran from the climax of episode two until the beginning of episode four, where the Doctor entered the Matrix Data Bank computer and engages in a surreal mental battle with Chancellor Goth, the high ranking Time Lord under the Master's control. Everything from a vintage biplane to a miniature railway was needed, so extensive recce work was carried out while *The Hand Of Fear* was being made.

Less than a week after completing that story, Baker joined Maloney's crew at Betchworth Quarry near Dorking, on 26 July. For the second day there the team moved to the goods yard, where the train shots were staged.

Work on 28 July moved from the Quarry to the Royal Alexandra and Albert School in Surrey, where the vast gardens and natural pond area stood in as the jungle sequences in the computer. This work, including the famous drowning shot (at the climax of episode three, the cliffhanger involved Tom Baker's head being held underwater and it caused uproar from the National Viewers and Listeners group, resulting in editing on the scene for the story's repeat screening), was completed on 29 July, and the next day was spent at Redhill Aerodrome, where the biplane scenes were staged.

Holmes:

"You have to look at *The Deadly Assassin* as a thriller. It's not a normal, run-of-the-mill *Doctor Who* story, nor was it ever intended to be. We were able to use a political edge that was normally beyond the limitations of other stories, and in doing so, we alienated a lot of the long-term viewers, but nothing can be achieved without change. I deliberately set out to overturn all the established rules and myths that had been set up with the Time Lords."

The Deadly Assassin moved studios to TC8 for a final two day studio session on at the beginning of September, leaving only a few insert shots uncompleted, which Maloney oversaw on an extra day on 7 September. The season had now started transmission, with the first episode of *The Masque Of Mandragora* being broadcast on 4 September with over eight million viewers tuning in. The ratings would steadily increase between that instalment and the end of *The Deadly Assassin* , whereafter there was a short break before broadcasting resumed with the next story in the new year (*The Face Of Evil*). *The Deadly Assassin* part three would reach a high for that run with thirteen million viewers.

The Face Of Evil was written by Chris Boucher, a new writer to the programme who had submitted several ideas to Holmes, who recognised the fact that there was a talent at work here, and finally won a commission with the rather luridly titled *The Day God Went Mad*, which had to be changed for obvious reasons. Part of his brief was to introduce a new companion for the Doctor.

Holmes:

"We wanted a character who would be far more positive and would actually stand up and deal with things herself. The Doctor was essentially very much a pacifist and would never incite any violence, so we thought it would be an ideal type of contrast to have someone that would do exactly that, and that's where Leela came from."

The name was created by Boucher and the role was taken up by Louise Jameson. She had been cast by Hinchcliffe and Pennant Roberts, who had been hired as the director for the story. They saw dozens of actresses and compiled separate lists of who they would make as their choice, and through a session of comparing notes, it was whittled down to Jameson, who was offered the part.

Holmes:

"Leela was very much a primitive, a savage who was quick to stab someone in the back with her dagger and then start asking questions. There was a bit of friction in the rehearsal rooms, because Tom was not at all happy about having such a violent companion. It wasn't Louise's fault, it was the concept of the character he objected to, and the thing about Tom was that he always made his feelings quite clear on such things!"

Tom Baker felt that the Doctor would never have been able to tolerate such aggression, and would surely have left her behind, rather than take her on board the Tardis.

Baker:

"I was appalled by the fact that she joined with the Doctor. She killed everything in sight, and there is no justifiable way to take life and death so lightly, but Louise modified her performance as she went along, and was superb. I'm afraid that Leela, as a concept, was never my ideal companion."

Holmes:

"The whole point of the plot was that Tom had been to this planet before and imbued a damn great computer with the Doctor's personality. Over the centuries, it had become schizophrenic. We had to have scenes of the Doctor talking to this thing, which had his own face (CSOed onto the screen with prerecorded material of Baker), so Tom was effectively talking to himself.

"Chris (Boucher) proved to be incredibly adept at churning out good *Doctor Who* scripts at a rapid pace, and there was barely any editing to do after he got to know the basics, so I gave him

Part of the elaborate studio set for **The Talons of Weng Chiang**.

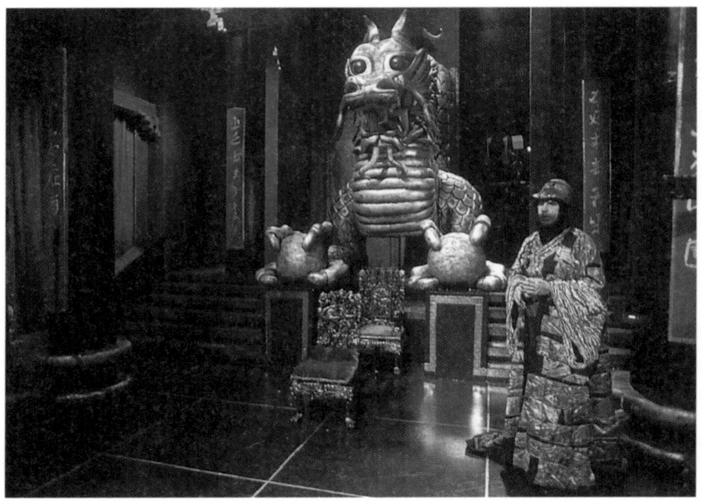

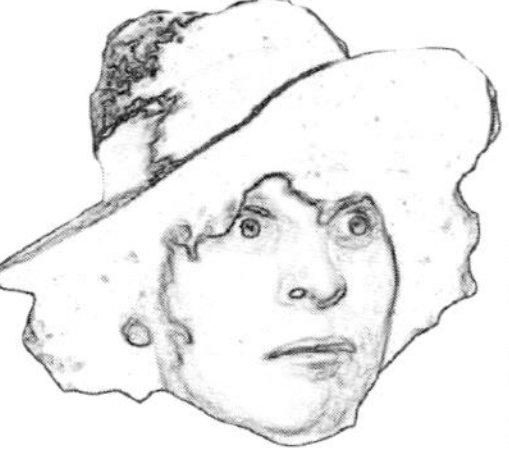

the next story to write, with a brief of, 'Do *Ten Little Niggers* (an Agatha Christie book) with robots', while I got on with the six -parter to wind the season up. Philip agreed that I should do it, as it was meant to be the swan song on the show for both of

The final session on *The Face Of Evil* ran from 25 to 26 October, again in TC3. Michael E. Briant was now in pre-production on Boucher's next script, called *The Robots Of Death*, with Kenneth Sharp returning as designer for the first time since *The Claws Of Axos* during season eight.

Briant:

"I think there comes a point where you can do just one to many *Doctor Who* stories, and I reached my limit with that one because as soon as I saw the script, all I could think was, 'Oh, no! Not more bloody robots!' So, I set out with Ken Sharp to try and come up with a different way of doing them.

"I had a notion of having their faces like Greek soldiers' helmets from ancient mythology, and Ken took it one step further by making both them, the crew and all of the interiors of the mining vessel they were on Art Deco in style. All *Doctor Who* robots didn't have to look like the Cybermen or Daleks, so we thought, 'What the hell!', and went for it."

The Voc Robots all had carefully hand-painted masks made for the actors, whose costumes were simple tunics with soft shoes. Sharp went and visited the *Queen Mary*, studying the Art Deco interiors on board to get ideas for the corridors and lounge areas of the sandminer, where all the action of the studio-bound story was due to take place.

The Robots Of Death also saw the last appearance of Newbery's wood-panelled Tardis console room, which was phased out as the new production team arrived at the end of the year.

Briant:

"The Robots all had a calm, smooth, reassuring tone to their voice, like the computer from *2001* (Hal), because that was very unnerving and I wanted to try and get the same effect. There were scenes where they were meant to be totally deranged, with glowing red eyes, and they still had a pleasant tone to their voices as they tried to kill

"Tom was well into his element by then, and was certainly more settled when compared to *Revenge Of The Cybermen* (Briant's last story). In rehearsal, when the script said something like; the Doctor runs past the robot, Tom would want to change it all around, and he'd take me to one side and say, 'Why don't I leap towards the light on the ceiling, swing over the robot's head, land on a trolley and speed down the corridor, before leaping through the doors at the end of the corridor and closing them, with the skill of the most accomplished of acrobats!'. And you would quietly reply, 'Well, let's try it as written, and if we get time (knowing damn well that you never would), we'll give it a go.'"

Holmes had actually asked Robert Banks-Stewart to write the finale for the season, but the writer was unable to take on the job as he'd recently accepted a long term contract with Thames Television. In a very short period of time, Holmes drafted up the first four episodes of *The Talons of Greel*, with the setting revolving around a Victorian music hall theatre, based loosely on an idea Banks Stewart had devised.

David Maloney had been brought in to direct the story, and Roger Murray-Leach was secured as the designer for his seventh and final *Doctor Who*. Typically, to avoid the chore of completing six part stories on the same plotline, Holmes completed the story with the final two episodes veering wildly from the narrative of the first four.

Holmes:

"Magnus Greel did not feature extensively in the original episodes, he was very much the background villain; the shadow waiting in the wings to be revealed in the final act - but as I started work on the final scripts, I got more and more fascinated with the potential he had, and moved him to centre stage. As a consequence, I had to tinker with the first few episodes to redress the balance, although in the finished version, he still doesn't really come into the forefront of the story until the final two episodes."

As work on *The Robots Of Death* was being completed, the title was changed to *The Talons Of Weng Chiang*, to reflect the Tong gang warfare element that Holmes had introduced into the scripts. The production team would face other pressures, apart from having to actually complete the story, a documentary team would be following the production unit for several days as work progressed. *The Lively Arts* series on BBC2 had approached Hinchcliffe with a view to covering rehearsals and pre-production work on one of the serials. *Who's Doctor Who?* was eventually screened a week after *Weng Chiang* had completed transmission.

Maloney carried out some early filming in the second week of December, with day and night shooting being set up around some houses and streets in Twickenham that looked suitably Victorian, while streets around the old spice docks at Wapping and a small dock off the Thames in that area were used for a day on 13 December. After this point, Jameson and Baker were released for their Christmas holidays but they were due to return in the last week of December when any outstanding scenes in London would be completed before moving on to the Northampton Rep Theatre.

A series of extensive recces had located the venue, and it proved to have a stage and scenery gantry on the roof that were basically the same type that would have been used at the turn of the century. The cast and crew worked for six days from 8 January.

Holmes agreed to stay on to tide things over, as there were several scripts he'd already commissioned which he wanted to oversee with the new producer in case there were any problems. The head of the department, Bill Slater, offered the post of Producing *Doctor Who* to Graham Williams, who had been due to produce a thriller series called *The Zodiac Factor*, which had fallen through due to financial difficulties. He trailed Hinchcliffe during the latter stages of work on *The Talons Of Weng Chiang*. The production unit manager for that year, Chris D'Oyly John, was sounded out about taking over from Hinchcliffe initially, but he turned the job down, deciding to stay in the administrative side of television production.

Five days of studio work was needed to complete *Talons*, and this was divided into two sections. The first was carried out following a short rehearsal period after returning from Northampton, on 24 and 25 January while the final three days of recording ran from 8 February.

Tom Baker:

"We had a giant rat in that one, which had to chase Louise down a sewer tunnel in the studio. She had to time running away from it, because the poor man inside could barely move, as he was on his hands and knees, and I had to stand and be rather heroic and kill him with an elephant gun. I rather liked that one."

The ratings continued on a regular high for the second half of the season, with episode three of *The Robots Of Death* gaining over thirteen million viewers. After *Talons* had been completed, Baker and Jameson were released for their holidays, while Holmes stayed on to start work with Williams.

Holmes:

"Tom was not exactly happy with the thought of having Leela stay on as his companion, and he'd been told by someone that she would only be there for three stories. Just before Philip left, I asked him whether he'd told Tom that Louise had signed on for another full season, and he shrugged and said, 'Graham's the producer now, he'd better tell him!'

Hinchcliffe had created a very distinctive style with his three years on *Doctor Who*, and led the programme into an area of controversy with some of his story content, but he stood by his writers and directors no matter what. He went on to produce *Target*, a thriller series for the BBC which starred Patrick Mower, and called on familiar *Who* directors he'd worked with, such as Douglas Camfield. The series faced extreme criticism over the level of violence in some of its stories, and when asked about this, Holmes said:

"Philip believed in presenting uncompromising reality for the viewers. He didn't want to hide in the shadows, or shy away from themes or stories that might alarm some people. Douglas Camfield had a theory about producers, specifically the ones on *Doctor Who*, saying that they were either 'hawks' or 'doves'.

"I think 'doves' were the ones who stuck to the rules and did anything for a quiet life, never daring to cross the line into dangerous creativity. 'Hawks' were the ones who flew head-on into the set rules and broke them. They were the ones who set new precedents, the ones who fought for what they believed in. One thing I certainly agreed with Dougie on, was that Philip was definitely a 'hawk'."

One critic, who had grown up watching *Doctor Who* when Hartnell was in the role, looked back over the last three years as Hinchcliffe's era came to an end.

"It used to be a cliche to say that *Doctor Who* sent the children scurrying behind the sofa where they would only watch peering round its corner, or from the safety of behind a soft cushion, which they could easily bury their head in when alien creatures loomed forth, but it didn't seem to be like that when Jon Pertwee strode across the screens in his varying shades of velvet jackets. That *Doctor Who* had an adult logic behind it and the explanations were careful and scientific, and it suited the generation watching it perfectly. But now? Now we have *Doctor Who* according to Bram Stoker and Poe, chilling and frightening, enough to nearly send the adults diving behind the sofa, with its giant rats and vegetable men. I eagerly await its return in the autumn, with yet more horrors. Surely it can only get better?"

Michael Spice as Weng Chiang.

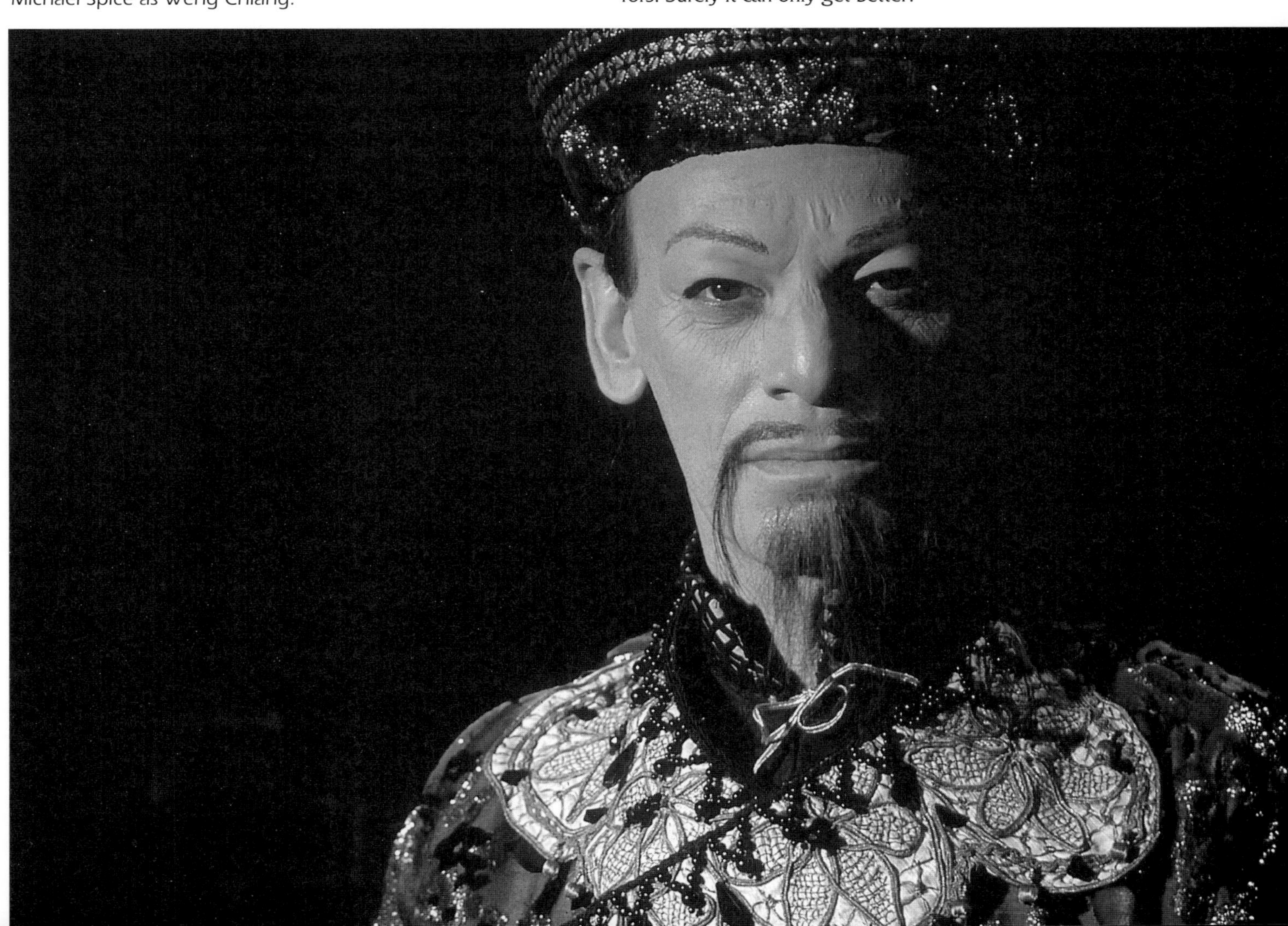

CHAPTER 6

WHISPERING CHAMBERS OF IMAGINATION

WHISPERING CHAMBERS OF IMAGINATION
WHISPERING CHAMBERS OF IMAGINATION

"Rehearsals always saw extraordinarily well known actors peeping through the doors, spying on us and laughing. I don't think it was ever derisive. It was just the joy of seeing overacting on such an immense scale."

TOM BAKER Unpublished interview – September 1988

"There was a mass defection going on. It was almost as though everybody was sick and tired of *Doctor Who*, and was going out of their way to avoid it, and finding an ideal excuse in the shape of *Blake's Seven*."

Pre-production started in the spring of 1977 as Graham Williams formally started work on the fifteenth season and, as he says, many of the familiar names from Hinchcliffe's tenure as producer had moved across to this new science fiction show. David Maloney moved straight on from directing *The Talons Of Weng Chiang* to become the series producer taking directors such as Michael E. Briant, Douglas Camfield and Pennant Roberts with him.

Williams:

"None of the old names, be they designers or directors, wanted to know, so I had to try and find some new ones and that wasn't the least of the problems. Bob Holmes was stuck on *Weng Chiang* for ages and couldn't start commissioning anything for some time, so all the scripts were coming in late for that first year, and when we did get Terrance Dicks' vampire one up and running, we were told we couldn't do it!"

Dicks was given the vampire legend to work on as he'd covered Frankenstein with *The Brain Of Morbius*, and it was one of the horror movie cycles that Holmes had yet to bring into the programme. *The Witch Lords* would have been a four part adventure, and was scheduled to open the new season.

Holmes:

"Graeme McDonald had just taken over as the head of the department, and he would have been told what we were planning for our 'opening night'. He came into the office and said, 'I don't think so chaps. Philip Saville's about to direct a *Dracula* for us (Starring Louis Jordan as the Count and Frank Findlay as Van Helsing), it's costing a small fortune, and I don't think we'll want people thinking *Doctor Who* is taking the mickey out of it. Do your one next year, OK?'

"Graham's heart hit the floor, because there was barely any time to get a new story in, but I knew Terrance could work like lightning because he'd probably been in the same sort of jam when he was *Doctor Who's* script editor, so I got him to do *Ten Little Indians* in a lighthouse."

Dicks was drafting up *The Monster of Fang Rock*, which was also known as *The Beast of Fang Rock*, while work began on the first season fifteen story to go before the cameras.

Williams:

"The scripts were late, so I'd found Derrick Goodwin, who had a lot of experience with sitcoms, but not much else, and I landed him with what was probably the most complex story we ever did."

Bob Baker and Dave Martin took on Holmes brief to play around with the concepts used in the *Fantastic Voyage* movie, and came up with *The Enemy Within*, which introduced a robot dog as one of the supporting characters.

Williams:

"One of the visual effects guys, Ian Scoones, came up with this wonderful design for K9, as a sort of metallic Doberman, but it was too big. I wanted something where the audience wouldn't be able to point and say, 'That's a midget in a robot suit', so I asked for something a bit more sophisticated, and they came up with the radio controlled metal terrier look that eventually went up on screen...

"The reason we made him a companion was simple, in that we wanted to give Tom a second sounding board that could be left behind. If you have a human sidekick, the Doctor had to take them with him whenever they landed, but with K9, you could leave him behind once they've landed if he didn't fit into the story. He was sort of an optional extra for the writers. We liked him to be used because he proved to be incredibly popular, but he wasn't vital if he made things awkward for them."

Robert Holmes noted that there was a certain degree of tension between the Doctor and his new pet.

Holmes:

"Tom used to love it in rehearsals, because John Leeson (who provided the voice of K9), used to get down on his hands and knees, crawling around the place, pretending to be the dog, and it gave him something more tangible to react to. When we got into the studio, and the dog wouldn't work, it used to drive Tom spare, and more often than not he'd kick it out of frustration."

There were problems with the mechanics of the creation, as attempting such things on television was rare and precautions had to be taken in case it proved impossible to use the device in the long-term. This resulted in two different endings being filmed for *The Invisible Enemy*, as it was retitled, when production began at Bray studios in April 1977.

Williams found that one of the 'old guard' was certainly willing to work on the show in the design department, and Barry Newbery returned for his thirteenth *Doctor Who* story. Tom Baker and Louise Jameson started rehearsing with the guest cast at the

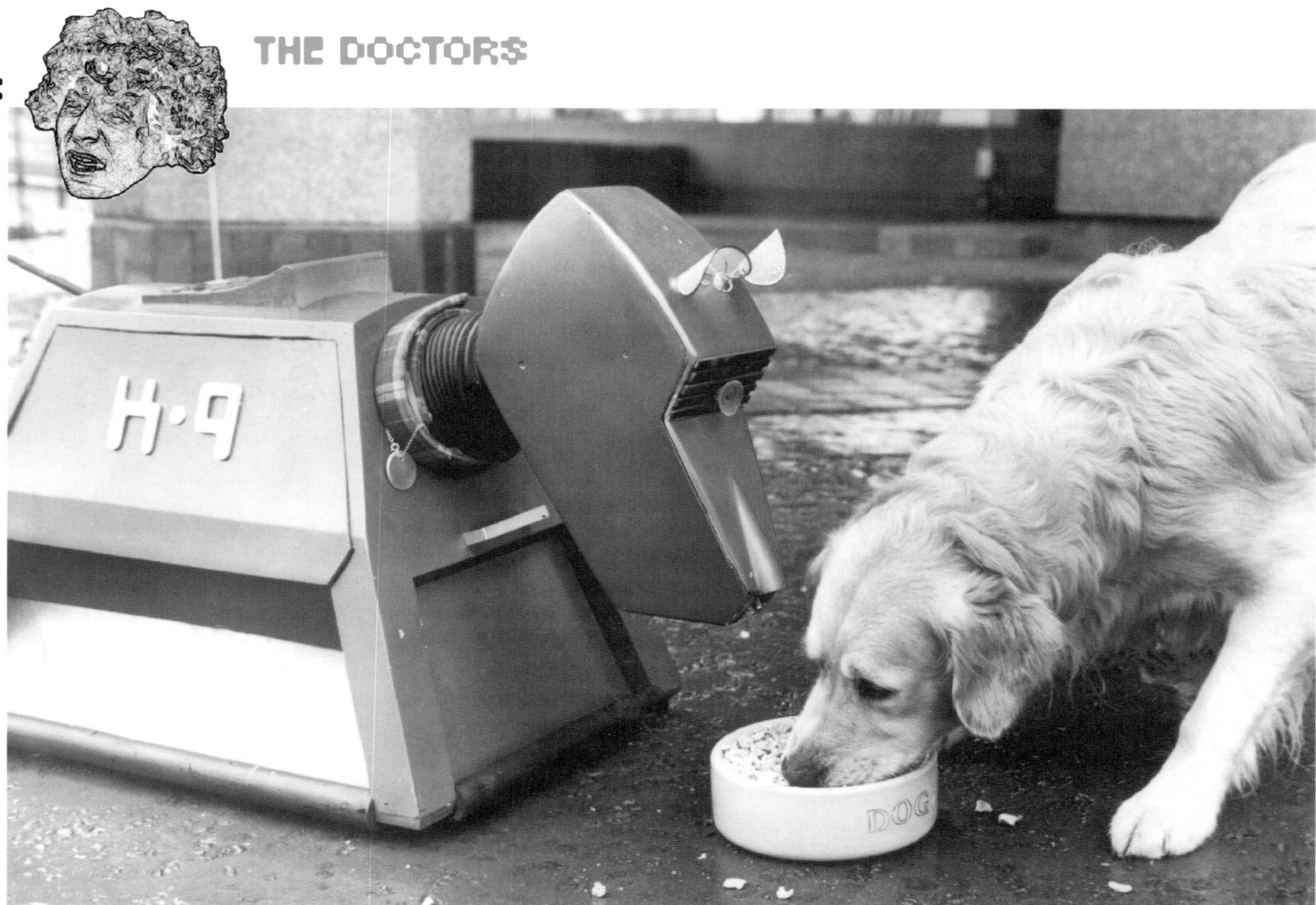

end of March, with the first of two three day studio sessions beginning on 10 April in TC6 at TV Centre.

Because of the time spent concentrating on getting K9 to work properly, very little time was allocated by the special effects team on the Nucleus, the alien parasite that invaded the Doctor's mind during the course of the story.

Tom Baker:

"The Doctor had been having brainstorms of considerable magnitude, and set about wandering around in his own head to find the villain, which was basically a rather large, pink prawn. Now, the poor prawn tried to be as threatening as he could, by occasionally waving a claw or some mandible, but other than that, he just sat there and looked prawn-like. I think a rather large deep-fat fryer would have put paid to his schemes!"

K9, in the context of the story, was created by Professor Marinus at the Bi-Al Foundation, a vast space station medical research centre. One ending was filmed with the robot staying with his creator, and the other with Marinus asking the Doctor to look after him. The decision would have to be made as to whether he stayed with the series or not because, as Newbery explains:

"K9 would go haywire whenever radio signals interfered with his circuits, and it was difficult for him to move across anything other than a flat surface. Something as small as a matchstick could bring him to a grinding halt, so the camera cables had to be repositioned so that nothing got in his way. It was all a bit chaotic."

A huge problem was about to hit the production team as they started work on Dicks' lighthouse story, now called the *Horror Of Fang Rock*. The studio space that had been booked for *The Witch Lords* had been lost and as a consequence, there was no way that *Fang Rock* could be recorded in any of the studios at TV Centre as they were all fully booked. One of the outer regional facilities had to be used as an alternative, and director Paddy Russell settled for the relatively new Pebble Mill complex in Birmingham.

Holmes:

"There was a throwaway line in *The Time Warriors*, where Linx bluffly boasted about how the Sontarans were mightier than the Rutans, against whom they were waging an unending war, so it seemed like a good idea to finally bring them into the series. The Sontarans had spent two stories eying up the earth for its strategic potential, so it was hardly unfeasible for the Rutans to have done the same at some point.

"In the end, after the build up running through the entire story, waiting for them to appear, all we got was a green jelly fish with a lisp, and it was a considerable let down. I don't blame the special effects boys, though. In all fairness to them, they were in an alien territory in Birmingham, and there weren't the same facilities as they had in London, so it wasn't really their fault."

Horror Of Fang Rock was completed with a three day recording session between 7 and 9 June, after which Baker and Jameson had to return to London to begin rehearsals on *The Sunmakers*, with Pennant Roberts as their director.

Holmes:

"Graham Williams asked me to do a four-parter for the middle of the season, and later the six part finale, but I just couldn't cope with a workload like that. I'd been on *Doctor Who* since about midway through *Death To The Daleks* some four years earlier, and I was just burnt out. I couldn't find an original idea in my head as far as *Doctor Who* was concerned, and just wanted to get away. I said I'd try and come up with the four-parter. The whole thing was a skit on the Inland Revenue System, because we had a Gatherer and a Collector, and there was the odd dig at income tax forms, like having Corridor P45. The ending, where the Collector turned out to be a lump of green seaweed vanishing down the plughole on the seat of his wheelchair, was something I dearly wished some of the real IRS men would do!"

Williams had brought in an old colleague, Anthony Read, to trail Holmes as his replacement script editor from this point onwards, with Read having already had extensive experience in such a capacity on the long running thriller series, *The Troubleshooters*

With Roberts working with Tony Snoaden, his designer, several locations had to be scouted out for the story, with the first outdoor filming of the season being done on this story. A very high building was needed to achieve shots where nothing could be seen on the horizon, and the Imperial Tobacco Factory in Bristol was found to be ideal, with the interior of the complex offering wide, pristine white corridors for several chase sequences that had to be staged.

Roberts had worked extensively on Terry Nation's grim apocalyptic series *The Survivors*, and remembered one of the locations he used for that which would be ideal for the lower tunnels of the city in the story. From 13 to 18 June, location work moved from Bristol to the Camden Deep Tunnels in London.

Image Of The Fendahl had been submitted and accepted by Holmes before the production team were told to tone down the horror content of the stories, so it was effectively the last story to be made in the 'gothic' tradition that Hinchcliffe had established. The story touched on similar themes of occult worship that had been used in *The Daemons* in Season Eight.

Five days of location filming saw the programme return to Stargroves, where *The Pyramids Of Mars* had been shot, between 1 and 5 August. The director was George Spenton Foster, working with Anna Ridley as his designer.

Holmes:

"The Fendahl story was quite unsettling with these creatures that were meant to be malevolent dark shapes, like some horrific creation from an H.P. Lovecraft story, but money was tight and we ended up with a couple of viscous rolls of carpet. It sounds as though I'm being a bit flippant about the whole thing, but it was frustrating because there just weren't the resources to make anything that was truly spectacular."

The original running order for the season, as Williams had planned it, would have been *The Invisible Enemy*, followed by *The Vampire Mutations* (the alternative title for *The Witch Lords*), *The Sunmakers* and *Image Of The Fendahl*.

With the production problems with Terrance Dicks' story, and the resulting delays, it was altered to *Horror of Fang Rock, The Invisible Enemy, Image Of The Fendahl* and then *The Sunmakers*, with the final two stories of the year following on in their production order. David Weir was drafting up the final six episodes as *The Killer Cats Of Ginseng*, while the next story saw Bob Baker and Dave Martin complete a four- parter called *Underworld*, based on the legend of Jason's quest for the Golden Fleece.

Former long-time BBC production manager Norman Stewart was hired as director for *Underworld*, with Dick Coles as his designer. Coles overspent considerably on the spaceship interior that was needed for the story, as Graham Williams recalled:

"We lost a vast amount of money on this elaborate control room, that took up practically all of TC8, with its gantries and doorways. Poor Norman Stewart had an awful time trying to get the angles he wanted on the actors because there just wasn't enough room on the control deck so he had to do a lot of it from the ground level looking up towards the characters, which looked a bit odd.

"There wasn't enough money to build the huge caves that the scripts called for, so we had to compromise and have them built in miniature, with the backgrounds CSOed against a blue backdrop. Tom wasn't happy with all that, because there were just one or two boulders and it became a bit mime-heavy. The studio was a bit tense on that one."

Williams had further problems to solve when the scripts for The *Killer Cats Of Ginseng* were submitted.

"It was just totally different from the plotline Anthony Read had planned out with the writer. The finale had this trial by combat scene with the Doctor and a huge panther creature, which was fine, but it was set in some place as big as Wembley with 96,000 extras dressed up as cat people. It was impossible, so I stopped the costume people we had working on it (some of the Killer Cat designs were actually completed), and told Gerald Blake, who was going to direct it, to hold on, while we had a rethink."

The voice of K9, actor John Leeson, takes the troublesome robot for a walk.

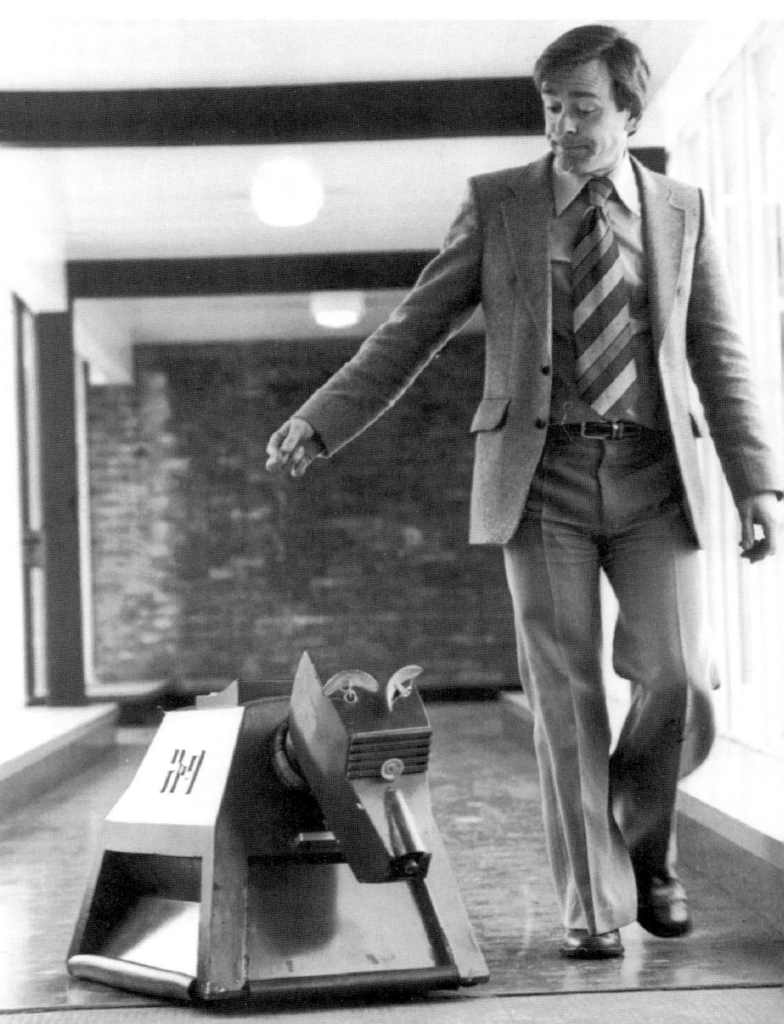

Williams had wanted Robert Holmes to come up with a sequel to *The Deadly Assassin*, exploring the societies on Gallifrey, with the theory that not all the inhabitants of the planet were necessarily Time Lords, hence the Killer Cats. Holmes backed out, Weir stepped in, now Williams and Read had to salvage the situation, still intent on doing a Gallifrey story, and basically turned to Robert Holmes to seek advice.

Holmes:

"Graham was in a frantic state of that *Killer Cats* fiasco, so I told him to use the same routine we'd done with *The Seeds Of Doom*, having what was basically a four-part story, which had a plot twist, leading into a sub-plot two-parter, which utilised some of the same characters. I heard from him a bit later, when they'd got something like the first four parts done, that he wanted to use the Sontarans, and bring them in as a surprise twist for the final two episodes."

Read had completed six episodes in two weeks, which were then rewritten by Williams over six days with very little sleep (this was when the Sontarans were brought in). So, after a three week delay, Blake had a story to work on, and Barbara Gosnold came in as the designer, after the initially signed Roger Murray-Leach became unavailable - but that was not the end of the problems the production team had to contend with.

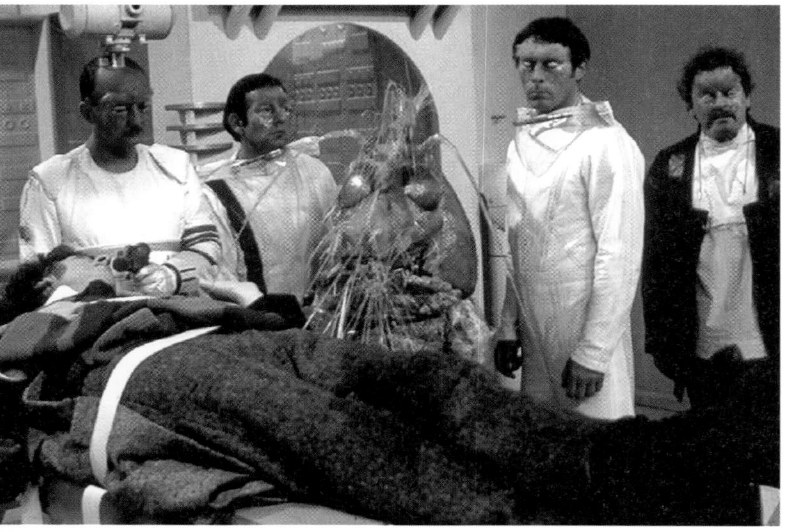

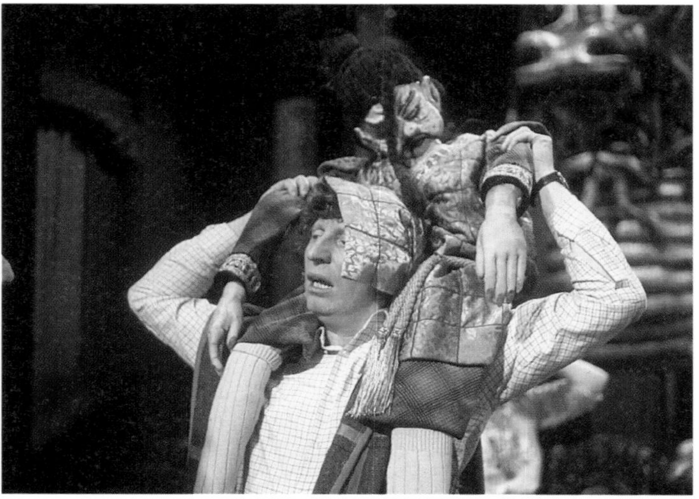

ABOVE: **Invisible Enemy**.
BELOW: The Doctor toys with a malevolent marionette during rehearsals for **Image of the Fendahl**.

Rehearsals for the rearranged first studio session started its two week run on 26 October, just over a week after completing *Underworld*. Then the regular 'Crackerjack Clock' strike kicked in.

Williams:

"It always happened towards the end of November, and it was basically a dispute between the props department and the electricians' department over whose job it was to turn the clock on at the start of *Crackerjack* every Friday. Studios were all blacked out, and only the important shows, of which *Doctor Who* was not deemed to be one, got the floor space when it ended. We were given one studio block, a couple of days' filming and all the rest had to be done using Outside Broadcast cameras."

Apart from that crisis, another last minute rewrite came when Louise Jameson told Williams that she wanted to leave the show.

Williams:

"Things were a bit tense between Tom and Louise and I'm certain it was nothing to do with her but with the character of Leela. She wanted to go, however, and there was little we could do about it. I vetoed the idea of killing her off, because it would have ended the season on a grim note, so we married her off to one of the characters on Gallifrey and had her stay there."

The production began with a couple of days' shooting all the model sequences that were needed at the Bray studios at the beginning of November. The one three-day studio block the story had, which went from being *The Invaders Of Time* to *The Invasion Of Time*, started on Sunday 6 November in TC8. Location work began in mid-November with two days being spent at a sandpit.

After that, the unit moved to Saint Anne's Hospital, an abandoned building in Surrey where the old Mental Wing was suitably redressed for both filming and recording. The old lift, stairs and various corridors were used, before the crew moved on for a day spent at the swimming pool in the British Oxygen Headquarters in Hammersmith. A two week break followed while Williams and Blake planned out where to do the rest of the story.

Blake:

"It was a nightmare all around, tempers were frayed and Tom was getting angry over the way the show was being treated by the BBC, saying, 'Anybody would think we were a flop', or words to that effect. We didn't have any studio time left, so after a couple of weeks' break, we went back to the Hospital. It had worked out for the first few days, so it only seemed logical to go back."

The editing was completed four days before Christmas, just managing to work within the rule that the entire season had to be finished before the end of December.

With Jameson now gone, the team broke up for their holidays over Christmas, returning in January 1978 to start work on the next season, with Tom Baker due back in March. There had been a distinctive slump in the ratings for the year as a whole, which had begun with *Horror Of Fang Rock* on 3 September. It was now dipping as low as just under seven million viewers, although by the time *The Invasion Of Time* hit the screens, it got over eleven million viewers in the first two episodes.

Williams had wanted to run an interlinking theme through the stories of season fifteen, but the problems with *The witch Lords*

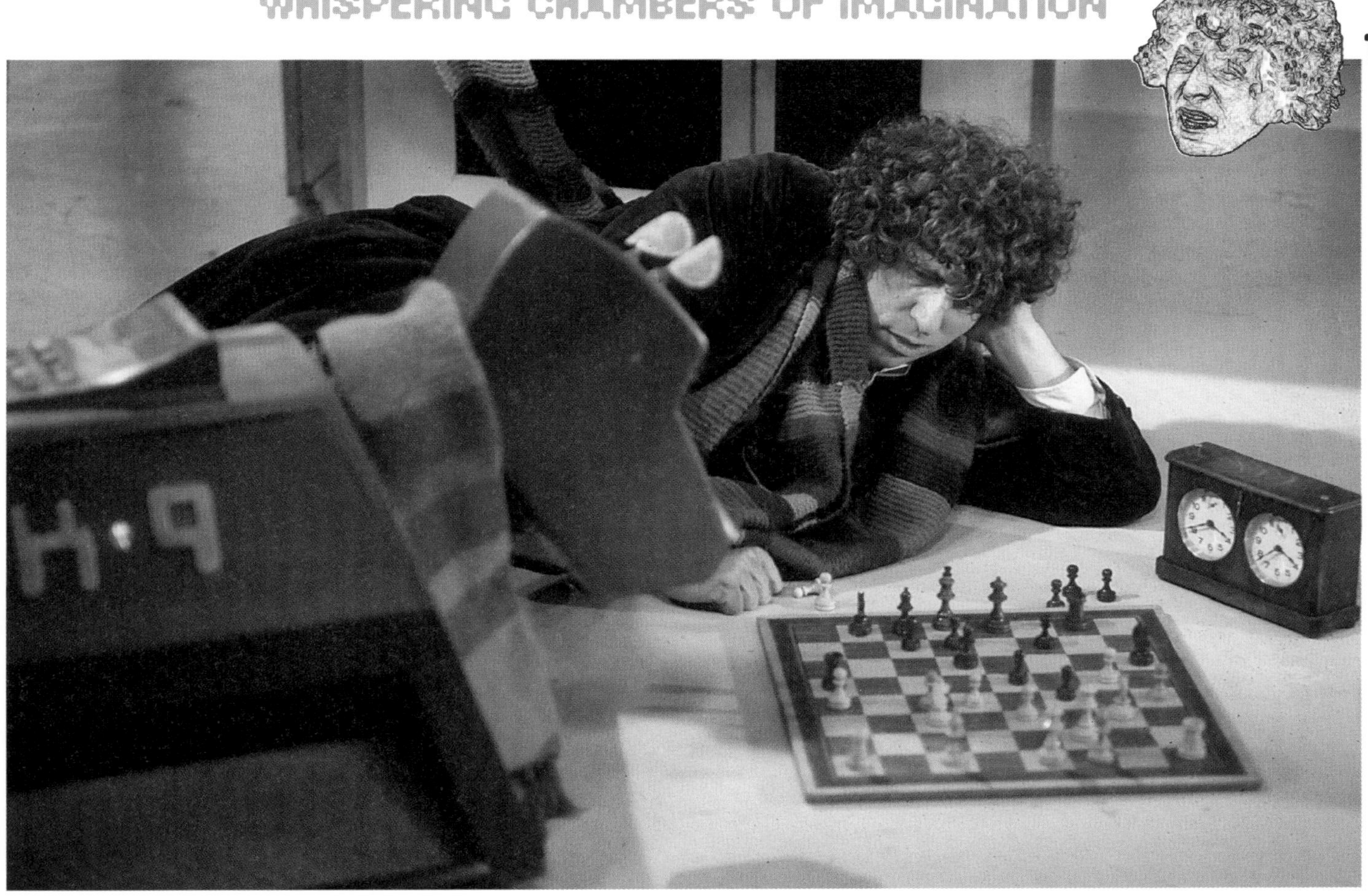

Master and hound at play in ***The Ribos Operation****.*

had prevented him from doing this. When Anthony Read joined the production team, Williams worked with him on drafting up a plan for the sixteenth season that would involve this idea, and came up with the plan of having each of the six stories act as part of a quest that the Doctor had to fulfil.

Williams:

"I'd always been fond of epic serials, and I wanted to try and run what was effectively a 26 part story throughout the year. By bringing in the White Guardian and the Black Guardian, and the task of having to assemble the bits of the Key to Time for the good guy to right all universal wrongs before the baddie got hold of it, we gave the Doctor a strong purpose.

"The immediate problem that I caused for myself was that the entire season had to be made in story order as broadcast. With each story leading straight into the next one, you couldn't juggle any of them around if one needed more work than the next, and shift episodes to later on in the year. It became restricting and as a consequence, by the middle of the year, it was driving all of us mad, especially Tom."

Robert Holmes was by now available to write for the show again, and agreed to start the season off with *The Ribos File*, which evolved into *Operation*, and then the final *The Ribos Operation*, which would introduce a new companion.

Williams:

"I had a brainstorming session with Tony Read and we decided that there had been enough screaming girls, and that the new one would have to be the exact opposite of Leela, because there was no way that Tom would have tolerated having another killer on board the Tardis. We went for an 'Ice Maiden' approach with a woman who was cold, totally aloof and totally detached.

"We saw literally hundreds of hopeful girls, who were all wonderful and awful in equal proportions, and in a way, Mary Tamm, whom we eventually chose, was not ideal. This is in no way intended to imply that Mary is not an exceptional actress, she's just too nice a person in real life and we ditched the idea of Romana's cold character."

George Spenton Foster was brought in to direct the first studio-bound story, with Ken Ledsham as his designer, who came up with the snow-bound 'gothic' look that Holmes' scripts called for.

Holmes:

"The thumb-nail rule that Anthony Read was working on was not to directly introduce jokes into the scripts, but to bring elements of pastiche and subtle parody into the stories, which would lead to a humorous edge. I mean, it was quite clear that whatever you gave Tom, he would play to the hilt, so when you brought in the larger-than-life characters, the sparks started to fly between the actors.

"When you watch Tom, there's a look on manic glee in his eyes on screen which I don't think was acting. It was him enjoying the duel of acting styles with the other actors. That *Key To Time* Season brought in people like Peter Jeffrey, John Woodvine and Simon Lack, who were equally as strong as Tom, and I think he enjoyed that element, if nothing else."

The Ribos Operation was completed over the next three day studio session in TC4, which ran from 23 to 25 April. Pennant Roberts was waiting to begin rehearsals on the next story, *The*

Pirate Planet, with a few days of rehearsal for the location sequences the story required, before the cast and crew departed for South Wales. The fields, caves and the interior of a power station had all been found in and around Gwent.

Filming took place for five days from 1 May, working around the Brecon Beacons, Abercave Caves and the Berkley Power Station. Designer Jon Pusey had to disguise the entrance to a disused railway tunnel to act as the way into the Pirate Captain's city. The original plotline, about a Time Lord being held inside an aggression absorbing machine, which powered a vast structure that could materialise around worlds and absorb all their natural energy, was penned by a new writer to the series by the name of Douglas Adams. His workload at that period was pretty intense, as he'd won a commission at exactly the same time to draft up scripts for a radio series, which he'd title *The Hitchiker's Guide To The Galaxy*.

Graham Williams.

"Bruce Purchase (who played the Pirate Captain) took the idea of the character to quite an extreme. It was tactfully pointed out that he was turning into a sort of robotised Captain Bligh, which was probably exactly how Douglas had written it, but Pennant let him practically imitate the Charles Laughton version from *Mutiny On The Bounty*. That was fine in itself, but it got a bit competitive between Bruce and Tom - there was a bit too much eye-rolling going on for that one!."

The story was finished, again working in TC6 on June 5th. Exactly a week later, cameras began to shoot the location material needed for *The Stones Of Blood*, which Read had commissioned David Fisher to write as *The Nine Maidens* while *The Invasion Of Time* was being rewritten. Darrol Blake was directing what was effectively a landmark for the show. *Doctor Who* was now fifteen years old, and *The Stones Of Blood* was the one hundredth serial.

Williams:

"We did go through rehearsals for a scene where the Doctor and Romana had a birthday cake with a hundred candles on it, with K9 wearing a party hat, but when we got to the studio it was just a case of, 'on second thoughts...' It struck me as being a bit self-congratulatory, slapping your own back, that sort of thing."

Fisher was on a double commission at the time, so he was effectively drafting up the final versions of the next story's scripts while *The Stones Of Blood* went down to Oxfordshire for five days of filming from 12 June. Blake needed a stone circle, and after the legendary Stonehenge in Wiltshire had been ruled out due to the fact that it was open to the public and only a couple of hundred yards from a major motorway, Rollright Stones was found as an ideal substitute, and was suitably augmented with a few extra BBC polystyrene rocks.

Additional filming was carried out at a nearby quarry, which doubled as a cliff-edge for scenes where Romana is meant to fall down the rock face, and Professor Rumford's cottage exteriors were shot at Redd Cottage in Little Crompton. Tom Baker remembers the late Beatrix Lehmann, who played Rumford in her last television performance, with great affection:

"She was a wonderfully eccentric character, who seemed to have been in showbusiness since the term was invented. I don't think many people realised she was as old as she was, because the energy and vitality she displayed for a woman of her years put the rest of us to shame."

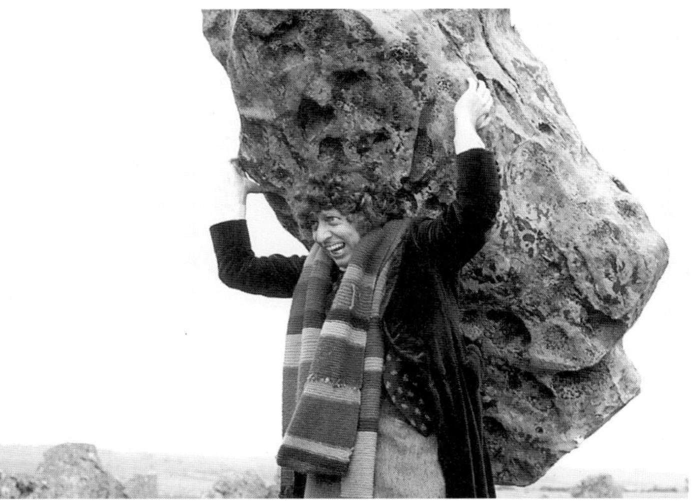

Baker demonstrates a feat of strength, albeit with a prop boulder, on location for **Stones of Blood**.

Fisher's next script, which director Michael Hayes was now working on, had gone from being called *The Seeds Of Time* to a title that revealed its inspiration, *The Prisoners Of Zenda* (Fisher was using a classic movie/book as his inspiration, in a tradition established by Robert Holmes). The production team felt this was painfully obvious, so it entered production as *The Androids Of Tara*. The designer was Valerie Warrender.

The scripts called for a fortress of some kind to be used, and Hayes secured permission to use Leeds Castle and it's grounds for the five days of location work that the story had been given. The cast arrived on 23 July, and recording began on the 24th, running until the 28th.

Williams:

"We had this ancient fishing rod that was worth a fortune and a much valued treasure by it's owner, who was all to happy to have Tom using it in the story - happy, that is, until Tom cast off his first line. Tom being Tom, he swore blind that he was a maestro with the rod and line, but he didn't know what the heck he was doing, and this thing that was worth about £500 took off from his hands, slowly sailed through the air as everyone's jaw hit the ground, and landed in the river. While the PA's were diving in to retrieve it, Tom just stood there, eyes bulging, put a hand over his mouth in mock horror and said, 'Whoops!'"

Robert Holmes completed his second script for the season, and felt that he was 'drying out' as far as ideas were concerned on *Doctor Who*. This came to a head with *The Power Of Kroll*.

Holmes:

"I just couldn't get it to work at all. Graham wanted to do a story with the largest monster that had ever been seen in *Doctor Who*, I mean, it had to be as big as the Albert Hall, and that was a near impossible brief to begin with. I knew we were going to get in trouble from that moment onwards, because Tony Read didn't want a repeat performance of the Ribos script with more, as he put it, 'outlandish rogues', so I had to produce a straight drama with a scenario that was ideally suited for being one of the more humorous stories.

"The whole idea of the *Key TO Time* season as whole was by that point becoming very restrictive. Each story had to basically be a quest to find where a particular segment was, and then the Doctor had to resolve how he was going to get at it. Tony wanted the monster to be the segment in my one, so I literally had to have the Doctor find a way to poke a hundred foot high squid in the guts with his locator device. It was a nightmare, and I didn't really want to do any more after that. It was about five years before I went back to do another script."

Michael E. Briant, now shooting *Blake's Seven*, knew the story's director, Norman Stewart, very well socially and found that he was not at all happy working on *Doctor Who*. He found the technicality of the show very demanding, and found handling the complex CSO work on both *Underworld* and *Kroll* near impossible.

Stewart took the cast and crew down to the Iken marshlands in Suffolk. A large part of the filming was carried out on the River Alde, and the crew had to move on continually because of the rising water levels, which were caused by the ever changing tides in the area.

Williams:

"There were a hell of a lot of problems on *Kroll*. All of the shots had to be lined up ensuring that nothing blocked the horizon, so that the model shots of the creature could be put in during post-production, and that took up a hell of a lot of time. And then there were the Swampies, who Norman Stewart decided he wanted to be green, so these poor sods had to be sprayed the colour of wet grass every day, and the stuff just wouldn't come off. The make-up girls had to scrub them down, and their skin was red raw every morning, only to be painted again for the next shots that they were needed for. I really felt for the extras on that one."

Stewart went on to the Bray studios during the following week to work on all the scenes where the Kroll was actually seen on screen. Some scenes were put together using stop motion animation. The story had a couple of working titles while Holmes was developing the scripts, moving from *The Shield Of Time* to the far more apt *The Horror Of The Swamp*, before finally settling on the one used for broadcast.

Bob Baker and Dave Martin's *Armageddon* had the difficult task of winding the Doctor's quest up, and they were working to specific plot points that Anthony Read laid out clearly in his brief to them. So far the segments had been solid matter, with the Kroll, they became living. For a final twist, the last one was going to be a human body. Don Giles moved on after designing the sets for *Kroll*, and Richard McManan-Smith took up that post as he joined Michael Hayes, who had been brought in to direct the six-part finale, his second story that year.

Hayes carried out several days work filming at Ealing before beginning on the studio sequences. With no location work, *The Armageddon Factor*, as it was finally called, would be entirely studio bound and completed in nine days.

Williams:

"*The Armageddon Factor* worked surprisingly well, because I think Mike managed to put together an extraordinary cast and gave the whole thing a doom-laden look that was really dark. We didn't know it at the time whether Mary (Tamm) was willing to stay on for a second full year because we were also going to lose Tony (Read had only ever wanted to stay for one full year), so when she said she wanted to leave, it was a clean sweep all round.

"Lalla Ward was playing the Princess, and she seemed to spark with Tom, which was unusual. He was getting slightly predatorial and some of the directors were beginning to get a bit nervous of him, because in fairness to him, he carried the show and had been doing so for a hell of a long time, so if it wasn't right or a scene wasn't working, he blew his stack. He was a perfectionist to an alarming degree."

The first three day studio block ran from 5 November in TC3, with the second running from 20 to 22 November in the same facility. With Tamm now wanting to move on, Ward's work was effectively becoming a protracted audition piece.

Williams:

"Bearing in mind that Mary might jump ship, we kept an eye on Lalla to see whether she had the right qualities for being a companion, and more importantly, whether she could keep up

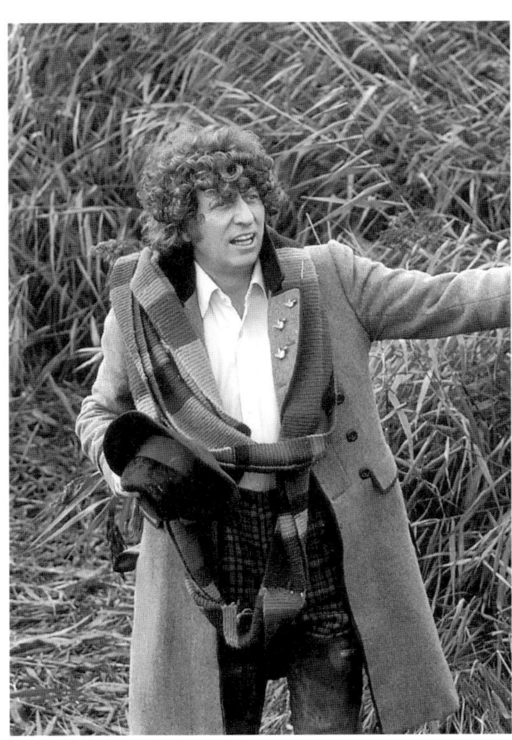

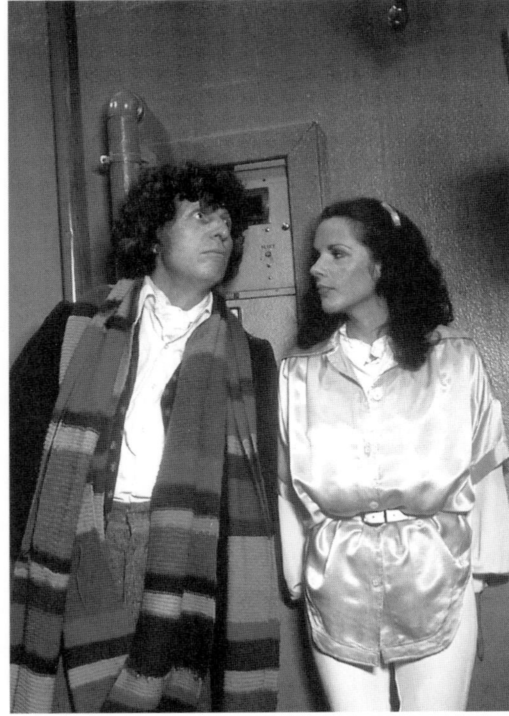

RIGHT: Suffolk's Iken Marshlands was the location for **The Power of Kroll**.
FAR RIGHT: Mary Tamm, as Romana, was the Doctor's companion for season sixteen.

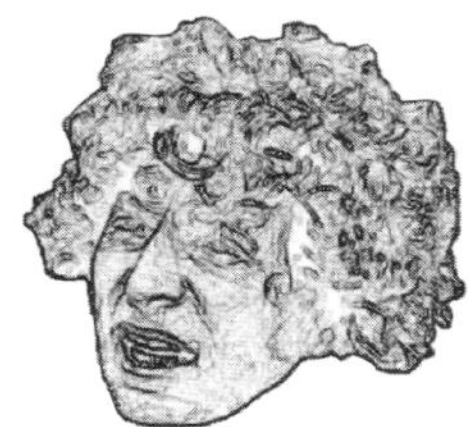

with Tom's frenetic pace. She passed with flying colours and became everybody's ideal choice to take over."

The final three days took place from 3 to 5 December, once again in TC3, with the story completed on time and on budget, which had been extremely tight as there had been considerable costs entailed from the extensive location work that was done on the earlier stories.

Williams had also found a new script editor:

"Douglas Adams had produced an intriguing story with *The Pirate Planet*, and seemed to understand the mechanics of how science fiction operated, which was exactly what we needed in a script editor. Tony had planned out several stories, keeping well away from any linking themes, as the *Key To Time* had nearly driven us insane, so Douglas basically had to come in and keep things rolling along."

Several ideas were toyed with over what to do with the Doctor's new companion, including making her a roving archaeologist, but Williams eventually hit on the idea that seeing as she was a Time Lord, why couldn't she just regenerate like the Doctor? A decision was made to have her taking on the form of Princess Astra (Ward's character in *The Armageddon Factor*), reasoning that seeing as she was dead, there was no harm in taking on her form.

Season sixteen started transmission on 2 September, with episodes averaging between seven and a half to nine and a half million viewers. Strangely, the most disappointing story as far as the production team were concerned, *The Power Of Kroll*, hit the ratings high for that year, when episode two achieved close to twelve and a half million viewers. On the whole, there was a noticeable, steady decline in the popularity of the programme, which only two years previously had been scoring an average of over ten million viewers per episode.

Williams:

"We were all too aware of the ratings and how they were falling, because the annual review always pointed this out all to clearly. Every year, a bit more seemed to be carved off the budget for the season, and we became more and more restricted in the scope of what we could do.

"When my final year's worth started to go out, one of the other producers in Union House wandered past in the corridor and said, 'Saw the show, getting a bit wacky, isn't it?' and I didn't see what he was getting at - but, in retrospect, we were going way over the top with the comedy, and I should have pulled in the reins, but I didn't and I have to admit that I had a far better time with season seventeen than any of the others. By that time I'd settled in, and was actually began to enjoy myself in the job."

The only script that was ready for production when Baker returned from his holiday was by David Fisher, and Christopher Barry returned for a final time as director to helm *The Creature From The Pit*, with Valerie Warrender joining him as the designer for the story. Adams had to call in scripts as quickly as possible, and one idea to boost the ratings was to bring an old foe back.

Williams:

"I hated the thought of doing a Dalek story, but there was a lot of pressure to wheel the damn things out again, so I agreed and we asked Terry Nation to do one. They struck me as being a bit hopeless; if they hadn't realised after so many defeats that this Doctor chap was pretty bad news as far as the guys from Skaro were concerned, then perhaps it was time for them to take up a different career - but, no, they were as stubborn as hell, and kept coming back for more. I thought that was ridiculous."

As with season sixteen, David Fisher was asked to come up with a second story in a row, and was drafting up *The Gamble With Time* as *The Creature From The Pit* began filming. Barry had planned out several days of filming at Ealing so that a sufficient space was available for the jungle sets that the scripts called for. Ward arrived for the rehearsals, with the plan being to establish the changeover of bodies for Romana in the Dalek story, which would be the first to be screened when transmission began in September.

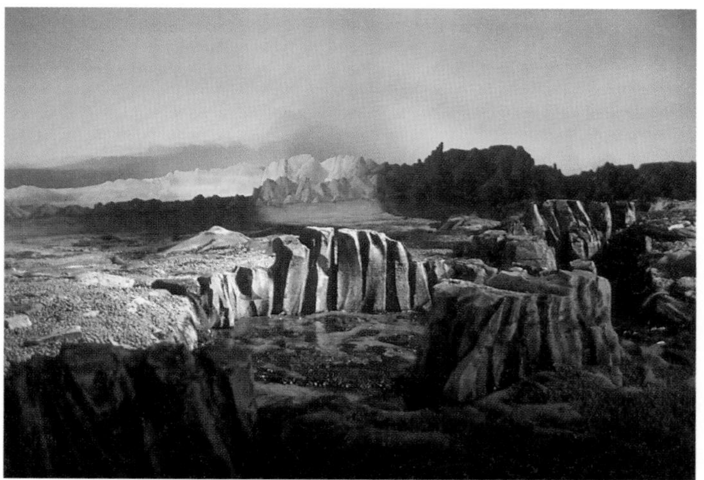

Prehistoric backdrop for **City of Death**.

The first appearance of the 'Creature' of the title in studio reduced the cast to tears, when they were confronted with what Williams described as a "Gigantic, puce green, decaying phallus..."

The monster was meant to be a vast, shapeless blob, with a single tentacle. Williams blames a breakdown in communication between Barry and the visual effects designers for what resulted.

Tom Baker:

"When it came to the point where the Doctor is bravely trying to communicate with the creature, the script said, 'He picks up the tentacle and blows on it, to see if anything registers'. Well, with the resulting tentacle being the shape that it was, and being an actor of great tenacity, I got through it, but the comments from the studio floor and the control gallery are barely printable, let alone repeatable..."

Subtle changes were made to the creature by the time the second studio block was staged so that it didn't look so suggestive when actually filmed. One of the minor parts in the cast was played by Morris Barry, who had directed three Troughton stories, and had by this point retired and taken up acting as a career instead of sitting behind the camera.

John Leeson was unavailable for the recording sessions for the entire season, so another voice artiste was hired to bring K9 to life. David Brierly completed five stories before Leeson returned for season eighteen. Williams had been costing out whether it was possible for foreign location filming on the tight budgets the production team were contending with for each adventure, and concluded that with only a skeleton camera crew and essential cast, it was possible, and it was to this end that *City Of Death* was created.

When *The Gamble With Time* had been drafted, both Adams and Williams found that the Bulldog Drummond elements that Fisher had wanted to incorporate far outweighed the number featuring the Doctor and Romana. It just didn't work as a *Doctor Who* story, so both producer and script editor had to start again from scratch, and penned the resulting four-part serial in a matter of a couple of weeks under a joint pseudonym.

Michael Hayes returned to direct for the programme once again, working with his *Armageddon* designer, Richard McManan-Smith. The *City Of Death* unit left for Paris on 30 April, with the basic plan being to cover as many of the famous landmarks as they could in four days. Williams had promised his head of department that the whole exercise could be done for the same costs as filming for the same period at Ealing, so it was essential that everything went according to plan.

The scenes that had to be completed had been planned out and rehearsed carefully in London, and the cameras started to run practically as soon as they arrived in Paris, with the afternoon of the 30th spent working outside an art gallery in the Boulevard St. Germain. On one of the final takes, the alarms were accidentally set off by Baker when he pushed against the doors (the gallery was shut for May day celebrations). Williams recalled that the production unit manager, John Nathan-Turner, was left to explain what had happened when the authorities arrived, because everybody else had fled.

All the cafe exterior scenes were completed at the Cafe Notre Dame on Tuesday 1 May , while the action on the following day moved from the Rue de Vielle du Temple, to both the top and bottom of the Eiffel Tower, before completing a brief sequence outside the Louvre Gallery.

Tom Baker:

"The memory of filming in Paris is one of haste and speed, blurred into one fast journey form one location to another. Very tiring, very energetic, full of colour and light, and tremendously enjoyable. We apparently achieved some record for the amount we shot in the amount of time we were there. Nobody recognised us, so there were few delays."

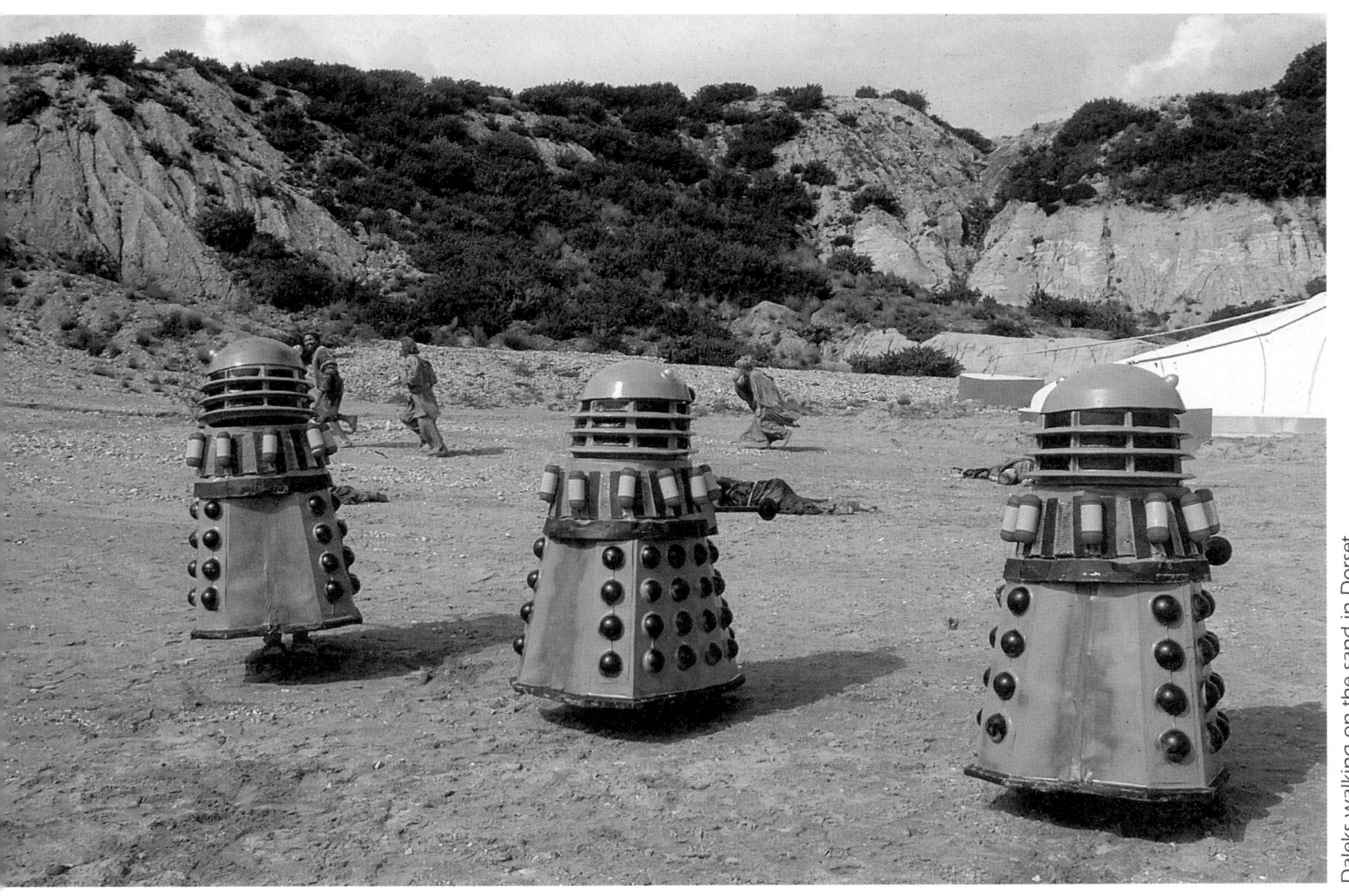

Daleks walking on the sand in Dorset.

On the final day, 3 May, the crew went back to the Boulevard St. Germain, on to Rue St. Julien le Pauvre and Rue St. Jacques, before finishing at the Boulevard St. Michel. The cast and crew then flew back to London.

Williams:

"I seem to remember that Tom wanted to give us a guided tour of some particularly fine wine cellars he'd heard about, but much as I'm sure everyone would have loved to have joined him,

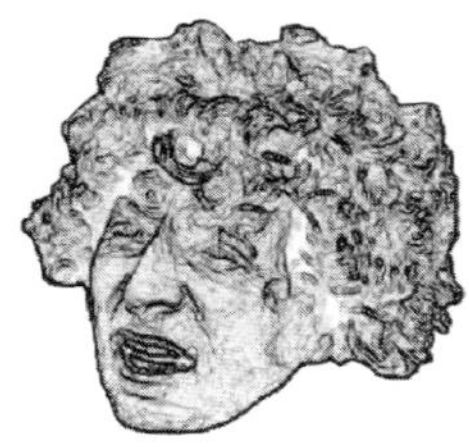

there just wasn't the time. We got back on our knees. Mike Hayes had worked minor miracles on that one."

City Of Death was finished on 5 June with John Cleese and Eleanor Bron making brief cameo appearances during an afternoon on the Louvre Gallery set. This resulted in one of the most notorious 'staged' out-takes from the entire series, with Baker standing on the set as Cleese approaches him with one of the BBC postcards of the Doctor, which were the standard issue for sending out whenever anyone wrote in asking for an autograph. He asks Baker to sign it for his nephew. Baker says he'd be happy to, but is unable to find a pen in his voluminous pockets and asks Cleese if he has one. After a pause, Cleese tells him not to worry, saying he'll tell him it's been signed, and that he won't know the difference because he's blind!

A week later location filming started on *Destiny Of The Daleks*, which Nation had completed. This adventure saw the return of Davros, from *Genesis Of The Daleks*. Michael Wisher was sounded out about playing the character, but was touring in a play in Australia, so the role went to David Gooderson, an actor with considerable radio experience. He was hired by director Ken Grieve in the hope that he could do a passable imitation of Wisher's characterisation but this did not work that well.

Five days of location work started on 11 June, with the production team moving around Dorset from the Winspit Quarry in Swannage to nearby Binneger Heath. The Daleks had deteriorated dramatically since they were last used, with the casings now looking broken, chipped and cracked. There was no time to set up any tracks for the operators to move them along as Michael Briant had done in *Death To The Daleks*, so it was up to the operators to physically lift the casings up from inside and walk them across the sand as best they could. Whenever they were seen moving, the cameras were positioned in such a way so that the feet sticking out from underneath could not be seen.

Williams:

"I honestly didn't think that it was worth carving a big chunk out of the budget to build new ones. There wasn't the time, and I didn't particularly want to use them that much on screen, so we genuinely had to sellotape the ones we had left to get them through the shoot."

The Daleks arrived at TC3 for the studio recording on 2 July, with the first session finishing the next day. All the scenes with Davros were completed on one of the blocks as the character was not used on location. The Tardis scenes saw the regeneration of Romana, with three different actresses playing different 'bodies' as she selected her new form, before settling on the likeness of Princess Astra.

Williams:

"Douglas came up with the idea of having a different regeneration for each story of the season, with the joke being that she could never make up her mind which one she preferred. When we asked Tom what he thought, he said he'd quite like to have a parrot as his companion so it could sit on his shoulder and listen to the Doctor's 'infinite wisdom'."

Destiny Of The Daleks was completed in TCl on 17 July, leaving Baker and Ward free to begin rehearsals on *Nightmare Of Eden*, which marked the first solo script for the series by Bob Baker. *The Time Warrior* director Alan Bromly was hired by Williams to direct with Roger Cann as his designer.

Williams:

"I think Alan had a pretty rough time with the last one he'd done, and said as much in fact while he was in prep, but I reckon he must have thought that things had moved on and got a lot better, when in actual fact, they'd got worse.

"Alan basically resigned and walked out on the whole show midway through that first block in the studio. The whole camera script for the first three days had been done, so I sat in the director's chair and called all the shots, so all of his planned sequences were recorded. I had to take over fulltime, because he didn't want to come back, so I had to rehearse the cast for a couple of weeks and do the next block, although I let Alan's name stay on screen as there would have been a few political problems if Graham Williams went up as both producer and director. Adams had brought Anthony Read back to fulfil an ambition of his, never realised during his time as script editor, to write an adventure based on the mythological legend of Theseus and the Minotaur. The title went from the rather lurid *Lair Of The Dark Lords* to *The Horns Of Nimon*.

Williams:

"It was all rather extravagant and bizarre, and was the atypical example of how our designers tried to twist the human form beyond recognition and ended up making it patently clear that the villains really are just men in monster costumes. It just didn't work.

"The best villains in any science fiction literature are always humanoid. It puts them on an equal level with the hero, so they are equally matched. I was put under a hell of a lot of pressure to bring back the Master, after Philip had used him, but we never got the right kind of script, so it never happened."

The Horns Of Nimon was entirely studio bound, with Kenny McBain directing and Graeme Story working as his designer, with all his sets for the city corridors that the story featured being based on the designs of computer circuitry.

*Davros returned in **Genesis Of The Daleks**, seen here in rehearsal.*

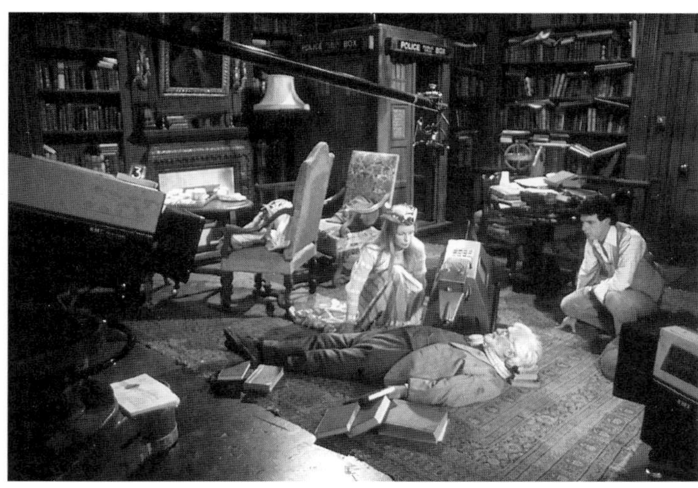

Professor Chronotis' study in **Shada**.

Williams:

"We got a choreographer in to try and co-ordinate the movements of the Nimon, but no matter how hard they worked, they still looked like men in high heels and black tights, wearing rather bogus bull-masks."

The story was completed over three final days running from 7 October. Pennant Roberts was in pre-production with the season's finale, which would mark the last work on the series by Williams, who had decided to move on after three stressful years. Victor Meredith was working as the designer, and the scripts were by Adams, who called upon his college years at Cambridge for the setting of *Shada*. The working title was originally *Sunburst*.

Adams had wanted to write a script where the Doctor's mood swings finally getting the better of him as he goes into a self-imposed retirement, having grown sick and tired of having to save the universe every day of his life. The producer intervened, with Williams feeling that it would go against everything the programme had established about the character by turning him into such an anti-hero. Redrafting ensued, and *Shada* took shape.

The main setting for the story was the rooms of a Cambridge professor, who was in reality a Time Lord with his chambers being his Tardis. There was little choice other than to go to the place itself, and have Professor Chronotis's environment be as accurate as possible. Following a couple

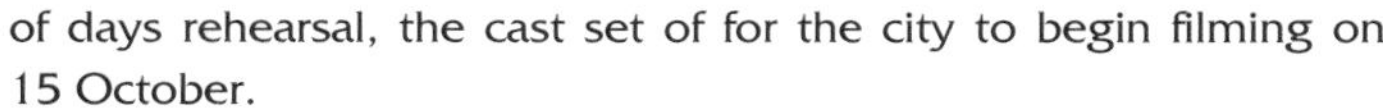

of days rehearsal, the cast set of for the city to begin filming on 15 October.

Over the five days there, the unit moved from Emmanuel College, for the exteriors of Chronotis's chambers, to the section of the River Cam behind the colleges, where Baker and Ward were filmed punting for an afternoon. A bike chase was shot around Botolph Lane, Trinity Lane, King's Parade, Saint Edward's Passage and the road and bridge leading off from Garrat Hostel Lane. Portugal Street and Portugal Place were also used, along with King's Parade.

For scenes around the villain's invisible spaceship, Skagra, the main high street and specifically the meadows around the nearby village of Granchester were used. The final day's work was completed on the 19th, after which everyone returned to London and studio rehearsals began. Only one was completed, from 3 to 5 November in TC3, before a technician's strike at TV Centre stopped any further work on the story.

Williams:

"The sets were about to go up, in fact several of them had already been built (In TC6), when we were told that we had to stop work. There was no way of salvaging the story, so we had to end with *The Horns Of Nimon*, which was a sad way for me to go out, but there was nothing that could be done."

Williams production unit manager for the past three years, John Nathan-Turner, had been suggested as an ideal candidate to act as associate producer for season seventeen, but internal politics prevented this from taking place. He was, however, offered the chance to take over from Williams when Williams left.

Williams:

"There were a lot of things we tried to do while I was working on *Doctor Who* that didn't work and, equally, there were a lot of things that we did that I feel proud of. It was a strange mixture, and it nearly drove me mad making the programme, but again equally, some days were the happiest of my professional life in television. It was a completely unpredictable mix. You never knew what was going to hit you next..."

Ratings wise, season seventeen picked up considerably, compared to season sixteen, with *Destiny Of The Daleks* and *City Of Death* both getting over fourteen million viewers for some of their episodes. It came to an end on 12 January 1980, with the new producer's plans for a major revamp for season eighteen being well underway.

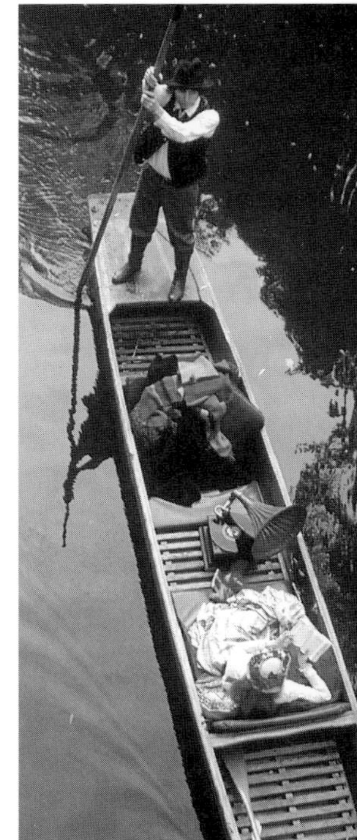

LEFT: **Shada** - Lalla Ward as the regenerated Romana, who had been with the Doctor since **Destiny of the Daleks**.
RIGHT: **Shada** - The Doctor punting with Romana.

CHAPTER 7

CHASING THE SHADOWS WITH LIGHT

CHASING THE SHADOWS WITH LIGHT

CHASING THE SHADOWS WITH LIGHT

"In one episode I actually shot Peter Davison but this was in no way an attempt on my part to get his job!"

COLIN BAKER interviewed – July 1985

"There is no law that dictates that when the Doctor regenerates, he shouldn't turn into a woman. I don't see any reason to suppose that the Doctor should always be played by a man."

Tom Baker's departure from *Doctor Who* made the headlines when it was confirmed on 24 October, 1980. In the ensuing mass of interviews he undertook, this simple speculation gave the reporters even more copy, but John Nathan-Turner had by this time already selected the actor he wanted to play the fifth Doctor. It was confirmed that the role would stay male on Tuesday 4 November, when confirmation of the casting was featured as one of the stories on the BBC's *Nine O'clock News*. Baker would make the news again a few weeks later on 13 December, when he married his former companion, Lalla Ward.

Peter Davison was already a familiar and popular figure with television viewers, thanks to his work on *All Creatures Great And Small*, in which he had been playing the role of Tristan Farnon since the series made its debut in 1978. Nathan-Turner knew him, having worked as the programme's production unit manager for three years, and felt he was the ideal choice to draw a wider audience to *Doctor Who*, as he had proved to be very popular with the younger and female viewers who followed *All Creatures*.

The offer was made to Davison via a telephone call one Saturday morning midway through October, which took the actor aback completely, as he could not visualise himself as being suitable for the role. Remembering that he had the same doubts about playing Tristan, he got back to Nathan-Turner after a few days and said, 'Yes'. The contracts had been finalised on the same day that the news broke - his first day in the studio in January 1981, when the regeneration scene from fourth to fifth Doctor was recorded.

Production was due to commence on his first full year, season nineteen, in March when Fielding, Sutton and Waterhouse would start work on the first story. With the first few storylines being commissioned in October, seven stories had to be produced to fill the 26 episode run with six four-parters and a single two-parter (to avoid having to make a six-parter, Nathan-Turner revived the format which had last been used in 1974 on *The Sontaran Experiment*), and Bidmead started to work with his replacement script editor, Anthony Root. Bidmead had only ever intended to stay for one full year, and Root was brought in for three months to act as a temporary replacement while Nathan-Turner looked for someone to take up the post full time.

One of the earliest decisions made was to record the first few stories out of broadcast sequence, to allow Davison time to settle into the role, before the crucial debut story was recorded. The first to go before the cameras would be *Four To Doomsday* which Terrence Dudley was drafting.

Dudley:

"I'd spoken to John Nathan-Turner about writing for the series while we were doing *Meglos*, and he was not adverse to the idea, so I came up with a storyline about a race of frog-like creatures, who thought they were gods. The whole notion was to play on how extreme authoritarianism can go whenever a Dictator gains not so much the control, but the trust of a race."

Christopher Priest was also working on *The Enemy Within*, which dealt with the revelation that the Tardis had been powered by a creature trapped in the core of its engines, which starts to fight back as it suddenly regains its will power. Eric Saward had been brought in to draft four episodes of *The Visitation*, and Christopher Bailey's *The Mara* underwent a title change to the more cryptic *Kinda* by the beginning of 1981. Dozens of other storylines and scene by scene episode breakdowns were accepted by other writers, and it was Root's job to sift through them for any workable material and turn the remainder down.

Work began on *Four To Doomsday* by the second week of March, with the story being planned out as an entirely studio-bound story,

One of the first problems that had to be overcome was to finalise the costume for the Doctor, with the idea being to give him the appearance of a Victorian Cricketer. This partly came from a photograph Nathan-Turner had of Davison playing in a charity cricket match, from his days on *All Creatures*, which had made the producer think of him for the part of the Doctor in the first place. With a cricket jersey, striped trousers, frock coat, question marked lapels and a cream panama hat, the outfit was completed with a stick of celery in the coat lapel – a last minute suggestion made by Nathan-Turner.

The creatures featuring in the story, the Urbankans, were described by guest actor, Stratford Johns (famous for playing Charlie Barlow in *Z-Cars* and the subsequent spin-off series, *Barlow At Large*) as being, 'Bloody big frogs', with the elaborate facial make-up alarming the actor when he first arrived to start work in the studio.

TC6 housed the sets for the first three days of recording, which started on Monday 13 April, with Davison's first scenes in the Tardis control room being completed and finished on Wednesday 15 April. The next day, the new Doctor's costume was unveiled before the press, with the actor carrying a cricket bat, standing outside the Tardis prop, which had wickets chalked onto one of it's doors to complete the effect.

Problems started to arise with the scripts for the rest of the season at this point, as *Zeta Plus One* proved unworkable, with the writers unable to fulfil Nathan-Turner's revised brief of bringing

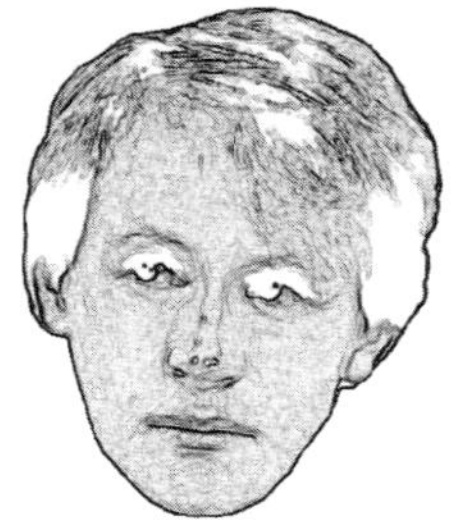

the Master back in the story. Anthony Ainley had proved to be popular, and the producer wanted to carry through the plot thread left open ended at the end of *Logopolis*. To this end, a new story was quickly commissioned, with Bidmead returning to start work on *The Visitor* which was due to be finished by the end of the month.

Root was now moving on, and Eric Saward, who had just completed writing *The Visitation*, joined the production team as the new full-time script editor. *Four To Doomsday* was completed on Thursday 30 April, and rehearsals began on Friday 1 May for *The Visitation* for a day, with the cast joining Director Peter Moffatt (which is, incidentally, Peter Davison's real name. He had to change it when he joined Equity) on location in Black Park in Buckinghamshire, for four days of shooting.

The first appearance by a Terileptil, Saward's new race of monsters featured in the story, with the name coming from a play on the words Territorial Reptile, came on the days spent at the second location for the story, Tithe Barn, also in Berkshire, which doubled for the exterior of the manor house featured in the serial.

The heavily padded body suit, with a scale-patterned latex exterior, concealed the actors completely. The heads were a complex radio controlled mechanism, with the lips and eyes being worked off camera by a visual effects operator. A microphone within the mask picked up the dialogue as the actors spoke, saving the problems that were normally encountered by the boom microphones being unable to pick up the voices which were slightly muffled under the latex.

With the finale of the story revolving around the great fire of London down Pudding Lane, it was obvious from an early stage that all the sequences actually involving flames would have to be staged in a controlled environment. So Moffatt and the crew worked for two days at the Ealing film studios with several glass matte shots being used to create composite images of the Tardis landing in the 17th century streets.

Kinda was now complete and Peter Grimwade had been appointed as the director, with Malcolm Thornton as his designer. Bidmead had changed *The Visitor's* title to *Castrovalva*, which was now a direct sequel to season eighteen's last story, picking up from the closing moments of *Logopolis*, and *The Enemy Within* had been scrapped altogether. Saward was writing a second story to take its place, with *Sentinel*, which Anthony Root was overseeing the editing for as a final duty on *Doctor Who*.

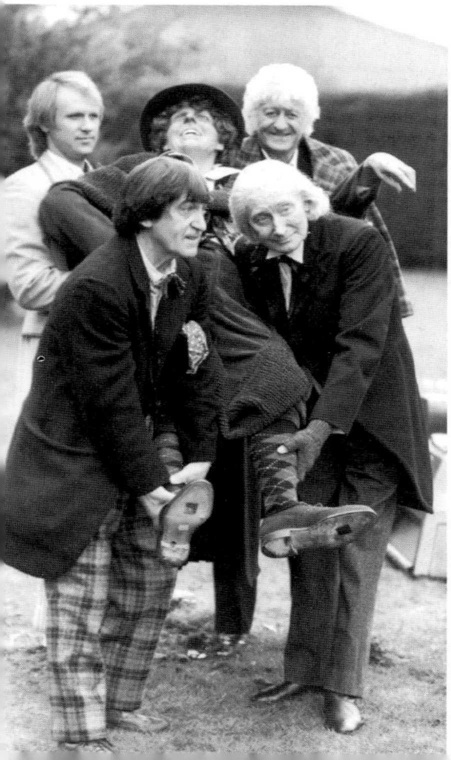

Peter Davidson joins his previous incarnations for a publicity photograph. Tom Baker was unavailable but Madame Tussaud's provided a substitute.

Work now began at the Acton Rehearsal rooms on *Kinda*, which would once again be a studio bound story. The money saved on having *Four To Doomsday* made in such a way had been ploughed back into the location budget for The Visitation. Any savings on *Kinda* would go towards the extensive shoot that would be required for Castrovalva, which was due to start filming at the beginning of September. By working this way, the budgets always balanced out in the end.

Grimwade's first recording block ran from 29 to 31 July 29th, with all the scenes inside the main dome being completed. Grimwade recalled the relationship between Matthew Waterhouse (Adric) and guest actor, Richard Todd:

"There was an idea to try and get a bluff, Colonel Blimp figure in to play Sanders, and it was a real stab in the dark to see if Richard Todd would come and do it. I mean, this guy was a huge film star in the 1950s and 60s, so I thought we'd get a polite thanks, but no thanks, but he said he'd be delighted to come and do it. I'll always remember Matthew taking him to one side, and giving him advice on how to react to cameras in a TV studio. Richard was very courteous and showed interest, Peter Davison's jaw hit the ground though."

A vast amount of real and fake foliage had to be brought into the studio to create the jungle sets required, which could easily be moved around between recording breaks to effectively create a new setting. Due to the fact that the script was never redrafted to accommodate for the late addition of Sarah Sutton to the regular cast, Bidmead wrote in some brief scenes for the beginning of the first episode, following on from her collapse at the end of *Four To Doomsday*, to explain that she would spend the duration of the story resting in the Tardis. This meant that Sutton was only needed for a single day in studio.

The second recording block ran from 12 to 14 August, with the final scenes of *Kinda* being completed with the appearance of the Mara itself, a gigantic snake. The resulting effect on screen was basically achieved by using a huge puppet, supported by wires on a pulley system rigged to the roof of the studio. No matter how complex the video effects were that Grimwade grafted on to the final edits, and no matter how fast he cut around the prop, the fact that it was no more than a puppet could not be disguised. A mental note was made to try and address this problem when production began on the sequel story, which had an early title of *Dreamtime*, which was commissioned while *Kinda* was still in production as both Nathan-Turner and Saward were pleased with the finished product and felt that the Mara should be brought back as quickly as possible.

Following two weeks of rehearsals with director Fiona Cumming, location filming began on Davison's debut story, with Janet Budden joining her as the designer for *Castrovalva*. Five days were spent in total, with the unit returning to Black Park in Buckinghamshire, to film all of the forest scenes, while the remainder of the exterior material was staged around Harrison's Rocks in Kent, with Davison's newly regenerated and injured Doctor scrambling across the climbing range to try and get to the planet's main city.

To create a highly stylised look, Budden based her sets on the extraordinary work of M.C. Escher, whose precise sketches of buildings constructed around forced perspectives and oblique angles had become famous during the 1920s.

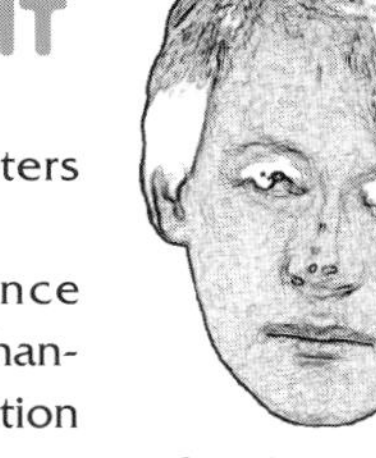

Castrovalva was completed with all the interior city scenes, including the vast town square set being erected in TCI, where various stairways and balconies were incorporated into the structure. Anthony Ainley was also present to record his scenes as the Master, with the three day block running from 29 September to 1 October. Saward, meanwhile, had changed the title of his next story to *Earthshock*, with Grimwade now working on the camera scripts for what he planned as a very cinematic story, determined to bring a fast pace to the serial which would basically be studio bound. Before that, however, a two part story by Terrence Dudley had to be completed.

Dudley:

"I sent in a storyline shortly after I'd finished *Meglos*, along with the proposal for *Four To Doomsday*, but Chris Bidmead didn't like *The Beast* much, as it was called then, but Eric did and I reworked the whole thing with him until it became *Black Orchid*. The whole thing was basically a bit of a showcase to show off the fact that the new Doctor liked playing cricket, so we put plenty of jokes about whether he knew the Master (a nickname of the famous W.G. Grace) into the dialogue, but I don't know whether everybody knew what we were getting at with that one..."

Black Orchid was technically the first purely historical story to be included in the programme since *The Highlanders*, and required several days of location work around a 1920s manor house. Nathan-Turner had spotted an ideal site in the shape of Blackhurst House in Kent, while *Castrovalva* was on location, so after a period of negotiation with the owners, the crew moved there with the story's director, Ron Jones, for four days from 6 to 9 October.

Prior to this, a day was spent on at the vintage Quainton Railway Station and at a nearby house down Quainton Road, which stood in as a Police Station, in Aylesbury. All the shots revolved around the Tardis materialising at the station, and then trying to get the Police Box back after it had been moved to the Police compound.

For the shooting at the house, designer Tony Burrough had to organise the construction of a false section of roofing for the fire sequence, as gas canisters had to be hidden to produce the required smoke, while a dozen or so extras were brought in for the party scenes for the earlier part of the story. Vanessa Paine was hired to act as a double for Sutton, as part of the plotline revolved around one of the characters being her exact double.

Castrovalva.

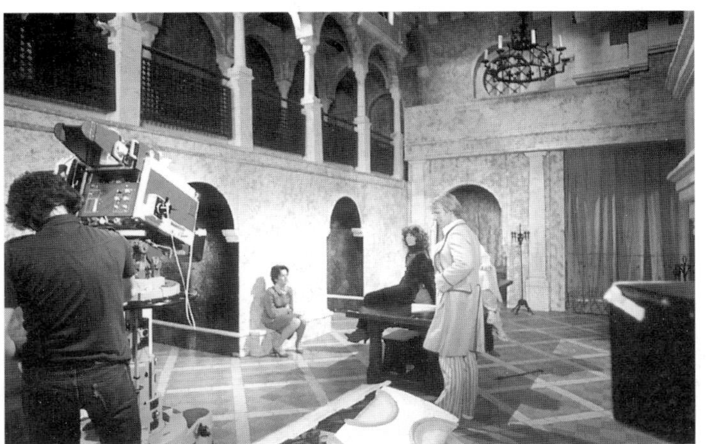

Seven years had passed since *Revenge Of The Cybermen*, and Nathan-Turner agreed with Saward's suggestion to bring them back when *The Enemy Within* fell through. A free-lance company made the new costumes, keeping only the distinguishing features that made the Cybermen instantly recognisable, and basically revamped the entire appearance of the creatures. A pilot's thermal insulation suit was used to cover the body, painted a suitable shade of silver with several additional pipes added, and the hands and feet were covered with padded gloves and moon boots, again, both sprayed with silver paint.

The head masks were cast in fibre glass and had the chin section cut away and replaced with a clear piece of plastic. The actor's chin, covered in silver make-up, could be seen moving whenever a Cyberman spoke, and rather than being a separate part of the costume that had to be fitted on separately, the chest units were now incorporated into a section that draped over the shoulders, and locked into the base of the mask. Several extras experienced extreme claustrophobia due to the fact that the masks had to be held onto the head by a back plate, which was screwed into place. The sound of the screws tightening behind their heads was more than enough to unnerve them, and it took at least fifteen minutes to get them out.

The Cybermen actors quickly found that there was an uncomfortable side effect to playing the creatures as the fibre-glass shell of the mask continually rubbed against their noses, leaving them red-raw by the end of the day. This soon gained the nick-name of 'Cyber-Nose', and there was little that could be done to reduce the problem. If any padding was put in the helmet to stop it, there was a danger that it could block the reception of the microphones within the costume, which slightly distorted the actors voices. The days of having a single actor perform all of the dialogue off-camera were now long gone.

TCI housed the vast freighter storage bay sets, where all the shots of the Cyber-army breaking out of their canisters were staged using a multiple-camera effect to create the image of hundreds of troops marching towards the screen, by spreading the image of the same eight actors across the picture three times. Designer Bernard Lloyd's sets were built so that sections of canisters could easily be moved around within the space available to create different areas of the hold.

Matthew Waterhouse completed his final scenes for the story from 24 to 26 November when Adric was killed off.

Time Flight began life with the working title of *The Xeraphin*, and Ron Jones, whose work on *Black Orchid* had impressed Nathan-Turner, was asked back to direct the new story, with Richard McManan-Smith working as his designer. With a plot involving a Concord being dragged back through time, the first thing the production team had to do was try and get permission to film around one of the aircraft, and luckily, Heathrow Airport were all too happy to oblige, They agreed to let the film crew work around one of the planes, and shoot material inside one of the Passenger lounges as well, over two days at the beginning of January. Negotiations with British Airways and the British Airports Authorities had taken many months to reach this stage, and now it looked as though the story might get affected by a BBC strike.

THE DOCTORS

After *Earthshock*, the regular cast broke up for their Christmas holidays for a longer period than usual, due to a dispute causing the studio blocks for *Time Flight* to be moved to the beginning of 1982. To make matters worse, the costs of *Earthshock* meant that there was only a very tight budget available for Jones to work with.

Due to industrial action, the second recording block was cut down to one single day, when in reality at least three would have been needed. This placed incredible pressure on production team but by by rapidly working through the material all day, rather than just recording in the evening, the story was completed in TC8 on 3 February.

With season nineteen completed, work continued through March as rehearsals began on *Snakedance*, Christopher Bailey's sequel to *Kinda*, which was planned as the second story for season twenty. Nathan-Turner was keen to bring back an element of the programme's past in each of the stories for the anniversary year, and the return of the Mara was apt as a representation of the most recent series villains. Fiona Cumming was set to direct, with Jan Spocyznski as her designer.

Several sequences were shot at Ealing, where several live snakes were used for scenes featuring the character of Dojan (played by Preston Lockwood) who had no dialogue but featured throughout the story and completed his work in a single day.

Plans were now underway for the next story, which Johnny Byrne had been commissioned to write, with *Arc Of Infinity* moving from the studio bound setting of Gallifrey to the location scenes set in Amsterdam. It was part of Byrne's brief to bring the character of Omega back, having been featured in the tenth anniversary story, *The Three Doctors*, in 1973. This was another of the returning elements that Nathan-Turner wanted to utilise.

While *Snakedance* was being completed, recce work was being carried out by Ron Jones and his production manager for the five day shoot that was planned for the beginning of May. Remembering the difficulties and resulting criticism of *Kinda* with the final manifestation of the Mara, the visual effects department created a far more sophisticated prop for the final scenes of *Snakedance*, with a slender latex creation which was operated with wires running up through the neck and air-bags, operated off-camera, which inflated and deflated to move the head on cue.

The Brigadier meets himself in **Mandryn Undead**.

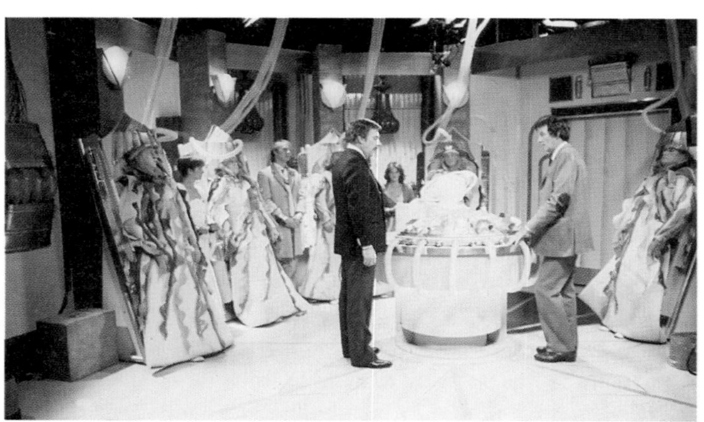

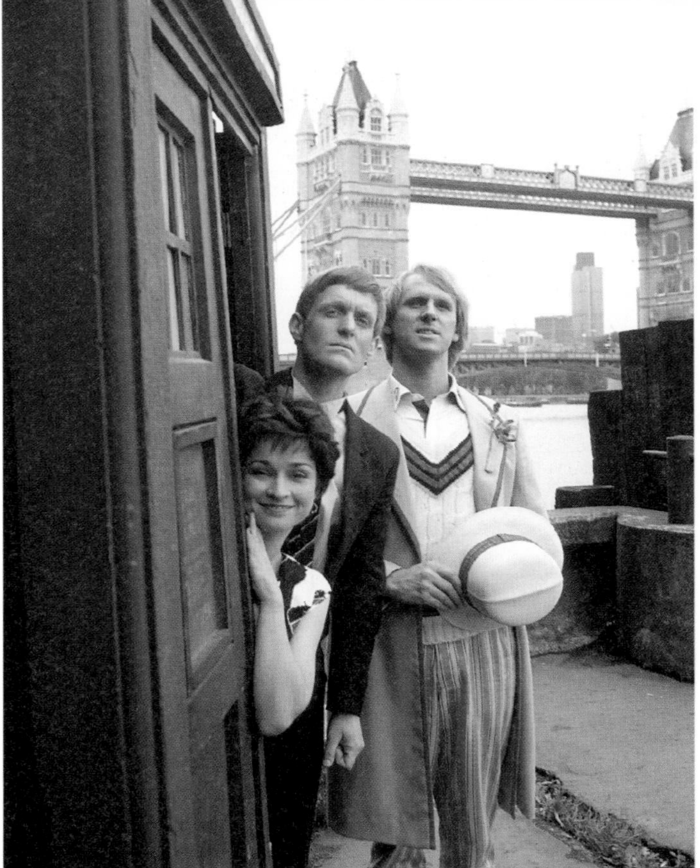

The Doctor, Tegan and Turlough, together for the last time in **Resurrection Of The Daleks**.

Following a brief runthrough on the scripts, the main cast and crew departed for Holland on Monday 3 May, setting up the camera equipment as they got there and staging all the scenes of Tegan's arrival at the Schiphol Airport. The rest of the day was spent working round the Muntplein town square and flower market.

Jones:

"The whole thing about going to Holland was that we had five days of shooting, with practically the free run of the place, so I tried to set out to make it look as though there was money well spent on that one. When I did the recce with John Nathan-Turner, we didn't have time to plan out the chase sequence between Omega and the Doctor at the end, so it was genuinely a case of figuring out where we could set up and shoot bits as we moved around the streets..."

Tuesday 4 May saw the completion of all the scenes around the youth hostels featured in the story, using Bob's Youth Hostel, before moving on to Singel, Herenstraat, a nearby Police Station, Blauburgwal, Hoopman Bodega, and finally a second Youth Hostel. Amstelveld, a nearby flower stall, and Huis Frankendael on saw Davison playing both the Doctor and Omega, with the renegade Time Lord's body print of the fifth incarnation of the Doctor rapidly decaying. Wearing a blue boiler suit with green latex plastered across his face, Davison had to charge through the streets with the camera crew well out of view, while the general public could only stare at the scene in disbelief.

The complex confrontation scene at the Lock gates, south of the Skinny Bridge, were staged on Thursday 6 May, with Davison changing costumes to play both characters. The final day was spent using a telephone kiosk, the Dam Square and Damrak, before finally flying home on the evening of Friday 7 May. Studio rehearsals began thereafter.

One of the actors cast in one of the minor roles, as Commander Maxil, was Colin Baker.

Jones recalled:

"Colin basically went for the part with his teeth, and made far more of it than I think anyone else would have done. He gave the character a very strange quality, making him very sinister and basically, you couldn't help but notice him. He had a helmet with plumes of feathers on it, which I think he called something like Esmerelda, because he thought it looked like a rather excited chicken. That's the kind of guy Colin is, and I was delighted to see him eventually take over from Peter."

Season Nineteen had finished on 30 March, with the ratings picking up considerably compared to season eighteen, with an average of between eight and ten million viewers, and a high being achieved by *Castrovalva* episode four, which hit ten and a half million.

Saward was now planning out the remaining five stories of the season, while Nathan-Turner was beginning to set plans in motion for a special anniversary story for the twentieth anniversary day on 23 November 1983. The basic idea was to make a 90-minute special which would reunite as many of the Doctors and companions as possible. The extra money that would be needed to make it had been agreed with his head of department, and he was sounding out both actors and directors. Patrick Troughton was one of the first to agree to appear, and Robert Holmes was asked to write the script.

Holmes:

"It was like one of those blank jigsaw puzzles, where there's nothing but white bits that you have to try and fit together. I had a go, and came up with this notion of the Nestenes invading the matrix on Gallifrey, and having a twist at the end with Pertwee's Doctor turning out to be an Auton, but I backed out soon afterwards. It seemed an impossibility, right from the beginning..."

Meanwhile, Peter Grimwade was completing the finished drafts of a story called *Mawdryn Undead*, which he had submitted as an idea to bring back William Russell as Ian Chesterton, with the action taking place around a boy's school where he was the resident history teacher. This was not the only element the story would feature.

Grimwade:

"John (Nathan-Turner) was fond of doing these interlinked trilogies (*Full Circle* to *Warrior's Gate*, and *The Keeper Of Traken* to *Castrovalva* both have follow-through plots), and wanted to bring Valentine Dyall back as the Black Guardian.

"So, I put all this together, and then at the last minute, the Chesterton thing didn't work out, so we brought the Brigadier into it instead. I changed his character to a maths teacher, but it still seemed off having him teaching, but there was no time to change it by that point..."

Nicholas Courtney was happy to return to the series, as was Dyall, who had previously appeared as the Black Guardian in the final episode of *The Armageddon Factor*. The cast returned to start rehearsals with Peter Moffatt as the director in the first week of August, with Stephen Scott as the designer.

Courtney had complex costume and make-up changes as he was playing two different versions of his character, in both 1977 and 1983. This plot thread was left over from the drafts of the script that featured Chesterton, with 1977 being chosen as a recognisable year from the recent past, as it had been the Queen's Jubilee year. The plot threw some of the past continuity of the programme into chaos, as it effectively claimed that the Brigadier had retired midway through his years with UNIT.

The system Moffatt used was to complete all of the scenes featuring one version of the Brigadier during the morning session, whereupon Courtney changed costume and donned his moustache to play the other Brigadier for the evening recording sessions. This was complicated at one point, where the two Brigadiers meet each other, and a double was brought in to help achieve this effect.

Regular *Blake's Seven* director Mary Ridge was brought in to helm the next story, *Terminus*, which had been written by *Warrior's Gate* author Steve Gallagher. With Dick Coles working as her Designer, she planned out the story as a simple six day studio bound shoot, with one day spent working at Ealing. Mark Strickson had now joined the cast as Turlough, having stayed on with the Tardis crew at the end of *Mawdryn Undead*. *Terminus* marked the departure of Sarah Sutton as Nyssa, who decided to move on after two years with the series.

Strikes within the BBC began to effect the whole schedule for the rest of the year, and there was a continual possibility that the season would be cut short with only three stories completed.

A severely battle-damaged Dalek.

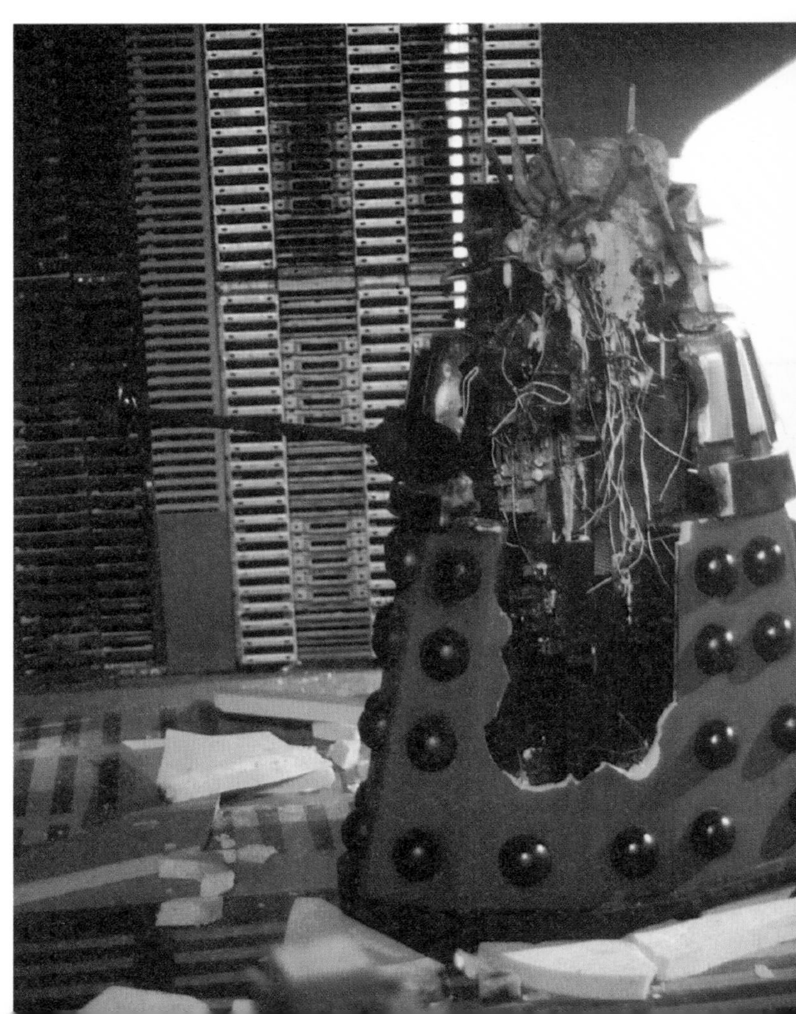

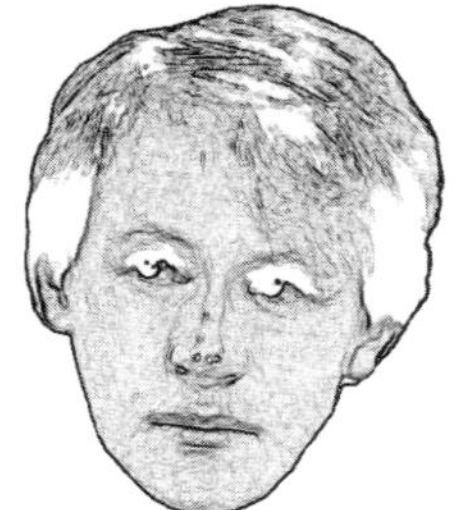

Terminus completed its first two days in studio on 11 and 12 October, and rehearsals began for the second block on the following week.

Recording continued from 25 to 27 October, but there were still several scenes that Ridge had not been able to finish, so the story was incomplete and Nathan-Turner had little choice other that to stage a remount. Fiona Cumming was now working on the next story, *Enlightenment*, by Barbara Clegg, which had the working title of *The Eternals*.

Dealing with a race through the space vortex in spaceships disguised as 19th Century clipper ships, scenes involving the cast on the decks of the vessels, and principally a sequence where Turlough falls overboard into space, had to be staged over two days at Ealing.

Rehearsals for the studio work on *Enlightenment* began on Saturday 6 November, and it was during this period that the electricians' strike at TV Centre kicked in, and the future of the remainder of the season suddenly looked doubtful. *Arc* through to *Mawdryn* were now ready for transmission, but *Terminus* had still not been completed, while *Enlightenment* had barely started. Saward had the final two stories ready for production as well, with *The King's Demons*, a two-parter by Terrence Dudley, and *Warhead*, a four-parter by Saward himself, which would bring the anniversary season to a close with the return of Davros and the Daleks. Tony Virgo was already working on Dudley's story as director, and Peter Grimwade was due to start pre-production to handle the Directing chores on WARHEAD just before Christmas.

No recording took place throughout November, but in an effort to try and salvage *The King's Demons*, three days of location filming were carried out. Three days of studio work was needed to complete the story, and this was due to take place from 18 to 20 December. In the end, the first day of this session was given over to completing *Terminus* and this had the knock-on effect of delaying *The King's Demons* . Consequently, *Warhead* was cancelled, the decision being made to use its allocated studio time in the new year to finish off the stories that were already underway, rather than start a new one altogether.

This brought the season to a premature close after only 22 episodes. The production team had to leave the problems of that season behind them, and start to concentrate on the anniversary special itself, *The Five Doctors*, which was due to start filming in March.

One of the main problems experienced on *The King's Demons* had been with Kamelion, a shape-shifting robot that was planned as being a new and unique addition to the Tardis crew. The character was a working animatronic prop, effectively a real robot, which was capable of many movements and expressions. The main difficulty was that one of the people who constructed the device had died shortly before studio work on the story had begun, and with him went the exact knowledge how to programme and operate the robot. As a companion, Kamelion was conspicuous by his absence from that point onwards, and would only make one more appearance in the programme.

Nathan-Turner had approached both Waris Hussein and Douglas Camfield about Directing *The Five Doctors*, but both men backed out, and the assignment was eventually given to Peter Moffatt. The script was by Terrance Dicks, who stepped in at very short notice to try and bring all the elements together that Nathan-Turner wanted the story to feature; a task that Robert Holmes had found to daunting to tackle.

All five Doctors had to play an equal part in the proceedings, while various companions and past adversaries also had to be included, but a major rethink had to take place when Tom Baker pulled out shortly before rehearsals were due to begin. Feeling that not enough time had passed between his departure and this new project, Nathan-Turner found a solution that would still enable him to include the Fourth Doctor in the story, by culling material from the Location work that was carried out for *Shada* in Cambridge.

Wasteland scenes were executed until 9 March 9th at Carreg Y Foel Gran in Ffestiniog, with all the cave and slate quarry material being completed after that in the nearby Manod Quarry up until 14 March, with 15 March being spent on the scene where the third Doctor and Elisabeth Sladen's Sarah Jane Smith are reunited along a country road near Gwynedd. The scenes of the second Doctor meeting Courtney's Brigadier Lethbridge-Stewart used the YMCA Hostel down Tilehouse Lane in Denham as the UNIT HQ (the same site used in *The Three Doctors*), and a aerodrome close by was used for shots of the third Doctor driving Bessie. Haylings House, also in Denham, was used as the Garden where the first Doctor is initially seen (Nathan-Turner had cast Richard Hurndall as a replacement for William Hartnell, having spotted the similarity when Hurndall appeared in an episode of *Blake's Seven* called *Assassin*).

In addition to Carole Anne Ford, who had returned to play Susan, other former companions asked to appear were John Levene, Deborah Watling, Louise Jameson and Katy Manning. In the end several ghosts were seen in the Dark Tower in the shape of Wendy Padbury's Zoe and Frazer Hines' Jamie, and Caroline John and Richard Franklin returned briefly as Liz Shaw and Captain Yates. Ainley's Master also returned, as a slight red herring for the story.

Troughton:

"It sounds like a terrible cliche, but suddenly being back with Frazer and Wendy, in the old costumes, and with the old Police Box in the corner, it genuinely felt as though we'd never left, yet something like fourteen years had passed."

Work began in TC6 on 29 March, with the Dark Tower Corridors and the tunnels where the first Doctor and Susan confront a Dalek being used, while all the main Gallifrey scenes were shot on 30 March. The interior of the Tomb of Rassilon, where all the Doctors would come together, and where the Master betrays the Cybermen (wearing slightly modified versions of the costumes from *Earthshock*, with lace-up footwear instead of moonboots) in the entrance hall, brought the story to its conclusion on 31 March. With the final edit finished by the end of April, it was eventually

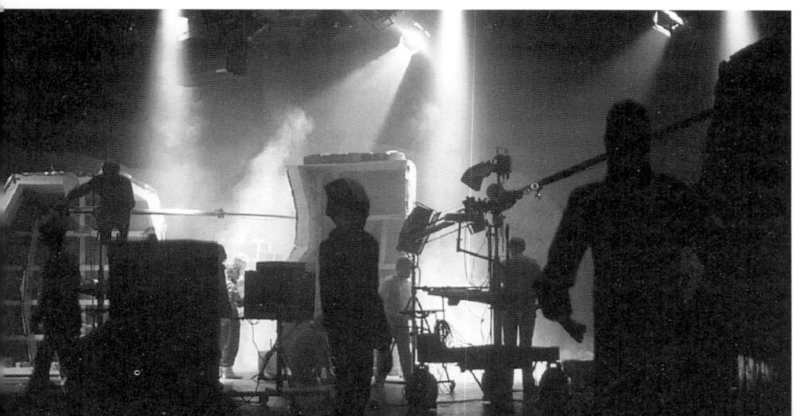

Atmospheric studio set for ***The Caves Of Andozani***.

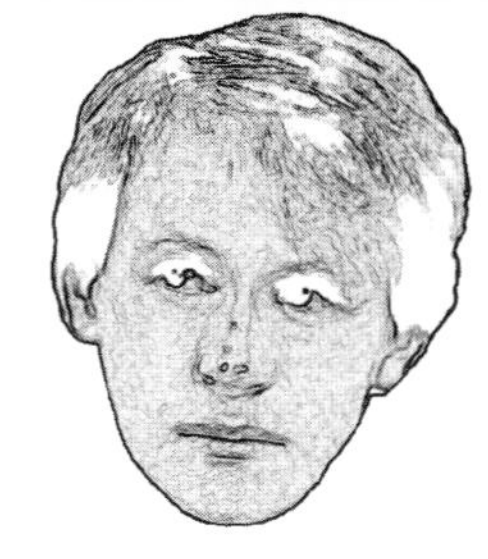

transmitted on 25 November as part of the evening's entertainment on the annual BBC charity appeal show, *Children In Need*, gaining a rating of over seven and a half million viewers, which was equal to the two highest rated episodes during season twenty,

Saward was now handling the first few stories of what Nathan-Turner wanted to primarily be a 'monster' season for the 21st year. Johnny Byrne was keen to write a story using Malcolm Hulke's creations, the Sea Devils, and Saward gave him the brief to write Hulke's other monsters, the Silurians, into the four part opening story for the following year, Pennant Roberts was brought back to direct, while Tony Burrough joined the team as his designer.

Both the Seas Devils and the Silurians were suitably redesigned, although their appearance was carefully based on their original 'look' from the early 1970s stories. The masks for all the creatures were made by a freelance company, with the Silurian heads equipped with a lever under the chin that moved the mouth as the actor inside said his dialogue, while the Sea Devils had two heads equipped with remote control eye-lids, enabling them to blink. The string-vest look was now replaced by a leather Samuri-like costume.

One of the more unfortunate aspects of *Warriors Of The Deep* was the Myrka, a giant sea creature that was operated in a similar way to a pantomime horse, but the special effects department were unable to complete the prop's construction in line with the standards they liked to keep, and made a formal request that it be withdrawn from the series. It was too late and Nathan-Turner had to insist that Roberts shot the creature as best he could. Nobody was pleased with the results.

Michael Owen Morris was already well underway working on the next story, a two-parter by Eric Pringle, which had started life as a four-part script called *Wargame*. It represented his directorial debut on television. Barry Newbery returned as the designer, marking his last work on the programme which he completed shortly before retiring from the BBC.

Four days of location filming was carried out around the villages of Shapwick and Blandford in Dorset, from Tuesday 19 July 19th to Friday 22 July. During the rehearsal period for the studio material needed for the story, the news broke on 28 July that Peter Davison was going to leave the series. He had never planned to stay longer than three seasons (Troughton had advised him to do as such when he told him he'd got the part in the first place), and planned to move on at the end of the 21st season.

Two days of location material had to be completed, so the cast were taken to the old spice dock area by Tower Bridge in London, where Sunday 11 September and Monday 12 September were spent working around Butler's Wharf, Curlew Street, Lafone Street and Shad Thames. Only one prop Dalek was needed, which was used for a sequence where it was pushed out of a loading bay in one of the warehouses, with the prop loaded with a suitable amount of explosives to cause a loud explosion when it hit the ground.

Michael Wisher was once again asked to play Davros, having agreed when *Warhead* was in pre-production, but this time he was unavailable, so Terry Molloy was brought in to take his place.

Four standard slightly repaired grey Daleks were used, with one of the casings being painted black during the story, so it could double up as the Supreme Dalek.

Resurrection Of The Daleks would undergo a slight alteration to its format before broadcast, with the scheduling of the Winter Olympics curtailing the programme's twice weekly broadcasts to one 45 minute slot. The result of editing them together and the subsequent high ratings the story won would have long term effects for the next season.

Peter Grimwade was now no longer directing for the show, but his script work continued with *Planet Of Fire*, which would see the debut of Nicola Bryant as the new companion, Peri, and the departure of Mark Strickson. The now annual foreign location shoot was allocated to this story, with Grimwade having to work from the holiday snaps of Lanzarote from its director, Fiona Cumming, to get an idea of some of the settings. Her Designer was Malcolm Thornton.

Following a couple of days of rehearsal, the cast, with Anthony Ainley present once more as the Master, arrived in Lanzarote off the Canary Islands and began working from Friday 14 October at Papagayo Bay. The next day saw them move to the Mirador del Rio and the quayside around the shores of Orzola, after which they spent the Sunday resting before carrying on for the next three days around various sites at the 'Fire Mountain'. Following that, everybody returned to London.

Studio work began in TCl on Wednesday 26 October with the story's final block moving to TC6 from Wednesday 9 November to Friday 11 November. The final appearance by Kamelion was recorded at this point, with Gerald Flood returning to provide the character's voice. The finale for the fifth Doctor's era now got underway with a mixture of both old and new talent, as Robert Holmes returned to write the four-part *The Caves Of Androzani*, while director Graeme Harper made what would go on to be his highly acclaimed debut on the series with the story.

Holmes:

"The whole thing I tried to do with the Doctor in *Androzani* was to put the Doctor through hell, to have a convincing reason for a regeneration. This was going to be a fight to the very last breath in his body, as I thought the fifth Doctor had the potential to be heroic that was never quite realised on screen, so hopefully I managed to redress the balance for his swan song."

Harper had very specific ideas about how he wanted to stage the regeneration scene on the final studio day, which brought Janet Fielding, Sarah Sutton, Strickson, Matthew Waterhouse, Kamelion and Ainely back to record an insert of their character speaking to Davison, as they swirled in a myriad of images before his eyes as he died.

Harper:

"I wanted the whole image to be a vast, swirling mass of colour, with the Doctor's body slowly splitting open, like the old title sequence until BOOM! the new Doctor suddenly sits up. It was a shame that we didn't have time to get it just right, but we got close to what I wanted."

One critic described Davison's Doctor as a wistful dreamer who looked like a benevolent teacher, but had the mind of a genius. His popularity had drawn the series back into the limelight after the slump at the end of the Tom Baker era, and he left just as his character was beginning to hit its stride. Nathan-Turner felt that just one more season would have cemented his reputation as one of the most durable Doctors, but it was not to be. The era of the sixth Doctor was about to begin.

CHAPTER 8

THE TUNNEL AT THE END OF THE LIGHT

THE TUNNEL AT THE END OF THE LIGHT

THE TUNNEL AT THE END OF THE LIGHT

"I now know Colin as a colleague and a friend, and it's interesting when you hear his side of what happened, because it was all rather strange!"

SYLVESTER McCOY Interviewed – April 1993

"Well, Tom was there for seven years and a hell of a lot of stories, so I'm hoping to give it my best shot and see if I can break his record. I'm going to have a smashing time ."

Colin Baker entered into the spirit of taking on the role of *Doctor Who* with admirable enthusiasm. It was a refreshing change of direction for him as far as television work was concerned, in that his last regular role in a long-running series had been playing the villainous Paul Merroney in *The Brothers* for the BBC, which was followed with a stint as a similar sort of character in the mid-afternoon soap, *For Maddie With Love*. Now he was set to play the hero for a change, and was clearly relishing every minute of it.

When Peter Davison made it clear that he intended to leave the programme towards the end of season twenty one, John Nathan-Turner had to go through the awkward process of finding an actor to take over once again, for effectively the third time during his run as *Doctor Who's* producer (if you count casting Richard Hurndall as a 'new' first Doctor in *the Five Doctors*).

He had last worked with Baker during the recording of *Arc Of Infinity*, from May through to June 1982, and a change meeting occurred when they both went to the wedding of one of the assistant floor managers, Lynn Richards. During the afternoon, Baker basically kept the entire group that had gathered for the event highly entertained, and it struck Nathan-Turner that if he could hold the attention of a group of 'hard bitten showbiz types', these qualities might translate to the small screen and work with a far wider audience, if he were to play the Doctor.

In order to discuss this possibility, Nathan-Turner called Baker in to see him at Union House, with the actor thinking that it was about something as simple as opening a garden fete, as he had recently been seen in the series and Peter Davison wasn't available. To say that he was taken aback when he was effectively offered the role was an understatement.

So that Nathan-Turner could assess what Baker's approach to the role would be, he supplied him with a number of video tapes representing stories from each Doctor's era and arranged for a further meeting to discuss Baker's thoughts after he had viewed them. They met with Nathan-Turner's approval on his return, and Baker was then taken to meet the head of the department, David Reid (allegedly approving of the choice of actor, according to Baker, due to the fact that they had a mutual interest in cricket. Reid was watching the Test Match when they arrived, and a conversation about the latest scores quickly overtook the topic of the new Doctor), after which, a four-year contract was signed. Nathan-Turner wanted Baker to stay for that length of time, as he felt that three years was too short a period and that Davison had not been with the programme for long enough.

Traditionally, the regeneration from Doctor to Doctor took place at the end of a season, with the new actor's debut story starting off the following year. The exception had been the regeneration from Hartnell to Troughton, which had taken place two stories into season four. Baker would now arrive in the penultimate season twenty one adventure, with his debut story acting as the finale for the year. His brief scene for *The Caves Of Androzani* was completed on one of the final recording days for that story, with director Graeme Harper calling him in for an evening's work to supervise the complex effects sequence planned for the change-over.

For the sixth Doctor's first formal story, Eric Saward was working with veteran script writer Anthony Steven on the script which was called *The Twin Dilemma* Steven had been working in television since the 1950s, with many of the Sunday afternoon classic serials to his name, such as *The Three Musketeers* and *The Return Of The Musketeers*, but he was not finding *Doctor Who* that easy. Due to the fact that Robert Holmes finale for the fifth Doctor needed practically no editing at all, Saward was able to step in and perform a series of major rewrites on Steven's material, with a lot of work being carried out on episode four in particular.

The decision had been made that Baker's costume had to be as strikingly different to Davison's one as possible, and its designer, Pat Godfrey, was given the brief to make it as 'bad taste' as possible. One idea was to have the sixth Doctor in a dark suit, somewhat akin to the type worn by Delgado's Master during season eight, but that was ruled out at an early stage.

The results, which were presented to Nathan-Turner for approval as soon as the designs were completed, were a blazing array of perfectly coordinated colours, which was exactly the opposite of what he wanted. This Doctor had to be one that you couldn't miss once you'd seen him, and Godfrey had to try again and come up with something loud and aesthetically insulting. She succeeded, and Baker donned the costume for the first time when *The Twin Dilemma* went into studio, nearly a month behind schedule because of a strike that was affecting the BBC.

Rehearsals had started when the cast came together after their Christmas break, with Peter Moffatt being brought in to direct, with Valerie Warrender as his designer. Nicola Bryant was now the sole travelling companion on board the Tardis, and struck up an immediate rapport with Baker.

Because of the delays faced by the production team, there had been no time to stage the two days of location filming that were

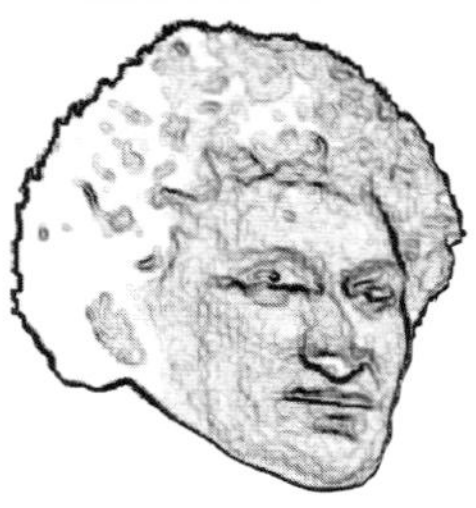

needed for the story. So in an unusual move, Moffatt had to break into his rehearsal time for the next studio block, and take the case and crew out midway through this period.

The simple requirements of a desolate landscape laid to ruin by the Gastropods, where the burning wreckage of a spaceship could be erected meant that one of the stock quarries had to be used. The team moved from Gerrards Cross Quarry in Buckinghamshire to Harefield Quarry in Rickmansworth, just on the outskirts of central London, from 7 to 8 February. It proved to be a difficult shoot, due to the fact that the wet weather turned the gravel into sludge and that because of the time of year, there were only five hours of suitable daylight each day. If the shots were not finished during that time, the set had to be abandoned because with the dark closing in rapidly, any thoughts of continuing filming were impossible. The Gastropods were used during this block. They were giant slugs, and the tubular costume only allowed the actors to shuffle along as their leg movement was heavily restricted. The lead creature, Mestor, required a detachable mask, as Edwin Richfield, the actor playing the role, suffered from claustrophobia and had to have it removed between takes.

Baker and Bryant were now given time off till May, when production was due to start on his first full year as the Doctor with the recording of season twenty two. Although the first episode of *The Twin Dilemma* drew over seven and a half million viewers, which was a slight dip compared to the conclusion of *The Caves Of Androzani*, its ratings continued to slide down to below six and a half million by episode four. Hopes were high for the sixth Doctor to make more of an impact with the opening night of the next season, and to this end, a decision was made to bring in one of the 'reliable' monsters as an added draw.

Earthshock had proved to be a popular hit during season nineteen and Nathan-Turner and Saward were keen to bring back the Cybermen. Gerry Davis had submitted a storyline called *Genesis Of The Cybermen*, which was effectively a prequel to *The Tenth Planet* but Saward rejected it, although the idea of making a sequel to an earlier story was used.

Work on *The Cold War* had begun towards the end of 1983, with Paula Moore taking the on-screen credit as the story's writer, although the actual text seems to have been heavily rewritten by Eric Saward. The idea of making it a sequel to *The Tomb Of The Cybermen*, with several other continuity linked references to past Cybermen stories, had come from Ian Levine who worked for several years with the production team as an unofficial continuity advisor on many aspects of the scripts. Two links with season twenty one's *Resurrection Of The Daleks* were also maintained, with the character of Commander Lytton being drafted into the storyline, Maurice Colbourne once again playing the role, while that story's director, Matthew Robinson, was hired to direct the new story, which underwent a title change to *Attack Of The Cybermen*.

The format of the programme itself was altered shortly before rehearsals began. The editing of *Resurrection Of The Daleks* into 45-minute episodes had been a great success, with the highest ratings of the season and a good audience response, so a decision was made to condense 26 25-minute episodes down to 13 45-minute ones, with the first one being *Attack*.

A certain degree of continuity was maintained in the casting of the story, with Micheal Kilgarrif returning as the Cyber-Controller, having originally played the part in *Tomb*, while David Banks was also brought back for a third time to play the Cyberleader. The story made the headlines during pre-production due to the fact that Koo Stark was cast as one of the Cryons, the native inhabitants of Telos where the Cyber tombs were built, but she pulled out of the production shortly before rehearsals began.

Kilgarriff:

"My death scene was rather spectacular with these severed pipes on my costume spitting green fluid all over the place, and I thought I'd better try and make it pretty impressive, so I literally went for it on the first take. I'm surprised I didn't kill Colin Baker in the process, but after I'd collapsed to the ground, with all this smoke and steam, they said it was all right, so I only had to do it once."

The Cyber-Controller was the only new costume made for the Cybermen, with the others reusing the ones from *The Five Doctors*. The Controller's head was basically the same mask mould used by the others, with a high dome on the top of the head and the 'handles' missing. The story was completed over three days in TC6 from Friday 5 July to Sunday 7 July.

Ron Jones was now casting around for an actor to play a highly unusual alien in *Vengeance On Varos*, which was due to start rehearsals a week later. The script had been completed by Philip Martin, who had originally submitted it as a story for Davison's Doctor featuring Tegan and Nyssa, called *Planet Of Fear*, which was later changed to *Domain* during its early stages of development, to avoid confusion with season twenty one's *Planet Of Fire*. Tony Snoaden took over from Marjorie Pratt as designer on the story as she finished off work on *Attack*.

Martin's original idea was to have the character of Sil, a representative from the Galatron Mining Corporation, as a small amphibious creature floating in a water tank. The use of puppetry was quickly ruled out, and Jones auditioned several midget and dwarf actors until he found Nabil Shaban and gave him the role. Shaban suffers from *osteogenesis imperfecta*, and as a result he is confined to a wheelchair due to his legs being underdeveloped. The costume department created a special body suit for him, with the head area being concealed within a hood, with a rim of latex make-up blending the skin of his face into it, while suitable colouring was used to blend his skin tones to match with the shades of his costume. Visual effects provided him with a mobile water tank to sit in, with a couple of 'Slave' extras continually dousing him down with a spray of the fluid as a link to keep the idea of the character as close to Martin's original concept as possible.

Martin:

"The whole idea revolved around trying to figure out what the entertainment industry of the future would be like and how the public's appetite could be sated. That evolved into having a prison planet where generations had passed and the original guards and prisoners had become the elite and their workers, who were pacified by continually being fed images of death and executions. The problem with the finished show was that the timing of the scenes was up the creek, and all the humour got trimmed out in the editing. To be honest, I thought it was far too grim in the end ."

While they were briefly reunited on *The five Doctors*, both Frazer Hines and Patrick Troughton found that enough time had passed for them to be able to enjoy making the programme again,

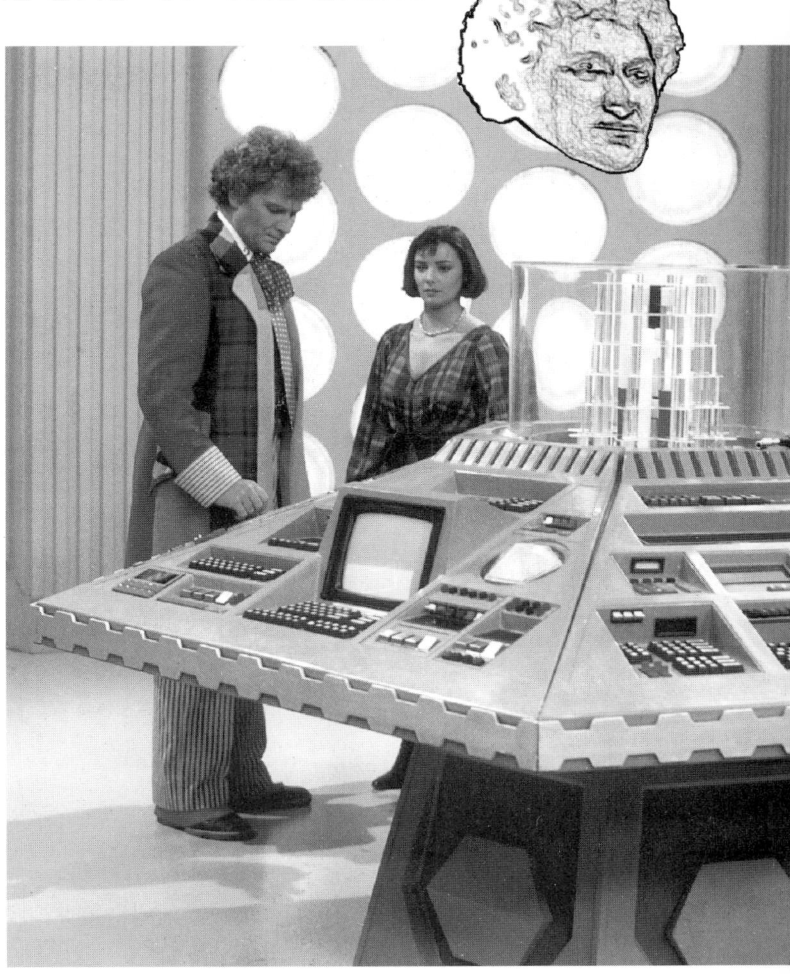
The new Doctor with Peni in **The Twin Dilemma**.

and they asked John Nathan-Turner whether it was possible for the second Doctor and Jamie to return for a one-off adventure. This brief was given to Robert Holmes to write as the equivalent of a six-part story, with three 45 minute episodes for *The Androgum Inheritance*, which was commissioned during October 1983.

Holmes:

"The idea was ancient, as I'd given it to Robert Banks Stewart while I was still script editing, saying, 'Do one where a race of alien gourmands come to earth to cull the population in order to eat them as fine cuisine'. I dusted it off as I really wanted to have another batch of aliens to write for, apart from the Sontarans, whom John Nathan-Turner was insistent on using in the story.

"My original brief was to set the whole thing around the jazz quarter of New Orleans and there was talk of having music obsessed aliens, but I realised how silly this was, and as New Orleans is also famous for its food, the gourmand idea worked just as well. When that fell through, there was talk of using Italy, but they ended up going to Spain. I found it far easier writing for Pat Troughton again than either Peter or Colin, as I knew how his Doctor ticked and I knew he loved rustic character parts, which is why I turned him into an Androgum at one point. If you rearrange the letters, that's actually an anagram of gourmand ."

The scripts were rewritten to match the requirements for location shooting around Seville with various sites scouted out by the production manager for the eight day shoot, which was due to start in the week following on from the completion of *Varos*. Peter Moffatt had been brought in to direct his second story with Baker, and Tony Burrough returned as the designer. The title was now confirmed for the serial as the more generic *The Two Doctors*.

After two days of rehearsal, the cast and crew flew to Seville on the 7 August. Moffatt and some of the team were already at work in Spain. The first four days were spent working around the grounds of a villa near Gerena, while the remainder of the shoot moved around the streets of Seville itself.

Troughton:

"There was a bit of a cock-up with the make-up and the wigs and such forth didn't arrive when we got out there, so poor old Jacquie Pearce (Jacqueline Pearce, of *Blake's Seven* fame as Servelan), John Stratton and myself couldn't shoot a dickie bird. We were being paid to lounge around in the sun by the hotel pool for a few days, which suited me just fine, until they got some fresh eyebrows and hair through.

"One night when we got back, there was no food, and I was starving, so I had to make do with the bag of wine gums I kept in my costume pocket and the contents of a hip flask, and I was what you could call a bit 'Uncle Dick' the next morning. Everyone got what was affectionately called 'Spanish Tummy' at some point while we were there."

Two new Sontaran costumes were made for the story, the uniforms closely based on the original *Time Warrior* designs, while the masks were sculpted with subtle differences that made both Varl and Styre look different. This was at odds with the original concept of the Sontarans being a cloned race. *The Two Doctors* crew flew back to London on Thursday 16 August, with all the material they needed 'in the can'. Studio rehearsals began the following week.

Holmes:

"There seemed to be a game going on between Colin, Pat and Frazer to see who could put the most revolting innuendo on a line of their dialogue. Colin invariably won, and Nicola just stood there trying to keep a straight face."

Holmes admits to enjoying seeing Troughton back, but had reservations about the story as a whole:

"Pat was basically Pat, and it wasn't as if he'd left the show over fifteen years earlier. I just felt it was all a bit constrained, there were so many elements to bring into the plot, and that held it up a bit here and there. I'd love to do a new solo adventure for either Pat or Tom, just to see how it would work today."

While a short break took place for the regular cast, planning started on the next story, *The Mark Of Rani*. *The Two Doctors* was swapped around with this story, so it would be transmitted fourth in the season, while *The Mark Of Rani* took its place as the third story. With the working title of *Enter The Rani*, and the earlier and more bizarre *Too Clever By Far*, the two-part script had been completed by the husband and wife team of writers, Pip and Jane Baker. Their submission had introduced the Rani, another rogue Time Lord, and their brief was expanded to bring the Master into the narrative, marking Anthony Ainley's first appearance with the sixth Doctor.

Set in 1830, director Sarah Hellings found an ideal location at the Blist Hill Open Air Museum in Shropshire, which doubled as a village during the Industrial Revolution. The cast and crew arrived on Monday 21 October, and started filming on the following day.

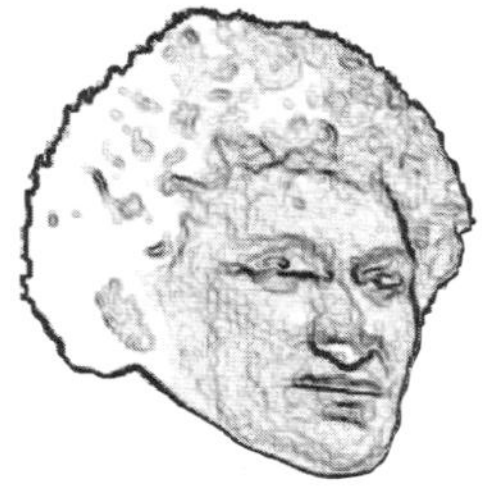

As the shoot took place in the late autumn, the weather was not exactly ideal and the final day was rained off with several scenes left unfilmed.

Kate O'Mara had been cast as the Rani, and it was a reunion of sorts between her and Baker as they'd worked together in *The Brothers*, only this time she was the villain. Following several discussions as to whether the missing shots could be staged in the confines of TV Centre, both Hellings and Nathan-Turner agreed that this was not feasible and booked a remount shortly before studio recording began. The Queen Elizabeth Woods in Harefield were used for a single day with Baker, Ainley and O'Mara present, along with Bryant, for the scenes where the Rani's chemical bombs turn several miners into trees.

Pennant Roberts was now waiting for Baker and Bryant to join him in rehearsal for the next story, *Timelash*, a studio bound two-parter to save on the overspending that *The Mark Of The Rani* had incurred with the remount. Writer Glen McCoy's submission had caught Saward's eye due to the fact that it brought H. G. Wells, the science fiction writer, and the Doctor together, but extreme problems with editing the material as it came in caused Saward to feel extremely disappointed with the finished product.

Admittedly, designer Bob Cove had very little money to work with on the sets, and the special effects department had very little time to create some of the creatures the story featured. This resulted in the Bandrils sole representative being seen on screen as a glove puppet, which some of the cast nick-named 'Sooty'.

Pennant Roberts recalls Paul Darrow (another one of the main actors from *Blake's Seven*) approaching him during rehearsals, asking if it was possible to play his character with a hump, like Laurence Olivier's version of RICHARD III. When he edited the material together, Roberts found that the second episode underran quite considerably, and Saward drafted some additional scenes that were not shot until the second recording block of the next story.

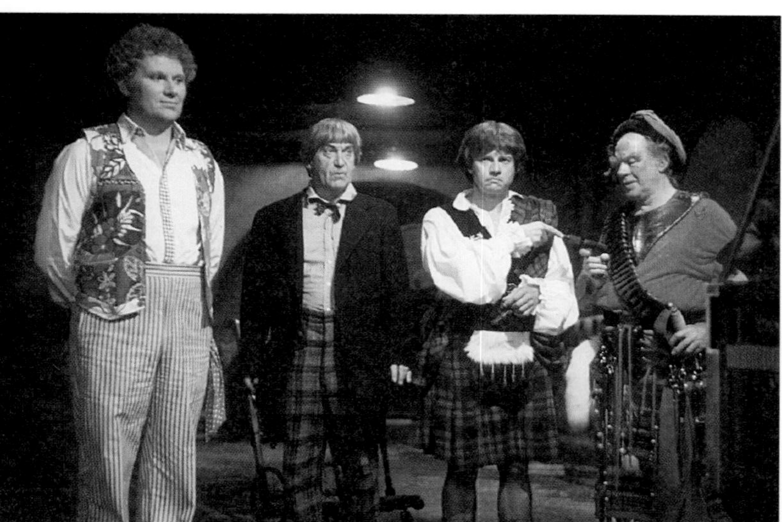

ABOVE: Colin Baker with Patrick Troughton, Fraser Hines and John Stratton in **The Two Doctors**.

RIGHT: Colin Baker cleaning quicksand out of his mouth in **The Trial of A Time Lord**.

David Chandler was rehired to play H. G. Welles again, and the Tardis set was erected in TC8 on Wednesday 30 January. Several extra minutes were completed with Roberts taking over in the control gallery from Graeme Harper, who was in the middle of directing *Revelation Of The Daleks*.

After working in a Christmas pantomime together, both Companion and Doctor started the readthrough for *Revelation Of The Daleks* on Thursday 3 January, two days before *Attack Of The Cybermen* was due to begin transmission, winning a reassuring figure of just under nine million viewers. Harper took his cast down to Portsmouth, where four days of location work began from Monday 7 January.

In the period between the crew arriving on the Sunday and preparing to start work on a vast hill near a nature reserve in Petersfield the next morning, a thick blanket of snow fell, making many of the planned shots impossible. One involved an elaborate sequence where the Daleks would be seen to fly, as Harper explains:

"We couldn't get to this valley we'd found, because of the weather. We had a catapult that could throw a Dalek casing twenty feet into the air, so it could be blown up, but we just couldn't do it."

Four new Daleks were built for the story, with a new gold and white paint scheme, and they appeared for confrontation scenes with the four old grey and black casings, bringing the total number of working props for the serial to eight. Several lightweight upper sections for the casings were also made and positioned on the standard bases for shots where Daleks were blown up. The bases suffered minimal damage when the explosion effects were executed.

Terry Molloy once again donned the Davros mask, playing two different versions of the Daleks' creator. One was the standard wheelchair bound character, now making his fourth appearance in the series, while the other was seen as a disembodied head in a life support system. To allow rapid turning movements, so Davros could effectively spin round to stare at people, Molloy had to be positioned on a turnstile with his legs strapped up behind his back. Between recording scenes, he had to be let out of the apparatus every so often as it was extremely uncomfortable. With *Revelation* completed, the cast broke up for their holidays, and plans got underway for season twenty three.

Saward already had several stories lined up; former *Doctor Who* producer Graham Williams was penning *The Nightmare Fair*, which saw the return of Michael Gough as The Celestial Toymaker,

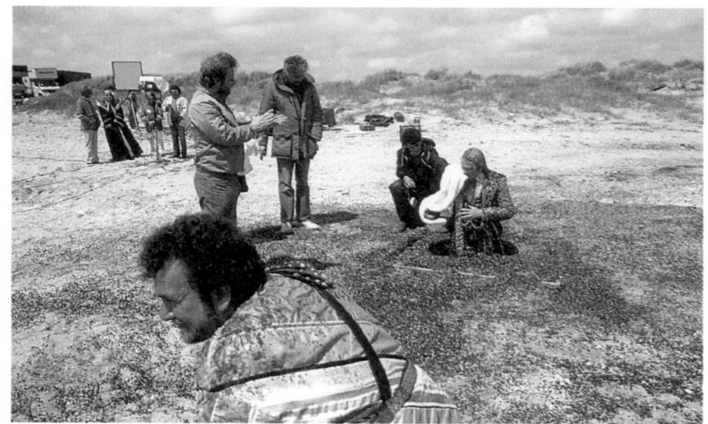

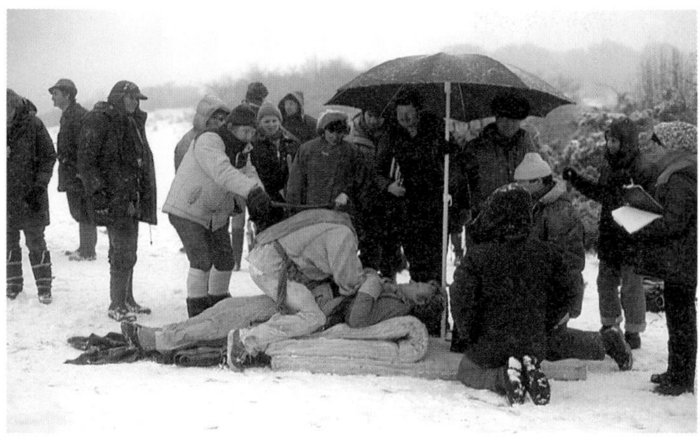

Wintry conditions on location for **Revelation Of The Daleks**.

and Matthew Robinson was due to direct. This was actually completed and handed out to the main cast, with five days of location work due to start at the beginning of May. The entire scenario would have revolved around the Toymaker using an amusement arcade on a pleasure beach to set deadly traps.

Fiona Cumming was signed up as the director for the second story, which was another two-parter, with the season continuing to follow the pattern of 45- minute episodes established with season twenty two. *The Ultimate Evil* had been completed by writer Wally K. Daly, and the story due to follow on from his tale of a ruthless arms dealer trying to instigate war between two peaceful races saw the return of the Ice warriors, with Philip Martin handling *Mission To Magnus*.

Martin:

"The whole idea was to bring the Ice Warriors and Sil together. They were meant to be the very last ones left in the galaxy, quietly trying to set up a base on the polar cap of Magnus, while Sil was trying to sell blankets and jumpers to the natives because he knew they were going to face an ice age if the Ice Warriors managed to freeze the planet over. I also brought in this villain, who was the old school bully from the Doctor's school days, with the mere mention of his name reducing him to a quivering wreck."

Ron Jones had been asked to handle the story, and thereby maintain a continuity with him directing the second story to feature Sil. After that, Robert Holmes was due to return again, with *Yellow Fever*.

Holmes:

"I got the location story again, because John Nathan-Turner had been to Singapore where he shot a load of footage and he wanted the entire thing to be based there with a load of old characters coming back. There were certainly the Autons, and I had some rather neat ideas of their hand guns firing bullets that could bounce round corners after people, and hands that melted over the mouth and nose suffocating people when they caught them. There was also talk of using the Master and the Rani. I'd have liked to have had the Rani using the Autons, and the Master trying to stop her through sheer jealousy as he'd always regarded them as his ally. There was even talk of having the Brigadier on holiday out there as well. I got a plotline done, but that's about all, really."

Christopher H. Bidmead had started to draft up *In the Hollows Of Time*, and the final story for the season was not confirmed, although plotlines were certainly being looked at from people as diverse as Michael Feeney Callan, Bill Pritchard, Peter Grimwade and even former companion Ian Marter, who once commented that his story involved "something in a very small box", with a title of *Strange Encounter*. By 25 January, however, things had changed considerably.

Concerned over the level of violence in the stories for the current series, the BBC management had decided to put the programme on hold for twelve months, while a major rethink over its format was instigated. This was an odd reason, as Nathan-Turner and Saward had to get scripts approved by their heads of department before pre-production could even begin. No criticism had been made, so they carried on with producing the stories under the impression that there were no problems. The production team was devastated.

On 27 January, the story hit the headlines, and it was then that the protests began. The BBC was flooded with thousands of letters and phone calls, frequently jamming the switchboards in the days that followed. The *Daily Star* launched a 'Save Doctor Who' campaign, and a protest record called *Doctor In Distress*, with all its proceeds going to Cancer Relief, was launched. The only reply that came from the BBC was that due to the disappointing ratings for the year (never below six million viewers, which was considerably more than the average figure for season eighteen), it was merely being 'rested', and that their was no foundation in the theories of both the press and the fans that it had been cancelled.

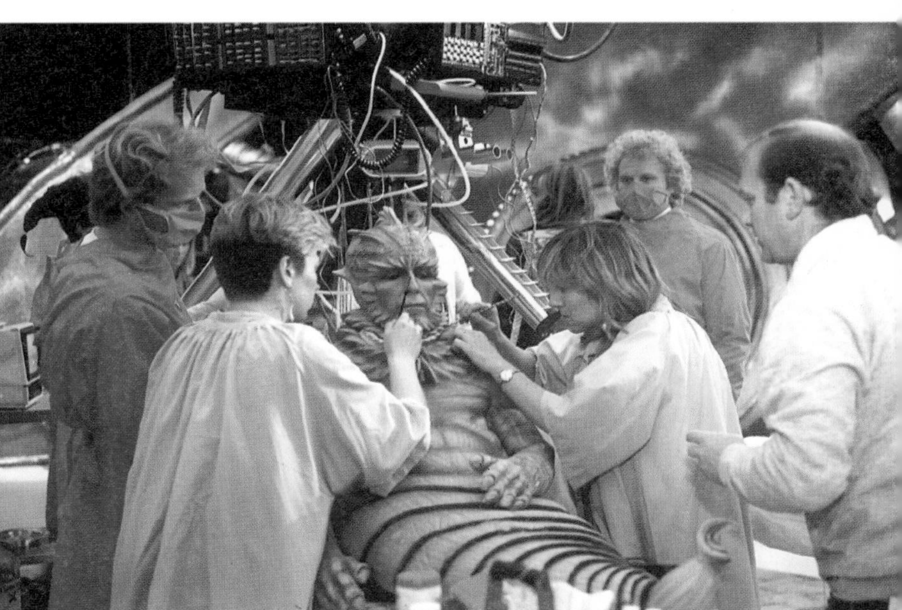

Last minute make-up in **The Trial Of A Time Lord**.

The BBC took a firm stand, saying that they had every intention of bringing *Doctor Who* back for the end of 1986, and that part of the reason behind the delay was to allow time to switch from winter to autumn schedules. This was again odd, as Philip

Hinchcliffe had to do exactly the same thing between seasons twelve and thirteen, and still had a new series starting within nine months. Whatever the case, there were plans to continue with the programme, although in a severely curtailed format. Rumours began to circulate that the episode count was going to be cut from 26 to 20, and possibly even 14 per year.

Michael Grade, in charge of the BBC's drama output, made an unusual move of criticising the production team on Radio 2, saying that they had become "complacent" and that the series had lost its imagination. He promised that *Doctor Who* would be back and on 18 December 1985, rumours were confirmed; season twenty three would only last for 14 weeks, making it the shortest one in the programme's history. The press had by now lost interest after ten months of speculation, and would only really pick up the *Doctor Who* theme again when the press call came during the first block of location work on *The Trial Of A Time Lord.*

Although some of the writers working on the planned season twenty three continued to draft new versions of their scripts, working to one of Grade's dictates that the show had to return to its 25-minute episode format, Nathan-Turner and Saward eventually wiped the slate clean, deciding to start again with a fresh batch of stories.

Saward called in a team of writers, comprising of Holmes, Philip Martin, Jack Trevor Story and David Halliwell. The idea was to create a series of stories with an interlinked theme that would be instigated with the first episode, and come to an end in episode fourteen, with the intervening stories playing a vital part to its narrative.

Martin:

"Eric told us that each story had to act as a part of the evidence presented at the Doctor's trial. This was ironic, as the programme itself was in exactly the same situation, having to prove itself to the jury, which in this case seemed to be Michael Grade. It was a hell of a responsibility because we were being told that it was effectively up to us to try and save *Doctor Who's* neck."

Robert Holmes, speaking in June 1985, just as the stories were being commissioned:

"It's all very Dickensian, with the Doctor being a bit like Scrooge. I'm handling his past, Philip's doing the present and Jack and David are handling the future. If we can come up with strong enough material, it should work quite well."

Holmes progressed rapidly with a four-part story called *The Mysterious Planet*, while Martin started work on *Planet Of Sil*, which would later have a working title of *Mindwarp*. Jack Trevor-Story never actually completed anything that was workable, and Halliwell's *Attack Of The Mind* was dropped quite early on. Saward had to quickly find another four-part and two-part story, and Christopher H. Bidmead was brought in to draft up *The Last Adventure.*

This met the same fate as Halliwell and Story's ideas and with time beginning to run out, Saward sought another script turning to the creator of *Sapphire And Steel*, P. J. Hammond, who started working on a script called *Paradise Five*. Holmes was now asked to write the final two-part story, in the absence of any other workable material, as soon as he finished *The Mysterious Planet. Time Inc.* was planned as the finale, while Pip and Jane Baker were brought in to write a replacement for Hammond's storyline which yet again proved unworkable so *The Ultimate Foe* was slotted into its place.

Baker and Bryant returned to the programme at the end of March 1986. Nick Mallett was hired to direct the first story, with John Anderson as his designer. The two central figures of the trial, alongside the Doctor, were cast by Nathan-Turner, with Michael Jayston as The Valeyard (who would be revealed at the end of the story to be a future incarnation of the Doctor), while Lynda Bellingham took on the role of the trial's judge, The Inquisitor. The atmosphere in rehearsals was somewhat tense to begin with as it was all too clear that the future of the show was hanging in the balance. The verdict on these stories would determine the future of the programme. All the working titles were dropped at this point, in favour of running the season as one long fourteen part story, called *The Trial Of A Time Lord.*

Robert Holmes' opening four episodes required a certain amount of location work with outside broadcast video cameras and recording began on Tuesday 18 April at the Buster Ancient Farm Project, before moving on to the Queen Elizabeth Country Park in nearby Horndean. The LI Service Robot was used at this point for the first time. The prop was made from a steel frame, with a fibreglass shell and moved on a small set of caterpillar tracks.

Roger Brierly, a tall actor noted for his radio work, had been hired by Mallett to play the giant robot, Drathro, which had all its scenes within the confines of TV Centre. The costume was built to his measurements, with a large anvil-like head supported on the neck and a viewing panel in the chest to create an even greater sense of height. At the last moment, he refused to wear the costume and one of the visual effects assistants had to climb inside and perform all the scenes, while Brierly recorded the dialogue off-camera.

The first section of evidence for the trial was finished over three days, from Saturday 10 May to Monday 12 May in TC3. The courtroom scenes started to be shot during this block, with the main set unfinished when Mallett started to work on it, leaving the main opening scenes of the Doctor's arrival on the space station unrecorded. The space station itself was a vast model, some six feet in diameter, which had a specially filmed computer controlled tracking shot circling around it.

Ron Jones was now working on episodes five to eight, with Nabil Shaban joining the cast to wear a slightly modified and repainted version of his Sil costume for his second story, which would feature other members of his race as the basic plot had retained Martin's original idea of setting the story on Sil's home planet. With only a brief sequence of location work needed, the four episodes were planned out as a studio bound story with six days of studio recording.

Three other Mentor costumes (Sil's species) were made for extras to wear, while two others were made for the other speaking characters; a guard Mentor and the high Lord Kiv, played by Christopher Ryan, who had a face cast taken so that a second body baring a similarity to his character could be made by the visual effects department. This enabled a convincing change to take place when Kiv's mind is transplanted into its body.

Nathan-Turner was keen to attract well-known faces to appear in the programme in order to attract a wider audience. This story saw Brian Blessed, famed for his long-running stint on *Z-Cars* and various other series, such as *I, Claudius*, making a guest appearance as King Yrcanos.

Martin:

"It was strange because when Eric Saward told me they'd cast him, it all dropped into place. The dialogue I'd written for the character was highly stylised, and he was probably the only actor who could pull it off."

Carry On film Regular Joan Sims had appeared in the first four episodes, and ex-*Avenger* Honor Blackman would arrive shortly to start work on the next four episodes, while *Coronation Street* regular Geoffrey Hughes was due to appear in the final two episodes.

Chris Clough was now working on the final six episodes with the director blocking them out as follows; working with the budget for a six-part story, the plan was to stage all of the extensive location shooting for the final two episodes first, followed by a two day studio block that would complete all the trial scenes that were needed, while two recording sessions after that would concentrate on the evidence featured in episodes nine to twelve. At this point, it's worth noting the various changes that were taking place behind the scenes.

Artistic differences had grown between Nathan-Turner and Saward to such an extent, that the script editor felt he could go on no longer and left the programme midway through recording *Mindwarp*. Robert Holmes had sadly passed away before he was able to complete the final two episodes of the story and Saward had undertaken the task of completing episode fourteen himself. Holmes had managed to finish the thirteenth, which Saward worked heavily on during the editing stages.

The story was originally due to end with the Valeyard and the Doctor tumbling through a vortex fighting each other, which Nathan-Turner felt was too 'downbeat' an ending, and asked Saward to make it lighter. Saward refused and withdrew his script, leaving the final episode unwritten with just over a week to go before location work was due to begin. As Nathan-Turner was now effectively script editing and producing, he got in contact with Pip and Jane Baker and asked them to try to complete a new draft in under a week, using only Holmes' version of episode thirteen as a starting point. They handed Chris Clough a working draft in three days.

Rehearsals began with a new companion, as Nicola Bryant had left at the end of Martin's story, and a controversial casting choice was made in the shape of Bonnie Langford, who came in to play Melanie Bush, or 'Mel' for short. The first two days of location recording were mounted at Camber Sands, in East Sussex, from Monday 23 June. From Monday 30 June to Friday 4 July, more scenes were completed around the grounds of the Gladstone Pottery Museum in Stoke-On-Trent. Anthony Ainley arrived to play the Master once again for this extensive period of night shooting. After this, rehearsals began back in London for the final studio-bound trial scenes, with only the courtroom sets and the interior of the Master's Tardis being needed. This was basically the same set used for the Doctor's time machine, but painted a suitable shade of black. The designer, Michael Trevor, now made way for Dinah Walker, who took over for the final four part section of evidence to be made which also had the more apt working title of *The Vervoids*.

Six Vervoid costumes were made. The bodies, simple body-suits covered with layers of plastic leaves and latex veins, were handled by the costume department while the heads were constructed by the visual effects department.

As it turned out, *The Trial Of A Time Lord* was a grave disappointment in the ratings, making its debut with just under five million viewers and ending on Saturday 6 December with just over five and a half, which was the peak for the entire run.

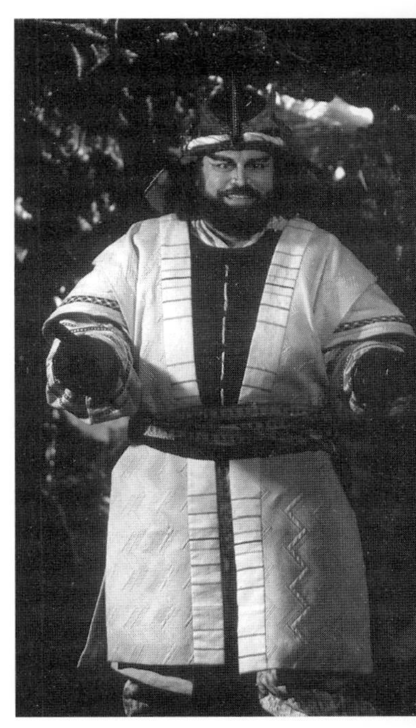
Brian Blessed as King Yrcanos.

At the beginning of November, Nathan-Turner was told by Michael Grade that the series could continue with a twenty fourth season, but there was a catch. He wanted to see a new actor in the title role. There was very little choice in the matter, and the sixth Doctor was effectively pushed out of the show. Colin Baker has always been someone who expresses his emotions very clearly and his anger was understandable when he was offered a chance to come and do just one four-part story to round things off and regenerate his Doctor. He said no, reasoning that he would have to keep himself clear of other commitments, such as a potential long run in a theatre play, just to wait for four weeks work at some point during the following year. He spoke to the press, and a rather sensationalised series of articles followed, taking his words wildly out of context.

Baker had joined the programme full of enthusiasm and had happily agreed to play the role for four years, and maybe even longer. He got his four years; after his initial four episodes for season twenty one in *The Twin Dilemma*, another whole year followed with season twenty two, then a year was missed before the final run of just 14 episodes. Like any actor who played the part, it haunted him and he donned the costume for a theatre play in 1989. In a way, perhaps he exorcised a ghost during this time, because the younger members of the audience who saw him backstage admitted to him that as far as they were concerned, Baker was their Doctor as they'd grown up watching him. So there will always be a core audience out there who 'grew up' with the sixth, and perhaps unluckiest Doctor of all.

Nathan-Turner now had to resolve the problem of presenting the audience with a convincing visual explanation as to why there would be a seventh Doctor on board the Tardis when the series returned the following Autumn. Season twenty four was confirmed as having another run of 14 episodes, and the hunt began for a fourth time to find a suitable actor to take over. Whatever the case, many producers and directors within the BBC would never forget the stigma that was now attached to the programme, due to the apparent 'cancellation', and the general opinion was that *Doctor Who* was living on 'borrowed time'.

CHAPTER 9

THE END OF INFINITY

THE END OF INFINITY

THE END OF INFINITY

"No matter how determined and resolute you may be, you can never leave *Doctor Who* . . . it will always be a part of you and when it eventually comes to an end something will surely die in all of us."

WILLIAM HARTNELL Unpublished interview – September 1967

By Christmas 1986, there were several factors that made the completion of season twenty four for transmission at the beginning of the following September look impossible. There was no actor cast as the seventh Doctor, there was no script editor, and therefore no scripts, production was due to begin in little under four months, and the producer was about to move on.

Whoever came in to take over would face a horrific schedule, and not have the fallback of a large budget to effectively 'pay' for things to be done faster. John Nathan-Turner agreed to stay on for another year as the producer to oversee the arrival of the seventh Doctor. He had originally wanted to leave after three years, but was now about to embark on his seventh.

Inevitably, with the departure of Colin Baker, agents began to flood the production office with requests for actors on their books to be considered as his replacement. One name that was put forward was Sylvester McCoy, which Nathan-Turner noted on his list of candidates and thought no more about it, until Clive Doig, a producer on various children's programmes, phoned to suggest McCoy as well. Doig had worked with McCoy on various shows, such as *Jigsaw* and *Eureka*, and recommended him as being ideal as McCoy was an eccentric in his own right. Taking in these words, Nathan-Turner went to see McCoy in a play in which he was then appearing. It was an adaptation of the folk-tale *The Pied Piper* with McCoy in the title role.

After a series of interviews and auditions, McCoy was one of the three actors who recorded a set audition piece. Janet Fielding returned to play the companion and work through the rehearsals with the actors before going into one of the smaller studios at TV Centre. The other two actors were relatively unknown, and McCoy's performance was strong enough to win him the role. On 27 March, the news broke, with one newspaper leaking the story the day before, and the actor signing up for an initial three-year run in the series.

The director who shot the auditions was Andrew Morgan, who was already working on the first story of the season before McCoy had been cast. Pip and Jane Baker returned to write *Strange Matter*, with Geoff Powell as the serial's designer.

Following on from her work on *The Mark Of The Rani*, Kate O'Mara was approached by Nathan-Turner with a view to her returning as the character for a second story, before the Bakers were even commissioned. He felt that the presence of the Rani would give McCoy's Doctor a strong opening night and the writers were given a copy of McCoy's audition on video tape to watch and give them some idea of his character. As with any Doctor, the first hurdle to overcome was designing a costume for him, although McCoy would wear a tailored version of Colin Baker's costume for a large part of the early stages of *Strange Matters*. The difference in physical statistics between the two actors meant that McCoy would be unable to wear the original version.

The approach that was chosen was to make the seventh Doctor's appearance far more sedate than number six's, with a cream jacket, straw hat and a jumper covered with a pattern of question marks. The outfit was finished off with a paisley scarf and an umbrella with a red question-mark shaped handle. For the third year of his run, McCoy would request a change of colour with his jacket, wanting something more in line with the darker direction in which the series storylines were heading, so from *Battlefield* onwards, he wore a dark brown version of the design.

Bonnie Langford returned to the programme to begin work with McCoy during rehearsals from the final week of March until Friday 3 April, after which location recording was due to begin on McCoy's debut, now retitled as *Time And The Rani*. A trio of quarries based around Frome in Somerset were chosen as being ideal sites for the planet of Lakertya, with the Bakers' original description of the world as being covered in forests rejected at an early stage. The Lakertyan actors were all carefully choreographed, so a uniform alien movement could be maintained by all of them whenever they were seen running. Their elaborate scale make-up, which had to be carefully layered across the skin of their faces, suffered in the weather conditions as continual drizzle caused the scales to slide off.

The main creatures for the story were the Tetraps, giant bat-like servants of the Rani, which were described in the script as having four eyes, and were designed accordingly. The heavily padded body-suits were lined with fur, with sections of sculpted latex representing the stomach and chest, while the heads and claws were also cast in the same material. The lead Tetrap's head was made as an animatronic working prop. It was capable of moving its eyes and its jaw, which had an extendible tongue. For the shots where the Tetrap's point of view was seen, four separate images of the surrounding area were overlayed so that they became one image on screen.

Studio rehearsals began as the cast returned to London, with the Tardis interior being one of the sets erected for these days. The traditional scene for any new Doctor, where he is seen trying on a variety of clothes, paid homage to past Doctors as McCoy's incarnation tried on a velvet jacket and ruffled shirt (Pertwee), the burgundy coat, hat and scarf (Tom Baker), the cricket pads, coat and hat of the fifth Doctor, and the fur coat worn by Troughton for *The five Doctors*. This scene was one of the first to be recorded.

Andrew Cartmel was now working as the new script editor, with the plan for the rest of the season being to have a second four-parter and two self-contained three- part stories, rather than a third four-parter and a two-parter. New writers to the series were drafting up the required material, with Stephen Wyatt working on *Paradise Towers*, South-African writer Malcolm Kholl handling *Flight Of The Chimeron*, and Ian Briggs was working on *Pyramid's Treasure*.

As Colin Baker refused to record a regeneration scene, the effect was achieved in the studio. The story had the Tardis make a forced landing induced by the Rani, and the resulting crash caused the regeneration. McCoy donned a baker-like wig, with his back to the camera lying face down on the floor, so that when he was rolled over by O'Mara, the image could be mixed to one of him without the hair-piece and at least show the final stages of the process.

From *Time And The Rani* onwards, a new version of the theme music arranged by Keff McCulloch would be used. This replaced a revised version by Dominic Glynn which was used only for season twenty three and was itself a replacement for Peter Howell's version that had been used from *The Leisure Hive* through to *Revelation Of The Daleks*.

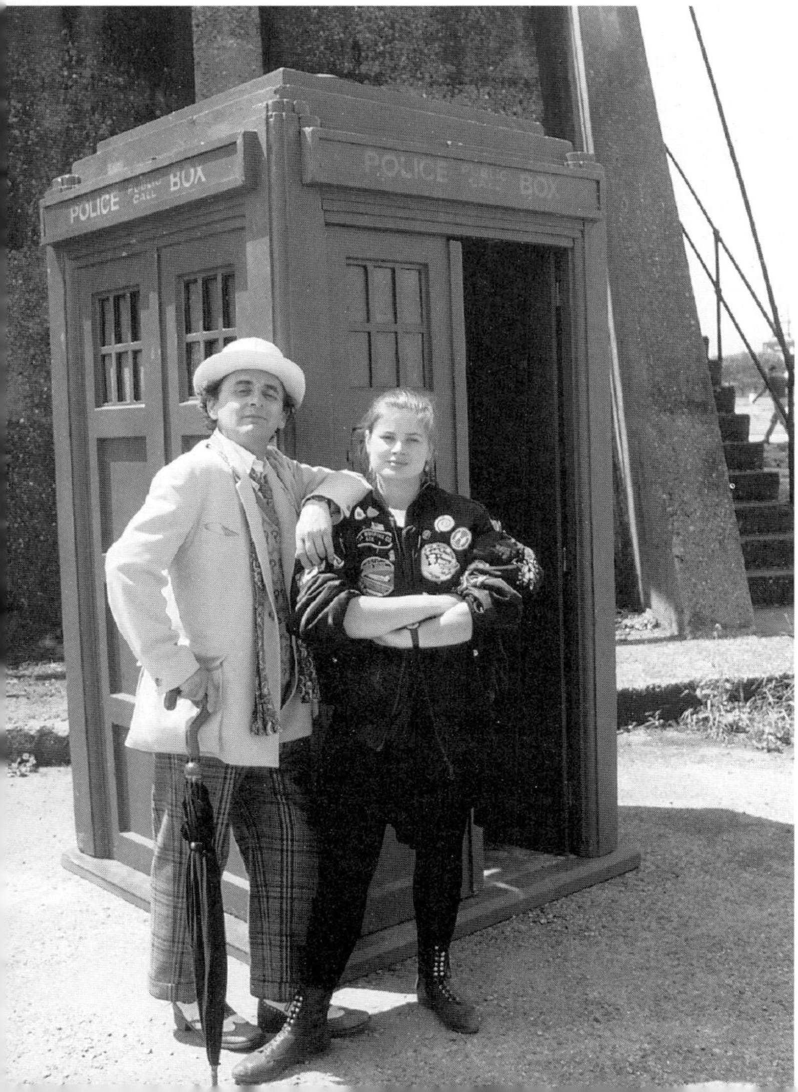

Paradise Towers entered production with director Nick Mallett taking several of the principal cast to Elmswell House near Buckinghamshire for one day of location recording, utilising a large indoor swimming pool there. designer Martin Collins suitably redressed the area for the scenes that had to be completed for part of the story's finale. The remainder of the story would be completed in the studio.

The vast street sets built in TCI for the first studio session, with overhead gantries and a town square, saw the first use of the Cleaning Robots. Large white creations, with a small motor, they could be driven around by the actor inside but the design did not exactly convey the air of menace that they were meant to have. Extendible arms operated from within held a variety of mechanisms, ranging from a drill head to a large metal pincer-like claw. Dump bins on wheels, again painted white, could be attached to the back of them, with the robots using them to carry bodies down to the basement, in the context of the story.

Money saved by having *Paradise Towers* relatively studio bound was ploughed into the budget for the next story, which was now called *Delta And The Bannermen*. This would be made back to back with Briggs' story, retitled *Dragonfire*, using the same director and designer (Chris Clough and John Asbridge). The basic production team would remain the same for all six episodes, with the first three being shot entirely on location, while the second three would remain studio bound.

Kholl's script revolved around a holiday camp in the 1950s, and rather than try to redress one of the more modern facilities that were available, recces were carried out to try and find one that had remained relatively untouched since that era. The Majestic Holiday Camp on Barry Island in Wales proved ideal, and the production quickly became nicknamed as 'Who-De-Who', parodying the sitcom title, *Hi-De-Hi*.

Scenes that were staged included a vintage 1950s coach being dropped from a crane to represent the fact that it was actually a spaceship crashlanding, with the BBC agreeing to suitably redress the flowerbed it landed on after subsequently blowing the vehicle up. The entrance to the holiday camp was actually the tradesman's entrance to the real thing, with a 'Shangri-La' sign over the gate completing the illusion.

Another major scene involved the Bannermen, clad in black jumpsuits and helmets, with Samuri-like flags strapped to their backs, thundering past on motor bikes shooting at the Doctor and Mel. The whole period at the camp was accompanied by glorious weather, which easily allowed the crew to complete all their material on schedule. To save any of the cast having to be rehired for studio work in London, a large hallway in the complex saw the interior of the coach and the Bannerman spaceship being erected as sets and the work for which they were needed was finished there.

The final day in Wales saw the arrival of Ken Dodd to shoot his scenes for the only nightwork executed on the story, at the Llandow Trading estate, where a World War Two aircraft hanger was redressed to become an intergalactic toll gate. After this, the

Sylvester McCoy with Sophie Aldred as Ace.

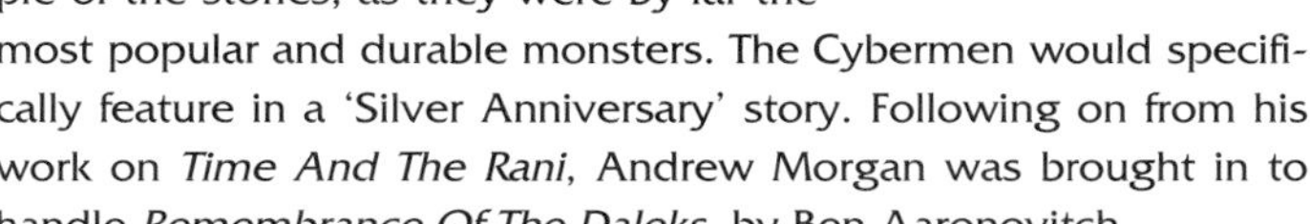

cast and crew were given a week off before rehearsals began on *Dragonfire*, which saw the return of Tony Selby to the programme. He had played Sabalom Glitz in six episodes of *The Trial Of A Time Lord*.

One of the first scenes to be recorded involved Sophie Aldred as Ace, a character quickly brought in as the new companion for McCoy's Doctor when Bonnie Langford decided to move on rather than sign up for another season. Last minute rewrites were carried out to draft in a farewell scene on board the Tardis. Aldred had nearly appeared in *Delta And The Bannermen* as Ray, having auditioned for director Chris Clough, but the part of Ray eventually went to Lynn Gardner. Like Aldred, Gardner was ideal for the role as she could ride a motorcycle, but fell off the scooter the character had to ride in some scenes whilst practising on it in a car park. Sara Griffiths was brought in to replace her, but Gardner was not forgotten and was used to record some tannoy announcements during the *Dragonfire* studio work.

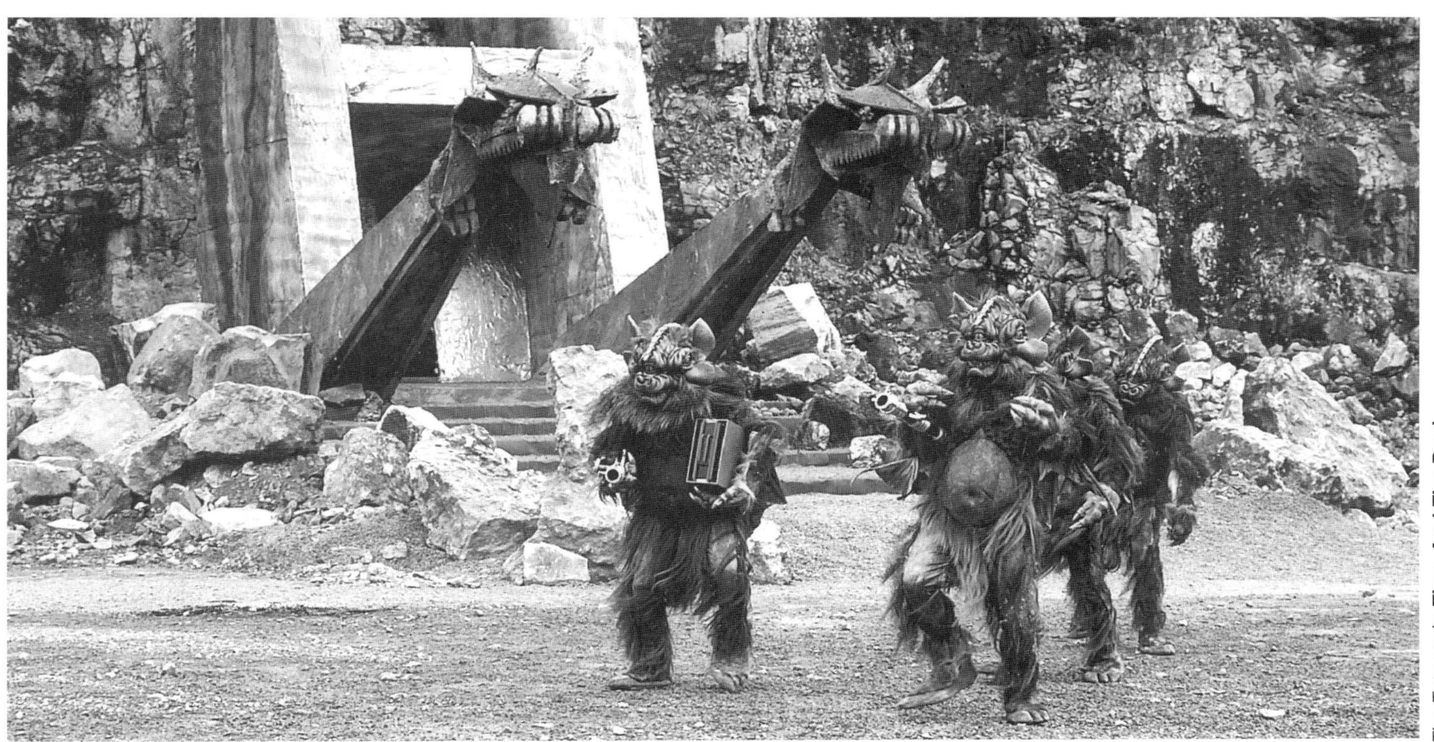

The Tetraps in **Time And The Rani**.

The dragon of the title, a bio-mechanoid creature, was played by Leslie Meadows, who was booked for both stories, playing a Bannerman in the earlier one. The carefully sculpted rubber body suit was topped by a vast headpiece for the head of the beast, with pipes running along its sides that could emit steam on cue. A replica of the head was built for scenes where the skull opens up like a musical box, revealing a crystal within.

Season twenty four started broadcasting from 7 September onwards, and the ratings were very low, due to the fact that the series had been scheduled opposite *Coronation Street* which dominated the top ten viewing figures every week. The highest figure came with episode one of *Dragonfire*, which scored five and a half million, while the lowest was just over four million, with episode two of Time And The Rani.

Nathan-Turner was now effectively starting to oversee a second major anniversary of the programme, as work began on season twenty five. From quite an early stage, he'd decided to bring back both the Cybermen and the Daleks for a couple of the stories, as they were by far the most popular and durable monsters. The Cybermen would specifically feature in a 'Silver Anniversary' story. Following on from his work on *Time And The Rani*, Andrew Morgan was brought in to handle *Remembrance Of The Daleks*, by Ben Aaronovitch.

Aaronovitch had initially been asked to come up with a three-part location story, following on from a submission called *Nightfall*, which had greatly impressed Cartmel. He came up with *Storms Over Avalon*, which proved unworkable but showed that the writer could produce a substantial action orientated script if needed. As a result, he was commissioned to write the Dalek story for the season. The scripts, which had a vast amount of continuity references to past stories and were set in 1963 (even including a scene where a television set is seen as a new science fiction series begins, termed in the scripts as *Professor X*), were ready by February 1988 as Morgan and his designer, Martin Collins, arrived to begin work.

An extensive amount of location work was called for, with both the grey and white Daleks needed for the exterior scenes, along with the black Supreme Dalek casing. For the brief studio scenes involving Davros, once again played by Terry Molloy, the character was seen in disguise as the Emperor Dalek, hidden within the large dome mounted on the white base of a Dalek. The front section was pulled back over the dome to reveal that only his head was now left, the last remnants of his human body having been removed.

Aldred and McCoy arrived to start rehearsals on the story from Monday 28 March, with nine days of location shooting in and around London beginning on 4 April. Theed Street, round the back of Waterloo railway station, was the main site for the first two days

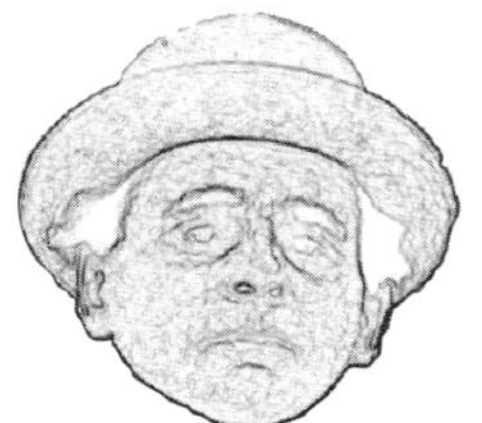

where a battle between white and grey Daleks under a bridge culminated in an explosion that was so big, it set off car alarms in the immediate area and could be heard right across London. It made the headlines of several newspapers the following day as the emergency services had been called. The blame was placed squarely on the Special Weapons Dalek. This had the lower casing of a white Dalek, whilst the upper half consisted of a specially-built gun turret. No other regular Dalek features were used on the character, with the familiar eye-stalk, gun and sucker arm all being absent. Aaronovitch had originally wanted this to be a vast, floating gun platform that hovered above the ground, but this proved impractical and would have been technically difficult to make it look convincing on screen.

From Wednesday 6 April, the crew moved to the Kew Bridge Steam Museum in outer London for two days where all of the sequences at the Totter's Lane junk yard were staged. Because of the sheer amount of work that had to be done, a second camera crew worked for the Thursday and Friday on insert shots and some of the Dalek battle scenes, with Nathan-Turner directing. For the main part of Friday 8 April, filming was done at the Paddington Cemetery, before moving on to the Saint John's School in Hammersmith to complete everything from 11 to 13 April. It was here that the landing of the Dalek shuttlecraft was shot. The large prop, complete with smoking pads, was lowered to the ground by a crane, the wires holding it being kept carefully out of view.

Studio rehearsals began at the end of the week, with a three day block planned out, running from 27 to 29 April. Sets included the interior of the school and shuttle craft. John Leeson returned to the series to provide a variety of voice work for the story, including the Dalek battle computer.

Alan Wareing was now working with designer David Laskey, as he prepared to start directorial chores on *The Greatest Show In The Galaxy*, which would nearly suffer the same fate as *Shada*, although for an entirely different reason.

The original idea had been to make Wyatt's scripts as an entirely studio-bound three-parter, with the interior of the circus tent set up in TCI, but this was altered when the production team decided to expand on the plotline and allow some location work to establish the fact that the serial was set on an alien planet. Rehearsals began on 6 May, and by Saturday 14 May recording began in and around Warmwell Quarry in Dorset. The slightly surreal prop requirements for this five day period included a vintage black hearse, driven by robot clowns dressed as Victorian undertakers, and a huge robot torso that could rise out of the sand. The first two days were spent shooting along the Skinner's Road, centering on the main arrival scenes of all the characters travelling to the Psychic Circus. Monday 16 May saw the action move to the centre of the quarry, where the main entrance to the tent had been erected. The main bulk of the circus site was due to be created with model work in post-production. The special effects crew rigged a massive explosion to detonate as McCoy calmly walked away from the tent flaps and to his credit, the actor didn't even flinch as a huge jet of flame blasted into the air only a few feet behind him.

The hippy bus encampment for the early and latter part of the story, with both old and repaired versions of the Bus Conductor robot, played by Dean Hollingsworth on both occasions, were staged at Golden Pond on Tuesday 17 May. Two different robot costumes were used as the character returned to the bus after being damaged by his own ticket machine laser in the first episode, only to be blown to bits in the fourth.

The final day, Wednesday 18 May, moved to the Blue Lagoon where all of the sequences involving the robot buried in the sand were staged, as was the Chief Clown's death scene. All of the clowns wore elaborate costumes based on traditional circus designs. The actors playing the undertaker robots all wore the same style of featureless white mask, with the exception of their Chief – the only human one amongst their number.

Having travelled back to London for the main studio block rehearsals the production team hit a problem when routine refurbishment at TV Centre revealed the ceilings of many of the studios to be lined with asbestos fibres. An emergency situation arose with all the facilities being closed down so that the asbestos could be safely removed. As a consequence, *The Greatest Show In The Galaxy* lost its studio. For a brief time the story was actually cancelled, but Nathan-Turner and Wareing came up with a feasible solution. If a Circus tent could be erected in one of the BBC Car Parks, all of the remaining material could be shot there instead. An agreement was made with BBC Elstree, and they began replanning the recording sessions around the sets that could be built within the tent. Recording finally began on Monday 6 June.

One of the last shots to be staged involved the character of Captain Cook, played by T. P. McKenna, falling down a stone

Remembrance Of The Daleks.

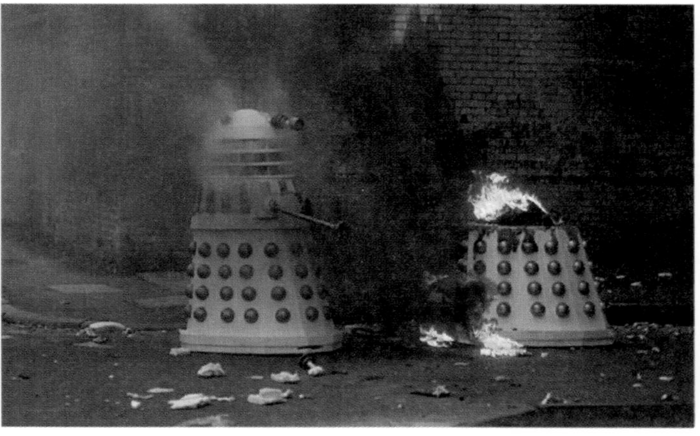

Cybermen on the rampage in **Silver Nemesis**.

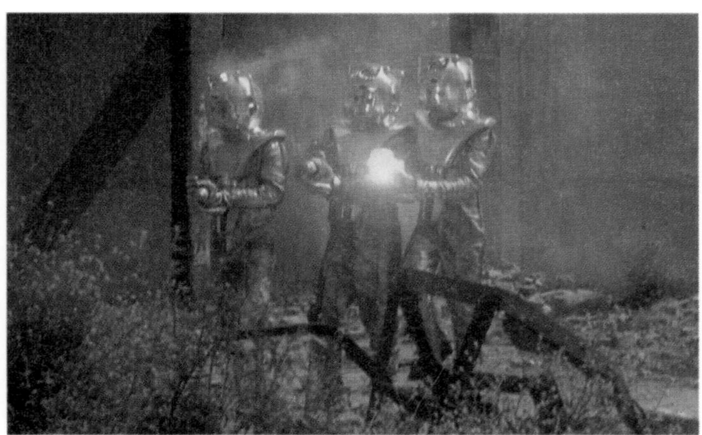

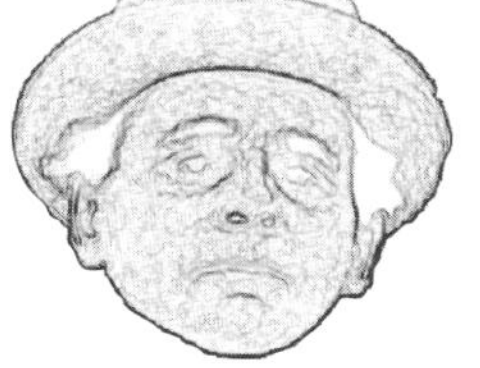

well. The well had been built about six feet above the ground, so that camera angles could be set up for shots of the Doctor and Ace looking down into the hole. As McKenna stepped over the edge, he fell badly and snapped an Achilles tendon, which put the actor out of action for some time afterwards.

With the tent work carrying on into a second week, four days were lost off the rehearsals for *Nemesis*, later retitled *Silver Nemesis*, the anniversary story featuring the Cybermen that had been written by Kevin Clarke. Aldred and McCoy arrived with only two days to block out all the material for this entirely location-shot story. Following on from the pattern set with season twenty four, the two three-part stories of the year would be made by the same production crew, one on location and one entirely studio bound. The team of director Chris Clough and designer John Asbridge were brought in for a second time to work with this system.

Location recording had to begin with a three day session around the Greenwich Gas Works in London, from Wednesday 22 June, while the latter part of the filming would have ideally been done around the ground of Windsor castle, where the rest of the story was set, but the authorities took a dim view of this request and a replacement had to be found. Arundel Castle in Essex seemed ideal and they had no major objections, so the story was scheduled to be completed there from Sunday 26 June to Sunday 2 July. A final day would be spent at the Black Jacks Mill Restaurant in Harefield on Wednesday 5 July.

For the anniversary story, the Cybermen (with David Banks returning for a fourth time as the Cyberleader) were suitably updated. New bullet-metal body suits and a shining finish to the head masks, which reflected the sunlight too much during recording and had to be 'buffed down'.

The final story of the season, *The Happiness Patrol,* written by Graeme Curry, went into rehearsal with the studio-bound story safely booked into studios at Television Centre. The first recording block took place in TC3 from Wednesday 26 July. One of the most elaborate creations for the story was the Kandy Man, who was originally detailed in the script as being a rotund scientist in a white lab coat with a large bow tie, but during the design period the character's name was taken literally and a creature made up from slabs of different sweets was made. With spinning eyes and tubes of different coloured fluids running round the robot's body, the tight- fitting heavy costume was extremely difficult to operate, and the actor inside frequently came close to collapsing. When the story was finally broadcast, the sweet manufacturers Bassett's were quite concerned about the malevolent Kandy-Man's striking similarity to their genial mascot, Bertie Bassett.

The other creatures featured in the story were the rodent-like Pipe People, living in the sewers of the city. The original idea of using puppets proved to be too expensive and was dropped in favour of using children wearing latex masks. Fifi, the dog-like pet of Helen A. (a character that was obviously a pastiche on Margaret Thatcher, then still the Prime Minister), was an elaborate fur-covered latex puppet. Three different versions were used during

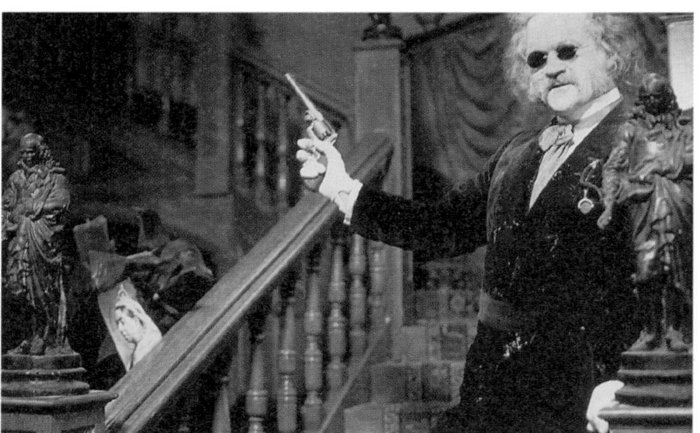

ABOVE: Ian Hogg as Josiah Smith in **Ghost Light**.
BELOW: The Heamovores in **The Curse of Fenric**.

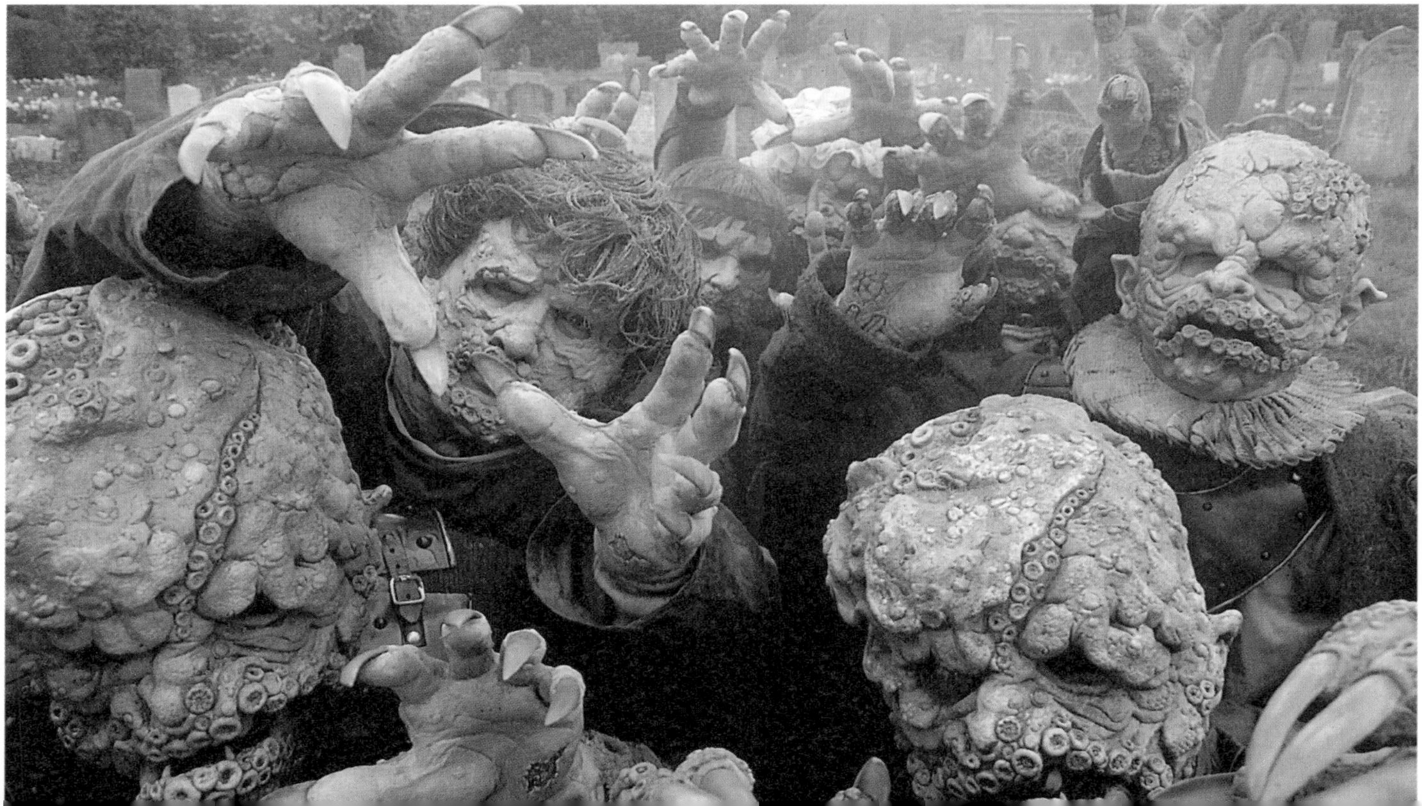

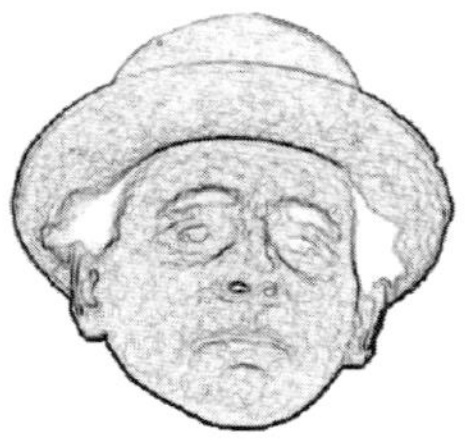

recording including one that could be pulled on a wire and be seen running across the floor with all four of its legs moving.

Remembrance Of The Daleks started transmission on 5 October, and once again the series was scheduled against *Coronation Street*. As a consequence it suffered in the ratings. The low was *The Happiness Patrol* episode two with just over four and a half million viewers, while *The Greatest Show In The Galaxy* part four managed to get a high of over six and a half million. By this time, work was already underway on season twenty six, with Ben Aaronovitch being asked to redraft *Storms Over Avalon* as a four-part adventure that would feature the return of Brigadier Lethbridge-Stewart and UNIT.

By November 1988, three scripts were being written, only two of which would actually see production. Aaronovitch's would soon become *Battlefield*, while Ian Briggs' new story went through various title changes from *Wolf Time*, to *The Wolves Of Fenric*, to *The Curse Of Fenric*. Robin Mukherjee's *Alixion* was dropped, possibly planned for recommissioning for season twenty seven. By April 1989, the final two stories for the new run of fourteen episodes were underway, with Marc Platt's *Life Cycle*, which had started out as *Lungabarrow*, and Rona Munro's *Blood Heat*.

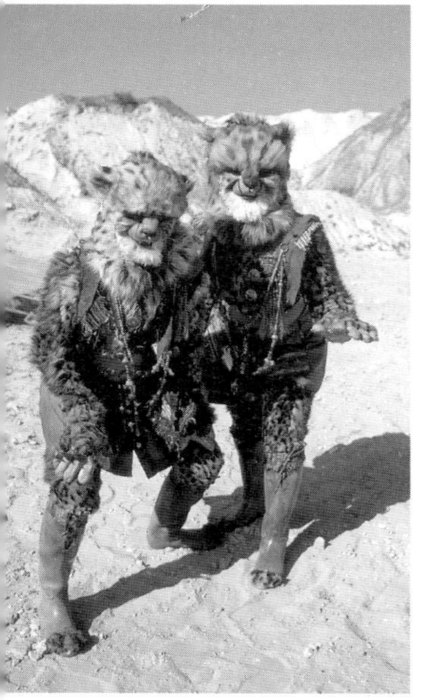

The Cheetah People in **Survival**.

Andrew Morgan would have returned for the UNIT story, but like Lovett Bickford and Tim Combe before him, the budget rule stopped this, and Nathan-Turner approached Graeme Harper about returning to direct for the programme, but he was unavailable. Michael Kerrigan was brought in at the beginning of April, with Martin Collins as his designer. Nicholas Courtney was vital to the production, and he was currently under negotiation for a role in a West End play, with an out of town tour before moving to London, which would have made him unavailable. To accommodate for this and ensure that the story would be made when he was around, Nathan-Turner swapped *Battlefield* around with Ian Briggs new story, so that *The Curse Of Fenric* went into production first. Nick Mallett was brought in to direct, with David Laskey as his designer.

The entire story was set around a coastal army camp during the Second World War and it was decided to make the serial entirely on location with all the recording centralised around one area. This was chosen as Hawkhurst in Kent for all the scenes outside the barracks. The barracks scenes were staged at Crowborough Training Camp in East Sussex, and shooting ran from 3 April through to 20 April.

Several scenes along the shoreline of the coast were staged at Lulworth Cove in Dorset, where the Heamovores were seen rising from the water. The original design for these vampiric creatures had their heads based on the mouth of a leech, but this was rejected, and a more decayed human flesh look was used instead. Masks were sculpted with blue skin covered in whelks and barnacles. The costume department came up with an array of clothing from different periods in history to show how the creatures came from varying points in history. The Ancient Heamovore was a heavy rubber suit, with moulded sections of latex fitting around an external costume. The mask was a complex radio controlled animatronic, with blinking eyes, mouth movement and continually undulating gills.

Battlefield began rehearsals as soon as McCoy and Aldred returned to London, with a variety of location work being carried out from 6 to 17 May. Courtney was now available, and the Brigadier was the only character returning from the original UNIT line-up. The crew moved around Buckinghamshire at first, shooting at the Fulmer Plant Park where Lethbridge-Stewart was seen buying plants with his wife, Doris, and then at a private house, Little Paston in Fulmer, which was used as the character's home. The main requirement for that location was that it should have a garden big enough for a helicopter to land in. When the Brigadier was coaxed out of retirement to rejoin UNIT on hearing that the Doctor had arrived back on Earth, he was picked up by an official copter. The subsequent crash scenes were completed in Black Park, last used for *Castrovalva*.

Work around the village of Hambleton was done with the Hambleton Old Hall doubling as the Gore Crow Hotel, while the village church graveyard saw the confrontation between the Brigadier and Morgaine (played by Jean Marsh, returning to the programme for the first time since *The Daleks' Master Plan*) around its memorial cross. The third Doctor's car, Bessie, was used for several days during this period, with dialogue establishing that the Brigadier had kept the vehicle in storage since he last saw the Doctor, just in case he ever needed it again.

Twyford Woods near Corby were used for scenes of the Knights of Morgaine and Ancelyn's rival factions confronting each other, while Rutland Water near Oakham saw major battle sequences being shot around an excavation site. Nathan-Turner stepped behind the camera to handle second unit work on these scenes for Kerrigan. Finally, several shots where wasteground was needed were set up at Castle Cement near Stamford. After this, the crew returned to London.

For the first time that season, recording took place in TV Centre, from Tuesday 30 May to Thursday 1 June in TC3. The interior of the Tardis was erected for the only scenes featuring the console room in for season twenty six. Once again, the final two three-part stories would be made by the same production team. The scripts were now called *Ghost Light* (Platt's) and *Catflap* (Munro's), which would become *Survival* shortly before rehearsals began. This location-based story was the first of the two to be completed, with Alan wareing as the director and Nick Somerville as the designer.

As work on *Survival* began at the Acton Rehearsal rooms, an investigation was instigated into an accident that had taken place during the last recording day on *Battlefield*. For one sequence, the last to be staged in the evening, Sophie Aldred had to stand in a water tank which was slowly filling with liquid as Ace is nearly drowned. The cubicle she was in had a thick transparent front, which suddenly shattered, flooding the studio floor. Aldred was quickly pulled out of the danger zone as water cascaded over the countless cables, wiring and live electrics around the studio. She was quite shaken, but soon recovered.

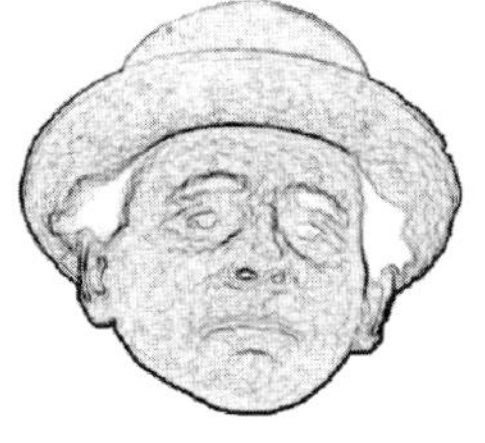

From 10 to 15 June, all of the 'earth-bound' material for *Survival* was recorded, the cast and crew working around the suburb of Perivale in London. Anthony Ainley was back for this story, playing the Master for the first time alongside McCoy's Doctor. Many scenes were staged around the Medway Parade, while the playground where Ace is pursued by one of the Cheetah People on horseback, was at the Ealing Central Sports Ground. The Cheetah People were full body suits, patterned with yellow fur complete with black spots. Their head masks left part of the face clear, to allow prosthetic make-up to be added to the actors' faces for the mouth and cheek areas. After 15 June, the team moved back to Warmwell Quarry in Dorset for all the sequences set on the home planet of the race.

Recording started there on Sunday 18 June, in a totally different area of the site to the ones used by Wareing on *The Greatest Show In The Galaxy*. By Friday 23 June, *Survival* was finished, just as industrial action that would have disrupted the production was due to begin. While they were on location, a few shots were taken of a vast Victorian house in Weymouth, to act as establishing shots for the next story, *Ghost Light*, due to begin rehearsals after a two week break.

Marc Platt's script was entirely set within the corridors and rooms of Gabriel Chase, and Nick Somerville created a set complete with a staircase and working lift in TC3 for the first recording block. The rehearsals began from 6 July when Aldred and McCoy returned from their short holiday.

As Josiah Smith, Ian Hogg had to endure long make-up sessions. His appearance had to change from that of a decaying, haggard version of the character to a younger, more refined version as he literally sheds his skin. Shots were carefully planned out to allow time for Hogg's costume and make-up changes.

The end of season party saw the regular production team and cast saying their farewells till the next season, which was already being planned out by Andrew Cartmel. Ben Aaronovitch and Marc Platt were certainly working on new scripts for the twenty seventh year. McCoy was planning to leave the series at the end of season twenty seven, and Sophie Aldred wanted to go halfway through. Aaronovitch was devising a new companion, who would be introduced in a story that was basically a crime-thriller, and after nine complete seasons as *Doctor Who's* Producer, John Nathan-Turner was waiting for his replacement to be appointed so he could move on. A new production team was due to see the McCoy era to its end and cast the eighth Doctor. Work was due to begin in March 1990.

Battlefield started on 6 September and was a ratings disaster. Placed against *Coronation Street* once again, a little over three million people tuned in. By episode four, with one of the most impressive animatronic creations yet seen in the programme making its appearance (The Destroyer was played by Marek Anton, who had to sync his dialogue in with the lip movements of a complex mask, which was controlled by an operator off camera), the figures only just reached the four million mark. *Ghost Light*, broadcast as the second story, fared little better. All three episodes hovered at the four million mark.

The heads of department realised what was happening and a second press conference, following the one at the season's launch, was staged to try and promote some public interest in the last two stories. *The Curse Of Fenric* suffered the same fate as *Ghost Light*, with little over four million viewers for each instalment. *Survival* reached a high of just five million for episodes one and three.

The decision for season twenty seven to be given the go ahead was suddenly delayed, and by the end of the year the BBC had formally announced that the series would no longer be made as an 'in-house' production. The BBC was farming out many of its more popular programmes to independent production companies, and it seemed that *Doctor Who* was about to follow this route.

A considerable number of companies started to make bids for the rights to the series, while all along, the BBC kept reassuring the programme's fans that *Doctor Who* was not dead. By the beginning of 1992, with no bids accepted, Sylvester McCoy and Sophie Aldred were resigned to the fact that their days with the series were over. It was looking extremely unlikely that Ace or the seventh Doctor would ever be seen again. The Head of Drama at the BBC, Peter Cregeen, had last given a clue to the programme's fate in November 1991, when he said that there would be a considerable gap between seasons. By implication, this meant that nothing would be made for the rapidly approaching thirtieth anniversary of *Doctor Who*.

Realising that there was nothing planned to mark this occasion, a script for an anniversary special was commissioned by BBC Enterprises. The plan was to make the story exclusively for video release. *The Dark Dimension*, written by Adrian Rigelsford with Graeme Harper returning to the show as its director, was to centre around Tom Baker's Doctor, with all of the other surviving actors who played the part also being featured in the storyline, but due to problems with the budget, formal production never actually began. The news that the project was being planned in the first place generated huge press interest, proving that there was still a great deal of enthusiasm for the programme.

By August 1994, five years had passed since the show had last seen production, and rumours began to circulate in the press that Steven Spielberg's Amblin Entertainment company was negotiating to acquire the rights to *Doctor Who*. The plan was to make the series in America with a multi-million dollar budget. Names were thrown up as speculation over the casting of the lead role began, with names as diverse as Eric Idle Alan Rickman, and former *Carry On* film star Jim Dale being press favourites. Whatever the case, it was clear that the U.K. based productions had ended with *Ghost Light*.

It would seem that 1995 will see the return of *Doctor Who* with the effects and style of the programme updated in line with the kind of quality achieved by *Star Trek; The Next Generation* and *Star Trek; Deep Space Nine*. In order to be able to compete in the modern television programme market place, where foreign sales are the lifeline of nearly every production, this was the way that the BBC felt it had to go. There will, however, always be the memory of what went before, and the tradition that was established of Saturday night viewing for all but six of its twenty six year run. *Doctor Who* defeated the Daleks, the Cybermen, and all manor of aliens and foes, but he couldn't overcome the growing expectations of his audience as their tastes became more and more sophisticated. To fight back, the new series will have to evolve and at least equal the competition on American TV to survive. If it fails, the Tardis may never be seen again . . .

WHO-OGRAPHY

D*octor Who* has not always been confined to television. Its popularity has led to the character being used in a variety of other ways, with movies, both radio and stage plays, and even the occasional appearance by the Tardis elsewhere.

At the height of the Daleks' popularity towards the end of 1964, the BBC were approached by Film Producer Milton Subotsky, with a view to his production company making a big screen adaptation of the first Dalek story. Terry Nation was keen for this to go ahead, and a contract was agreed, with Subotsky taking an option for an additional second film, if the first one was to prove successful.

A star with a worldwide audience appeal was needed and Subotsky found his Doctor in Peter Cushing, who was widely recognised for his work in the Hammer Horror Films, which had brought him international fame with *The Curse Of Frankenstein* in 1957, and cemented his reputation as a horror star with *Dracula* the following year.

Cushing:

"I was truly delighted to be able to break away from Christopher Lee and his fangs, and make something that the children would be able to see. Oh, they knew who I was because they'd tried to get in to see the Hammer films and been turned away, and now they wouldn't have that problem. It was also fascinating to work with robots like the Daleks. All my monsters up until that point had been positively humanoid!"

Subotsky cast Roy Castle as Ian Chesterton. Castle had worked with Cushing the previous year (1964), on *Doctor Terror's House Of Horrors.* Production ran from 8 March 1965 to 9 April 1965 at Shepperton Film Studios, with Gordon Glemyng directing a relatively faithful adaptation of Nation's *The Daleks*, which Subotsky had written himself. The co-production between British Lion and Regal productions opened on 24 June that year, just in time for the school holidays, and the opportunity of seeing the Daleks in colour on the big screen proved to be a huge draw. *Doctor Who And The Daleks* was an immense success and Subotsky was quick to secure the rights to *The Dalek Invasion Of Earth*, bringing David Whitaker in to supply what is credited on screen as being additional material.

Whitaker:

"I basically had to give the Daleks more scenes, as there was very little for them to do. Milton had got carried away with the subplot of the human rebels living on the old underground system and lost his way a bit. It was all done at very short notice, and very quickly, as I was still with the TV version at that time."

Whitaker was also under contract towards the end of 1965 with John Gale Theatre Productions, who approached Terry Nation to write a theatre play which they planned to stage at the Strand Theatre over Christmas that year. As the rights to the Doctor were tied up with Subotsky, the production company opted to use only the Daleks, feeling they had enough box office draw on their own judging by the takings on the first Dalek movie.

Whitaker.

"Terry had just finished his Dalek epic with Dennis (Spooner, co-writer on *The Daleks' Master Plan*) and was too tired to do it, and asked me if I'd have a go and take joint credit. The money was good, so I couldn't complain."

Using Daleks based on the TV variety, the show opened on 21 December 1965, and closed shortly after the new year with a healthy return and reports of many packed houses for the evening performances.

Cushing signed up for the sequel to the first film, when *The Dalek Invasion Of Earth* started shooting on 31 January 1966, with only Roberta Tovey joining him from the original cast. Bearing in mind the idea of using a supporting actor for comic relief, as had been done with Castle in the first film, Bernard Cribbins was brought in for the sequel, and Jill Curzon took over as the Doctor's other companion for the adventure.

With a title change to *Daleks: Invasion Earth 2150 AD*, filming was completed on 22 March, and it opened to a less than spectacular response across the country from 6 August. An idea to make a movie of *The Chase* as a third Dalek movie never materialised due to the poor box office returns on the second film. Subotsky, nevertheless, did plan out a third film towards the end of the 1970s, with *Doctor Who's Greatest Adventure*, which would have used both a TV and a movie Doctor (Subotsky once explained that he wanted to use Cushing again as he was now enjoying renewed recognition through his appearance in the 1977 blockbuster, *Star Wars*, and have Tom Baker handle all the action sequences), but this was never made.

Baker himself worked on an idea called *Doctor Who Meets Scratchman*, with Ian Marter, when they were both in the series. Ex-*Avengers* director James Hill was involved as the project's potential director. Horror star Vincent Price had provisionally agreed to appear as the villain of the title, the Devil himself. When finance couldn't be raised, Baker's appeal to the fans of the programme for help resulted in a flood of letters with various amounts of pocket money enclosed, but the actor had to return it all, as there was a ruling that prevented films being made in such a way.

Marter said in 1987:

"It would have been a lot darker than the TV show, and probably got into a fair bit of trouble, because we had these scarecrows coming to life and stalking through the dark after people. It was all set at night, and there were close-ups of them doing high-pitched screams like the things in *Invasion Of The Bodysnatchers*, and you had maggots pouring out of their mouths. Tom (Baker) loved the idea of subverting the everyday things around us, and making them dangerous, so he was all for these scarecrows."

Tom Baker in 1978:

"The Cybermen were in it, because I rather like them, and we were going to go down to Cornwall and have them slowly rising out of the sea, covered in barnacles, with their mouths jagged and dangerously grinning where the rust had eaten away at them. You see, Vincent Price would have woken them up from their crashed spaceship, without realising that a good whack with a cricket bat could shatter them, because they were so frail. It would have been hysterical."

There has always been talk of a *Doctor Who* movie, with Douglas Adams even completing an idea, again with Baker, for *Doctor Who And The Kricketmen*, but plans have always floundered. The last was in 1993, when Lumiere Pictures took over the rights from a company called Coast to Coast. Coast to Coast had held the movie rights for several years and had even gone so far as to complete a script on which TV writer Johnny Byrne worked.

Lumiere signed up Leonard Nimoy, more familiar as Mr Spock in *Star Trek*, to direct their project, and had a script by *Star Trek VI's* Denny Martin Flynn and Nicholas Meyer, but again, this fell through.

In 1974, the Doctor returned to the stage in *The Seven Keys To Doomsday*, which ran at the Adelphi Theatre in London for four weeks over Christmas 1974. With Jon Pertwee having just left the programme, a special regeneration scene was put together, showing him turning into the stage actor Trevor Martin. This was projected onto a screen before the actual show began. The script was by the script editor of the TV show, Terrance Dicks, and saw Wendy Padbury playing one of the stage companions, although not the TV character of Zoe Herriott.

Two years later, the character made his radio debut, in *The Time Machine* by Bernard Venables. Although Peter Cushing was due to record an extensive number of stories for the radio shortly after the second Dalek movie had been completed, the ill-health that had affected him during the latter stages of filming prevented him from recording any of the proposed scripts. It was up to Tom baker to bring the Time Lord to the airwaves.

Elisabeth Sladen, his current TV companion, also appeared in this twenty minute drama which was broadcast as part of the schools' series *Exploration Earth* on the BBC's Radio Four. Baker and Sladen completed another recording that year, but this time for Argo Records. *Doctor Who And The Pescatons* had been scripted by Victor Pemberton, another semi-aquatic adventure following his work on *Fury From The Deep* during the mid-1960s.

Narrated for the most part by Baker, the Doctor saved the Earth from gigantic amphibious creatures lead by the mighty Zor (voiced by Bill Mitchell). The adventure comprised of two 25-minute episodes, one on either side of the record. This was re-released years later on audio tape. The fourth Doctor was also heard in *Genesis Of The Daleks*, which was released as an LP at the same time, condensing the plot of the TV version with Baker narrating bridging material to fill in the gaps. An episode of *The Chase*, cut down quite extensively, had also been released as a single during the mid-1960s.

Although the Doctor was not featured, K9 and Elisabeth Sladen as Sarah Jane Smith did return in *K9 And Company* during Christmas 1981. This was a pilot for a possible spin-off series featuring the two characters. A single 50-minute episode was completed under the title of *A Girl's Best Friend*, scripted by Terence Dudley and directed by John Black.

Location filming was done around the Cotswolds from 12 November to 17 November, with studio recording at the BBC Studios in Pebble Mill following on the 29th and 30th. John Nathan-Turner oversaw the production between seasons eighteen and nineteen of *Doctor Who*. It was transmitted on 28 December 1981, achieving a respectable viewing figure of just under eight and a half million, but a follow up series never materialised.

As part of the *Jim'll Fix It* series in 1985, a young viewer by the name of Gareth Jenkins wrote in to the programme asking if he could meet Colin Baker and go inside the Tardis. The *Doctor Who* production team took it one step further and wrote a brief episode for him to appear in. Eric Saward completed the script, with Janet Fielding returning briefly as Tegan (Nicola Bryant, the companion at the time, was on holiday in America), while Marcus Mortimer directed using just the Tardis console set in TC6, on 20 February 1985. The title was *A Fix With The Sontarans*, and Clinton Greyn and Tim Raynham returned to don their Sontaran costumes from *The Two Doctors* for the nine minute playlet. It was shown a few days later on Saturday 23 February. Colin Baker found Jenkins' ability to memorise the most complex dialogue frustrating, as he couldn't get it right himself. This was effectively the last studio material involving Baker to be recorded before the hiatus kicked in midway through season twenty two's transmission.

During the year-long gap between that and season twenty three, a radio serial called *Slipback* was commissioned as part of a children's show called *Pirate Radio Four*, with both Baker and Nicola Bryant playing the Doctor and Peri for the six 10- minute episodes. Valentine Dyall was amongst the supporting cast, and shortly after completing this, he died. It was his last professional performance.

In 1989, Terrance Dicks completed his second major theatre script for *Doctor Who*, with *The Ultimate Challenge*, for Mark Furness Productions. Originally there had been talk of using a script penned between Ben Aaronovitch and Ian Briggs, but this failed to work out and Dicks was asked to write for his old Doctor, as Jon Pertwee signed up to play the third Doctor once again. During the nationwide tour, Colin Baker took over midway through the run, donning a new version of his sixth Doctor's costume. At one point, when illness prevented Pertwee from continuing with a show, his understudy, David Banks, stepped in to play a new Doctor for two performances. Banks had played the Cyberleader on television throughout the 1980s.

In 1993, Radio Five broadcast a five part radio serial written by Barry Letts, the former producer of the TV show, using one of the old ideas he had submitted to Gerry Davis for consideration as a TV serial in 1966. Suitably updated and reworked, *The Paradise Of Death* featured Elisabeth Sladen as Sarah Jane Smith and Nicholas Courtney as the Brigadier, with Pertwee as the third Doctor. An immense success on both broadcast and release as an audio cassette, a sequel was commissioned towards the end of 1994, with Letts once again scripting it, as a six-part adventure called *The Ghosts Of N-Space*.

With *The Dark Dimension* cancelled on 9 July 1993, there seemed little hope of *Doctor Who* being seen on television for the anniversary week. The *Children In Need* appeal stepped in, and John Nathan-Turner produced and co-wrote a fourteen minute, two-part special which was shot using a revolutionary 3D process. All the surviving Doctors, including a brief appearance by Tom Baker, and many of the companions were present and the locations ranged from the Cutty Sark, to Greenwich and Albert Square, the fictional residence of the *Eastenders* from the popular BBC soap opera. Expectations were high, and it made the front cover of the Radio Times, but many found it to be a major disappointment, only succeeding in making the critics nostalgic for when the series was still being made.

Following on from the *Whose Doctor Who* documentary in 1977, a new analysis of the series was made by the BBC's arts programme, *The Late Show*, producing *30 Years In The Tardis* with Kevin Davies skillfully directing and writing a homage to the show. It included many recreations of famous moments from the programme's past, with subtle touches to suitably update them. A recut 'director's edit' was released on video towards the end of 1994.

Doctor Who - A Basic Guide

A comprehensive listing of all the programme details for every story produced from seasons one to twenty six would take up a book this size in itself. This guide attempts to give a brief synopsis of each adventure, list the main cast of characters and production credits, and give the broadcast dates and ratings for each episode.

Glossary of Terms

Writer: Completes the initial script, based on an idea generated from a submission to the Production team, before handing it to the...

Script Editor: who works with the director and the producer to finalise the storyline and dialogue, until both these creative parties are happy to start pre-production.

Director: The director has to visualise the whole story in televisual terms, and guide the production team through every aspect of what he wants to achieve. He is responsible for what appears on screen at the end of the day.

Producer: The producer is in total artistic control, and looks after the budgets for the series. He has final approval of all aspects of the show.

Designer: Working with the director, he creates the sets and all the physical background details.

Special Effects: This department handles all the model work, special props, and in some cases the creatures needed for each story, although this task can fall completely into the hands of the . . .

Costume Designer: who either creates the monsters, or does it as a joint exercise with the special effects department. Other than that, they conceptualise the clothing for all the characters on screen and manufacture them if they are not readily available 'off the peg'.

Of course, there are countless other departments and individuals involved, but again, a more extensive guide is needed to cover those areas. One final aspect to take note of is the story production codes. These are noted in brackets after the story titles, and are basically used for reference by the production team. Each story has a code, and they are individual letters of the alphabet, e.g. *The Reign Of Terror* (H). Some letters are not used, like 'O', but in some cases this rule is broken. It can be as confusing as it sounds, but the general split between Doctors is as follows . . .

The first Doctor . -
Story A to Story DD
The second Doctor
Story EE to Story ZZ
The third Doctor -
Story AAA to Story ZZZ
The fourth Doctor-
Story 4A to Story 5V
The fifth Doctor . -
Story 5Z to Story 6R
The sixth Doctor -
Story 6S to Story 7C
The seventh Doctor
Story 7D to Story 7Q

As you can see, when the letters start to double up, they're put together, and by the time you get to Tom Baker's debut in *Robot*, rather than use 'AAAA', they abbreviate it to '4A'.

In the mid-1970s, many of the original prints of stories from the first three Doctor eras were destroyed in a mass junking session at the BBC film vaults, which also saw the wiping of many other classic series, such as *Z-Cars*, *The Likely Lads*, *Steptoe And Son*, etc.

Many Troughton and Hartnell stories only have selected episodes in the vaults today, and some are not represented at all. For stories where this applies, a suitable note has been made in the following listing, which is in broadcast order . . .

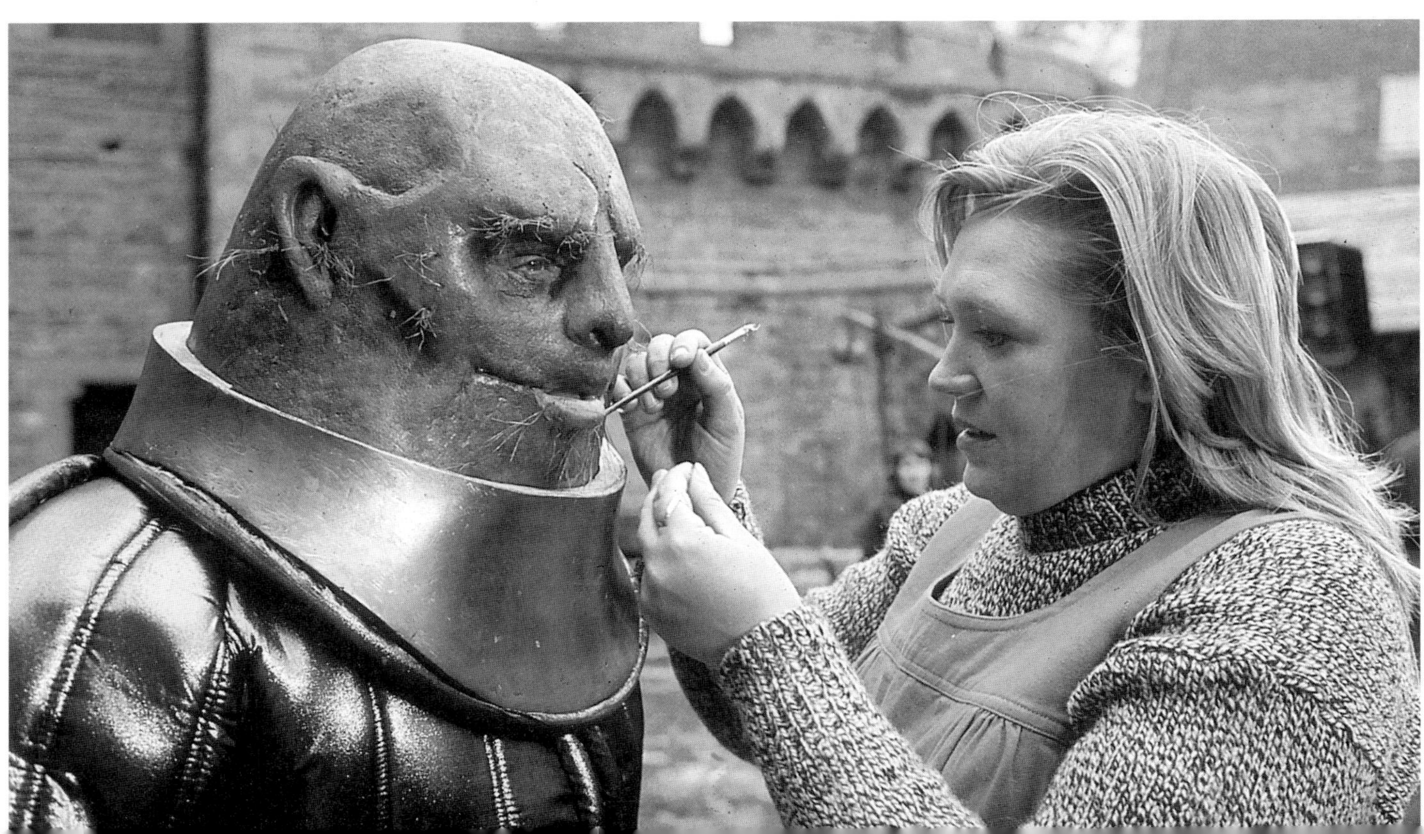

The First Doctor
(November 23rd 1963 – October 29th 1966)

Season One

Regular Cast
The Doctor . . . . William Hartnell
Ian Chesterton . . . . William Russell
Barbara Wright . . . . Jacqueline Hill
Susan Foreman . . . . Carole Anne Ford

Regular Production Team
Verity Lambert . . . . Producer
Mervyn Pinfield . . . . . . Associate Producer
David Whitaker . . . . Script Editor

100,000 BC (Serial A)
Written by C. E. Webber (episode one) & Anthony Coburn (episode one redraft & two to four)
Investigating the background of pupil Susan Foreman, her two teachers, Ian Chesterton and Barbara Wright, find that she lives in a time machine called the Tardis, with her grandfather, the Doctor. The Doctor is forced to take off with all four characters on board, and the ship arrives in 100,000 BC, where they are kidnapped by a tribe of cavemen, desperate to rediscover the secret of fire . . .

Episode One - AN UNEARTHLY CHILD (23/11/63) (4.4m)
Episode Two - THE CAVE OF SKULLS (30/11/63) (5.9m)
Episode Three - THE FOREST OF FEAR (07/12/63) (6.9m)
Episode Four: - THE FIREMAKER (14/12/63) (6.4m)

Kal . . . . Jeremy Young
Za Derek Newark
Hur . . . . Alethea Charlton
Old Mother . . . . Eileen Way
Horg. . . . . Howard Lang
Director . . . . Waris Hussein
Designer . . . . (& Vis Fx)(Pilot) Peter Brachaki . . . . (Pilot Remount & Episodes Two to Four) Barry Newbery
Costume Design . . . . . Maureen Heneghan

THE DALEKS (Serial B)
Written by Terry Nation (7 Episodes)
The Tardis arrives on the planet Skaro, where its crew encounters the Thals, a beautiful passive race, and the Daleks, mutations reliant on machine casings for mobility. The Doctor becomes involved in the unending conflict between the two races and manages to persuade the Thals that it's time to fight back after a Dalek trap sees their leader killed . . .

Episode One - THE DEAD PLANET (21/12/63) (6.9m)
Episode Two - THE SURVIVORS (28/12/64) (6.4m)
Episode Three - THE ESCAPE (04/01/64) (8.9m)
Episode Four - THE AMBUSH (11/01/64) (9.9m)
Episode Five - THE EXPEDITION (18/01/64) (9.9m)
Episode Six - THE ORDEAL (25/01/64) (10.4m)
Episode Seven - THE RESCUE (01/02/64) (10.4m)

Temmosus . . . . Alan Wheatley
Ganatus . . . . Philip Bond
Alydon. . . . . John Lee
Antodus . . . . Marcus Hammond
Elyon . . . . Gerald Curtis
Dyoni . . . . Virginia Wetherall
Dalek Voices by Peter Hawkins & David Graham
Director. . . . . (Episodes 1-2 & 4-5) Christopher Barry
(Episodes 3, 6 & 7) Richard Martin
Designer (& Vis Fx). . . . (Episodes 1-5 & 7) Raymond Cusick
(Episode 6) Jeremy Davies
Costume Design . . . . Daphne Dare

INSIDE THE SPACESHIP (Serial C)
Written by David Whitaker (2 Episodes)
A violent explosion knocks the Tardis crew unconscious, and when they regain their senses, the Doctor discovers that the ship is heading towards its ultimate destruction, and the others begin to suspect one another of sabotage. It's up to the Doctor to find out what has really caused the problem.

Episode One - THE EDGE OF DESTRUCTION (08/02/64) (10.4m)
Episode Two - THE BRINK OF DISASTER (15/02/64) (9.9m)

No supporting cast – Regular Cast only
Director . . . . (Episode One) Richard Martin
(Episode Two) Frank Cox
Designer (& Vis Fx). . . . . . Raymond Cusick
Costume Design . . . . Daphne Dare

MARCO POLO (Serial D) (No episodes exist)
Written by John Jucarotti (7 Episodes)
In the 13th century, the Tardis lands in China where it is taken by Marco Polo as a gift for the mighty Khublai Khan, and the journey the travellers embark on to get to his palace is fraught with danger, as the evil Tegana plots to steal the Tardis and sabotage Polo's expedition. On finally reaching Khan's domain, the Doctor gambles the time machine away in a game of backgammon and has to figure out how to get it back.

Episode One - THE ROOF OF THE WORLD (22/02/64) (9.4m)
Episode Two - THE SINGING SANDS (29/02/64) (9.4m)
Episode Three - FIVE-HUNDRED EYES (07/03/64) (9.4M)
Episode Four - THE WALL OF LIES (14/03/64) (9.9m)
Episode Five: RIDER FROM SHANG-TU (21/03/64) (9.4m)
Episode Six: MIGHTY HKULAI KHAN (28/03/64) (8.4m)
Episode Seven: ASSASSIN AT PEKING (04/04/64) (10.4m)

Marco Polo . . . . Mark Eden
Tegana . . . . Derren Nesbitt
Ping-Cho . . . . Zienia Merton
Khublai Khan . . . . Martin Miller
Ling-Tau . . . . Paul Carson
Chenchu . . . . Jimmy Gardner
Empress. . . . . Claire Davenport
Director . . . . (Episodes 1-3 & 5-7) Waris Hussein
(Episode 4) John Crockett
Designer (& Vis Fx) . . . . Barry Newbery
Costume Design . . . . Daphne Dare

THE KEYS OF MARINUS (Serial E)
Written by Terry Nation (6 Episodes)
The Tardis lands on one of the islands on Marinus, which is surrounded by an acidic sea, and the Time Machine is captured by Arbitan, a monk-like figure who is the Keeper of the Conscience of Marinus. The travellers split up to try and find the four keys that can energise the machine, which have been spread across the planet at different points, and have to return before the commando-like Voords take over the machine . . . . . .

Episode One - THE SEA OF DEATH (11.04.64) (9.9m)
Episode Two - THE VELVET WEB (18/04/64) (9.4m)
Episode Three - THE SCREAMING JUNGLE (25/04/64) (9.9m)
Episode Four - THE SNOWS OF TERROR (02/05/64) (10.4m)
Episode Five - SENTENCE OF DEATH (09/05/64) (7.9m)
Episode Six - THE KEYS OF MARINUS (16/05/64) (6.9m)

Arbitan . . . . George Coulouris
Altos . . . . Robin Phillips
Sabetha . . . . Katherine Schofield
Darrius . . . . Edmund Warwick
Vasor . . . . Francis de Woolf
Eyesen . . . . Donald Pickering
Yartek . . . . Stephen Dartnell
Director . . . . Raymond B. Cusick
Costume Design . . . . Daphne Dare

THE AZTECS (Serial F)
Written by John Lucarotti (4 Episodes)
Materialising in an Aztec High Priest's tomb, the Tardis becomes locked inside as the crew find a secret exit, and Barbara is proclaimed to be a reincarnation of the deceased, Yetaxa. The Doctor has to figure out how to get back to the Tardis before Barbara's attempts to convince the race to stop sacrificing human leads to danger . . .

Episode One - THE TEMPLE OF EVIL (23/05/64) (7.4m)
Episode Two - THE WARRIORS OF DEATH (30/05/64) (7.4M)
Episode Three - THE BRIDE OF SACRIFICE (06/06/64) (7.9m)
Episode Four - THE DAY OF DARKNESS (13/06.64) (7.4m)

Autloc . . . . Keith Pyott
Tlotoxl . . . . John Ringham
Ixta. . . . . Ian Cullen
Cameca . . . . Margot van der Burgh
Tanila. . . . . Walter Randall
Perfect . . . . Victim AndreÔ Boulay
Warrior Captain . . . . David Anderson
Director . . . . John Crockett
Designer (& Vis Fx) . . . . Barry Newbery
Costume Design . . . . Daphne Dare & Tony Pearce

THE SENSORITES (Serial G)
Written by Peter R. Newman (6 Episodes)
The crew of an Earth spaceship from the 28th century are found to be under the control of a race of creatures called Sensorites when the Tardis materialises on board. The Doctor finds the Sensorites are really passive telepaths who are terrified of how the humans on the ship might exploit their society, but there are already some trying to poison the creatures' water supply beneath their city. The Doctor intervenes . . .

Episode One - STRANGERS IN SPACE (20/06/64) (7.9m)
Episode Two - THE UNWILLING WARRIORS (27/06/64) (6.9m)
Episode Three - HIDDEN DANGER (11/07.64) (7.7m)
Episode Four - A RACE AGAINST DEATH (18/07/64) (5.5m)
Episode Five - KIDNAP (25/07.64) (6.9m)
Episode Six - A DESPERATE VENTURE (01/08/64) (6.9m)

John . . . . Stephen Dartnell
Carol . . . . Ilona Rodgers
Maitland. . . . . Lorne Cossette
First Elder . . . . Eric Francis
Second Elder . . . . Bartlett Mullins
Sensorite . . . . Ken Tyllson
Sensorite . . . . Joe Greig
Sensorite . . . . Arthur Newall
Sensorite . . . . Peter Glaze
Director . . . (Episodes 1-4) Mervyn Pinfield (Episodes 5-6) Frank Cox
Designer (& Vis Fx). . . . Raymond P. Cusick
Costume Design . . . . Daphne Dare

THE REIGN OF TERROR (Serial H) (Episodes 1-3 & 6 Exist)
Written by Dennis Spooner (6 Episodes)
Arriving in Paris during the time of Robespierre, the four travellers become separated. With the Doctor in disguise as an official, Ian is held as an English spy and Barbara and Susan are sentenced to death, and due to meet Madame Guillotine. The four have to plot to escape from the city and return to the safety of the Tardis . . .

Episode One - A LAND OF FEAR (08/08/64 (6.9m)
Episode Two - GUESTS OF MADAME GUILLOTINE (15/08/64) (6.9m)
Episode Three - A CHANGE OF IDENTITY (22/08/64) (6.9m)
Episode Four - THE TYRANT OF FRANCE (29/08/64) (6.4m)
Episode Five - A BARGAIN OF NECESSITY (05/09/64 (6.9m)
Episode Six - PRISONERS OF THE CONCIERGE (12/09/64) (6.4m)

Lerna Oitre . . . . James Cairncross
Jean . . . . Roy Herrick
Jules Renan . . . . Donald Morley
Robespierre . . . . Keith Anderson
Physician . . . . Ronald Pickup
Jailer . . . . Jack Cunningham
Leon Colbert . . . . Edward Brayshaw
Rouvray . . . . Laidlaw Dalling
Judge . . . . Howard Charlton
Webster . . . . Jeffrey Wickham
Danielle . . . . Caroline Hunt
Napoleon . . . . Tony Wall
Director. . . . . Henric Hirsch
With Uncredited Work by Timothy Combe
Designer (& Vis Fx) . . . . Roderick Laing
Costume Design . . . . Daphne Dare

Season Two

Regular Cast
The Doctor . . . . William Hartnell
Ian Chesterton . . (Serial J-R) William Russell
Barbara Wright . . (Serial J-R) Jacqueline Hill
Susan Foreman. (Serial J-K) Carole Ann Ford
Vicki. . (Serial L Onwards) Maureen O'Brien
Steven Taylor . . . . (Serial R Onwards) Peter Purves

Regular Production Team
Verity Lambert . . . . Producer
Mervyn Pinfield . . . . Exec Prod (To M)
David Whitaker . . . Script Editor (Serial J-K)
Dennis Spooner. . . Script Editor (Serial L-R)
Donald Tosh . . . . Script Editor (Serial S)

PLANET OF GIANTS (Serial J
Written by Louis Marks (3 Episodes)
The Doctor finally manages to land on modern day earth, but the Tardis is only an inch high, and the miniaturised crew try to foil the schemes of Forrester, an insecticide maker, facing all kinds of dangers along the way . . .

Episode One - PLANET OF GIANTS (31/10/64) (8.4m)
Episode Two - DANGEROUS JOURNEY (07/11/64) (8.4m)
Episode Three - CRISIS (14/11/64) (8.9m)

Forrester . . . . Alan Tilvern
Farrow . . . . Frank Crawshaw
Smithers . . . . Reginald Barratt
Hilda Rowse . . . . Rosemary Johnson
Bert Rowse. . . . . Fred Ferris
Director . . . (Episodes 1-3) Mervyn Pinfield (Episode 3) Douglas Camfield
Designer (& Vis Fx). . . . Raymond P. Cusick
Costume Design . . . . Daphne Dare

THE DALEK INVASION OF EARTH (serial K)
Written by Terry Nation (6 Episodes)
Earth has been conquered by the Daleks, with mankind almost wiped out by a space plague, and all but a handful of resistance fighters who survived have been turned into zombie-like Robomen, to work as drones for the aliens. As the Tardis arrives, Ian and the Doctor are captured by the Daleks, while Barbara and Susan join the resistance. The Doctor manages to foil the Daleks plan to hollow out the core of the planet and build a propulsion system to make the Earth into a type of giant spaceship. As he prepares to leave with Ian and Barbara, he decides to leave Susan behind

with David Campbell, whom she has fallen in love with, so that she can spend the rest of her life on Earth ...

Episode One - WORLD'S END (21/11/64) (11.4m)
Episode Two - THE DALEKS (28/11/64) (12.4m)
Episode Three - DAY OF RECKONING (05/12/64) (11.9m)
Episode Four - THE END OF TOMORROW . . (12/12/64) (11.9m)
Episode Five - THE WAKING ALLY (19/12/64) (12.4m)
Episode Six - FLASHPOINT (26/12/64) (12.4m)

Carl Tyler. . . . . Bernard Kay
David Campbell . . . . Peter Fraser
Dortmun. . . . . Alan Judd
Jenny . . . . Ann Davies
Larry Madison . . . . Graham Rigby
Wells . . . . Nicholas Smith
Dalek Voices by Peter Hawkins & David Graham
Director. . . . . Richard Martin
Designer (& Vis Fx) . . . . Spencer Chapman
Costume Design . . . . Daphne Dare & Tony Pearce

<u>THE RESCUE</u> (Serial L)
Written by David Whitaker (2 Episodes)
On the planet Dildo, the Tardis crew split up and Barbara is nearly murdered by a vicious creature called Koquillion, but survives and finds two survivors on board the wreckage of a crashed spaceship. Vicki is friendly enough, but Bennett sees Barbara as a threat. When the Doctor and Ian arrive, the mystery of exactly who, or rather what Koquillion is, is quickly resolved. At the end of the story, Vicki joins the Tardis crew.

Episode One - THE POWERFUL ENEMY (02.01/65) (12.0m)
Episode Two - DESPERATE MEASURES (09/01/65) (13.0m)

Bennett. . . . . Ray Barratt
(Also Koquillion as Sydney Wilson)
Space Captain. . . . . Tom Sheridan
Director. . . . . Christopher Barry
Designer (& Vis Fx). . . . Raymond P. Cusick
Costume Design . . . . Daphne Dare

<u>THE ROMANS</u> (Serial M)
Written by Dennis Spooner (4 Episodes)
On holiday in ancient Rome, the Doctor is mistaken for the recently murdered lyre player, due to appear at the court of Emperor Nero, where he is taken with Vicki. Barbara is taken by slavers and ends up working at Nero's Palace and Ian's journey on a slave ship is curtailed when it sinks, and he ends up as a Gladiator in Rome. Eventually the four of them are reunited back at the villa, oblivious to what has happened to each other . . .

Episode One - THE SLAVE TRADERS (16/01/65) (13.0m)
Episode Two - ALL ROADS LEAD TO ROME (23/01/65) (11.5m)
Episode Three - CONSPIRACY (30/01/65) (10.0m)
Episode Four - INFERNO (06/02/65) (12.0m)

Sevcheria . . . . Derek Sydney
Ascaris . . . . Barry Jackson
Delos . . . . Peter Diamond
Tavius . . . . Michael Peake
Nero . . . . Derek Francis
Poppaea . . . . Kay Patrick
Director. . . . . Christopher Barry
Designer (& Vis Fx). . . . Raymond P. Cusick
Costume Design . . . . Daphne Dare

<u>THE WEB PLANET</u> (Serial N)
Written by Bill Strutton (6 Episodes)
The planet of Vortis has been taken over by a parasitic intelligence called the Animus, which has enslaved the ant-like Zarbi, and caused the natural inhabitants, the Menoptera, to flee to another world. The Animus captures the Doctor and tries to take control of the Tardis so it can control all of time and space, but he manages to defeat it, and the Menoptera are able to take control of their home world once more

Episode One - THE WEB PLANET (13/02/65) (13.5m)
Episode Two - THE ZARBI (20/02/65) (12.5m)
Episode Three - ESCAPE TO DANGER (27/02/65) (12.5m)
Episode Four - CRATER OF NEEDLES (06/03/65) (13.0m)
Episode Five - INVASION (13/03/65) (12.0m)
Episode Six - THE CENTRE (20/03/65) (11.5m)

Vrestin. . . . . Roslyn de Winter
Hroster . . . . Arne Gordon
Prapillus. . . . . Jolyon Booth
Hlynia. . . . . Jocelyn Birdsall
Hilio . . . . Martin Jarvis
Zarbi . . . . Robert Jewell
Zarbi. . . . . John Scott Martin
Zarbi . . . . Jack Pitt
Zarbi . . . . Kevin Manser
Zarbi . . . . Gerald Taylor
Zarbi . . . . Hugh Lund
Animus Voice . . . . Catherine Fleming
Director. . . . . Richard Martin
Designer (& Vis Fx). . . . . John Wood
Costume Design . . . . Daphne Dare

<u>THE CRUSADE</u> (Serial P) (Episode 3 exists)
Written by David Whitaker (4 Episodes)
The Doctor becomes an advisor to Richard the Lionheart. His knights are ambushed by the Saracen hordes, and Ian sets out to rescue Barbara when she is kidnapped and taken to the court of El Akir. The situation becomes more complex when the Doctor accidentally reveals that Richard plans to marry his sister, Joanna, and the Saracen Saphadin learns of this information . . .

Episode One - THE WHEEL (27/03/65) (10.5m)
Episode Two - THE KNIGHT OF JAFFA (03/04/65) (8.5m)
Episode Three - THE WHEEL OF FORTUNE (10/04/65 (9.0m)
Episode Four - THE WARLORDS (17/04/65) (9.5m)

El Akir . . . . Walter Randall
Richard The Lionheart . . . . . . Julian Glover
Ben Daheer . . . . Reg Pritchard
William de Tornebu . . . . . Bruce Wightman
Saphadin. . . . . Roger Avon
Saladin . . . . Bernard Kay
Joanna . . . . Jean Marsh
Chamberlain . . . . Robert Lankesheer
Director . . . . Douglas Camfield
Designer (& Vis Fx) . . . . Barry Newbery
Costume Design . . . . Daphne Dare

<u>THE SPACE MUSEUM</u> (Serial Q
Written by Glyn Jones (4 Episodes)
On the planet Xeros, in a museum of the Morok Empire, the Tardis crew find it mysterious that neither the Moroks nor the subservient Xerons can see them, and are alarmed when they find a museum exhibit containing themselves. The Doctor deduces that time shifts experienced as they arrived have put them on a different time track, slightly in their own future, but this is suddenly rectified and a fight to avoid their future enslavement begins . . .

Episode One - THE SPACE MUSEUM (24/04/65) (10.5m)
Episode Two - THE DIMENSIONS OF TIME (01/05/65) (9.3M)
Episode Three - THE SEARCH (08/05/65) (8.5m)
Episode Four - THE FINAL PHASE (15.05.65) (8.5m)

Sita . . . . Peter Sanders
Dako . . . . Peter Craze

Lobos . . . . Richard Shaw
Tor . . . . Jeremy Bulloch
Morok Commander . . . . Ivor Salter
Dalek Voice by Peter Hawkins
Director . . . . Mervyn Pinfield
Designer (& Vis Fx) . . . . Spencer Chapman
Costume design Daphne Dare & Pauline Mansfield-Clarke

THE CHASE (Serial R)
Written by Terry Nation (6 Episodes)
The Daleks are pursuing the Tardis in their own Time Machine, moving from the planet Aridius, to the Empire State Building, the Mary Celeste, the Festival of Ghana and finally the planet of Mechanus, where the Doctor foils an attempt by the Daleks to destroy him using a robot double and a gigantic battle between the aliens and the Mechanoids takes place. At the conclusion, Ian and Barbara use the Dalek Time Machine to get back to present day earth, and the stranded space pilot Steven Taylor joins the Tardis crew as the ship leaves . . .

Episode One - THE EXECUTIONERS (22/05/65) (10.0m)
Episode Two - THE DEATH OF TIME (29/05/65) (9.5m)
Episode Three - FLIGHT THROUGH ETERNITY (05/06/65) (9.0m)
Episode Four - JOURNEY INTO TERROR (12/06/65) (9.5m)
Episode Five - THE DEATH OF DOCTOR WHO (19/06/65) (9.0m)
Episode Six - THE PLANET OF DECISION (26/06.65) (9.5m)

Rynian . . . . Hywel Bennett
Morton Dill . . . . Peter Purves
Captain Briggs . . . . David Blake Kelly
The Grey Lady . . . . Roslyn de Winter
Robot Doctor Who . . . . . Edmund Warwick
Dalek Voices by Peter Hawkins and David Graham
Mechanoid Voices by David Graham
Director . . . . Richard Martin
Designer (& Vis Fx). . . . Raymond P. Cusick & John Wood
Costume Design . . . . Daphne dare

THE TIME MEDDLER (Serial S)
Written by Dennis Spooner (4 Episodes)
Off the English coastline in 1066, the Tardis crew hear strange stories about a mysterious monk when they explore a Saxon village, and find artefacts from the future, such as a wristwatch and a tape recorder. The Monk is revealed to have his own Tardis, and enjoys meddling with history, his latest scheme being to change the outcome of the Battle of Hastings . . .

Episode One - THE WATCHER (03/07/65) (8.9m)
Episode Two - THE MEDDLING MONK (10/07/65) (8.8m)
Episode Three - A BATTLE OF WITS (17/07/65) (7.7m)
Episode Four - CHECKMATE (24/07/65) (8.3m)

The Monk. . . . . Peter Butterworth
Edith . . . . Alethea Charlton
Eldred . . . . Peter Russell
Wulnoth . . . . Michael Miller
Ulf Norman Hartley
Sven. . . . . David Anderson
Director . . . . Douglas Camfield
Designer.(&.Vis.Fx) . . . . Barry Newbery
Costume Design . . . . Daphne Dare

Season Three

Regular Cast
The Doctor . . . . William Hartnell
Vicki . . . . (Serial T-U) Maureen O'Brien
Steven Taylor . . . (Serial T-AA) Peter Purves
Katarina . . . . (Serial U-V) Adrienne Hill
Sarah Kingdom . . . . . (Serial V) Jean Marsh
Dodo Chaplet . . . . (Serial W Onwards) Jackie Lane

Regular Production Team
Verity Lambert . . . . Producer (Serial T-T/A)
John Wiles . . . . Producer (Serial U-X)
Innes Lloyd . . . . Producer (Serial Y-BB)

GALAXY FOUR (Serial T) (No Episodes Exist)
Written by William Emms (4 Episodes)
The Drahvins are stranded on a planet that is about to be destroyed, and want to escape by capturing the spaceship of the Rills, hideous walrus-like creatures, leaving them behind to die. The Rills exist in a special environment and use their robotic servants, the Chumblies, to carry out any maintenance outside their ship. The Doctor and the Tardis crew soon come to the conclusion that the Rills may not be as evil as the Drahvins say, and that the situation might be exactly the opposite.....

Episode One - FOUR HUNDRED DAWNS (11/09/65) (9.0m)
Episode Two - TRAP OF STEEL (18/09/65) (9.5m)
Episode Three - AIR LOCK (25/09/65) (11.5m)
Episode Four - THE EXPLODING PLANET (02/10/65) (9.9m)

Maaga . . . . Stephanie Bidmead
Drahvin One . . . . Marina Martin
Drahvin Two. . . . . Susanna Carroll
Drahvin Three . . . . Lyn Ashley
Garvey . . . . Barry Jackson
Chumblie. . . . . Jimmy Kaye
Chumblie . . . . Tommy Reynolds
Chumblie. . . . . William Shearer
Chumblie . . . . Pepi Poupee
Chumblie . . . . Angelo Muscat
Rill Voice by Robert Cartland
Director . . . . Derek Martinus
(initial Ealing work) Mervyn Pinfield
Designer (& Vis Fx) . . . . Richard Hunt
Costume Design . . . . Daphne Dare

MISSION TO THE UNKNOWN (Serial T/A)
(The episode does not exist)
Written by Terry Nation (I Episode)
On the planet Kembel, an agent of the Space Special Security Service, called Marc Cory, unearths evidence of the Daleks plotting to stage a concentrated attack on the solar system. His crew are killed one by one, by both the deadly Vaaga plants and the Daleks, and when the Daleks track him down he is exterminated, but the tape recording of his findings survives.....

No Regular Cast appeared – This episode acted as a teaser for what was to come in *The Daleks' Master Plan.*

Episode One: MISSION TO THE UNKNOWN (09/10/65) (8.3m)

Marc Cory. . . . . Edward de Souza
Jeff Garvey. . . . . Barry Jackson
Gordon Lowery . . . . Jeremy Young
Malpha . . . . Robert Cartland
Dalek Voices by Peter Hawkins & David Graham
Director . . . . Derek Martinus
Designer (& Vis Fx). . . Raymond P. Cusic & Richard Hunt
Costume Design . . . . Daphne Dare

THE MYTH MAKERS (Serial U) (No episodes exist)
Written by Donald Cotton (4 Episodes)
The Tardis is mistaken for the Temple of Zeus in Troy, in the midst of the Trojan War, and the Doctor is thought to be a God. Stephen, disguised as a warrior, takes on Achilles, whom the Doctor helps to defeat Hector, and bring about the fall of Troy. Vicki falls in love with Troilus, and decides to stay behind, while an unexpected new companion arrives on board the Tardis, as Katarina, a slave girl, helps the badly injured Steven on board the vessel.....

Episode One: TEMPLE OF SECRETS (16/10/65) (8.3m)

Episode Two: SMALL PROPHET, QUICK RETURN (23/10/65) (8.1m)
Episode Three: DEATH OF A SPY (30/10/65) (8.7m)
Episode Four: HORSE OF DESTRUCTION (06/11/65) (8.3m)

Achilles . . . . Cavan Kendall
Odysseus . . . . Ivor Salter
Agamemnon . . . . Francis de Woolf
Cyclops . . . . Tutte Lemkow
Menelaus . . . . Jack Melford
King Priam . . . . Max Adrian
Paris . . . . Barrie Ingham
Cassandra . . . . Frances White
Troilus . . . . James Lynn
Director . . . . Michael Leeston-Smith
Designer (& Vis Fx) . . . . John Wood
Costume Design . . . . Daphne Dare & Tony Pearce

THE DALEKS' MASTER PLAN (Serial V)
(Episodes 5 & 10 exist)
Written by Terry Nation (Episodes 1-5 & 7) & Dennis Spooner (Episodes 6 & 8-12)
From Plotlines by Terry Nation (12 Episodes)
Six months has passed since Marc Cory's death, when the Tardis materialises on Kembel, and his death is being looked into by SSS Agent, Bret Vyon. Mavic Chen, the Guardian of the Solar System, has betrayed his position and joined forces with the Daleks, who now have an awesome weapon in the shape of a Time Destructor, but need a Taranium Core to power it. Both Vyon and Katarina die in the early stages of the race to stop the Daleks, and Bret's sister, Sara Kingdom joins the Tardis crew as the Doctor successfully steals the core. The vast Dalek forces set off after him in pursuit. The chase moves through the earth of the 1920s and on to ancient Egypt, where the travellers come across the Meddling Monk. In the end, Chen is killed by the Daleks when his usefulness is at an end, and Sarah Kingdom sacrifices her life to switch the Time Destructor off, once it has been energised.....

Episode One - THE NIGHTMARE BEGINS (13/11/65) (9.1m)
Episode Two - DAY OF ARMAGEDDON (20/11/65) (9.8m)
Episode Three - DEVIL'S PLANET (27/11/65) (10.3m)
Episode Four - THE TRAITORS (04/12/65) (9.5m)
Episode Five - COUNTER-PLOT (11/12/65) (9.9m)
Episode Six - CORONAS OF THE SUN (18/12/65) (9.1m)
Episode Seven - THE FEAST OF STEVEN (25/12/65) (7.9m)
Episode Eight - VOLCANO (01/01/66) (9.6m)
Episode Nine - GOLDEN DEATH (07/01/66) (9.2m)
Episode Ten - ESCAPE SWITCH (15/01/66) (9.5m)
Episode Eleven: THE ABANDONED PLANET (22/01/66) (9.8m)
Episode Twelve: DESTRUCTION OF TIME (29/01/66) (8.6m)

Bret Vyon . . . . Nicholas Courtney
Mavic Chen . . . . Kevin Stoney
The Meddling Monk . . . . Peter Butterworth
Trantis . . . . Roy Evans
Malpha . . . . Bryan Mosley
Dalek Voice by Peter Hawkins & David Graham
Director . . . . Douglas Camfield
Designer . . . . (Episodes 1-2, 5-7 & 11) Raymond P. Cusick
(& Vis Fx) . . . . . (Episodes 3-4, 8-10 & 12) Barry Newbery
Costume Design . . . . Daphne Dare

THE MASSACRE OF ST. BARTHOLOMEW'S EVE (Serial W) (No episodes exist)
Written by John Lucarotti (4 Episodes)
Exhausted, and in need of a rest, Steven and the Doctor retreat to 16th Century France, and arrive in the midst of a bitter feud between the Catholics and Protestants. They rescue a young servant girl, who has overheard plans made by the Catholic Queen Mother to massacre all Protestant citizens. Steven gets confused when the Abbot of Amboise arrives on the scene, as he is the exact double of the Doctor. The Doctor is unable to alter history and stop the bloodshed, and the Tardis lands on modern day earth on Wimbledon Common, where a young woman charges in, mistaking the time machine for a real Police Box. Her surname is the same as the servant girl's, suggesting that she might have survived the massacre.....

Episode One - WAR OF GOD (05/02/66) (8.0m)
Episode Two - THE SEA BEGGAR (12/02/66) (6.0m)
Episode Three - PRIEST OF DEATH (19/02/66) (5.9m)
Episode Four - BELL OF DOOM (26/02/66) (5.8m)

Nicholas . . . . David Weston
Anne . . . . Annette Robertson
Abbot of Amboise . . . . . . William Hartnell.
Marshal Tavannes . . . . Andre Morell
Admiral de Coligny . . . . Leonard Sachs
Catherine de Medici . . . . Joan Young
Toligny . . . . Michael Bilton
Director . . . . Paddy Russell
Designer (& Vis Fx) . . . . Michael Young
Costume Design . . . . Daphne Dare

THE ARK (Serial X)
Written by Paul Erickson & Lesley Scott (4 Episodes)
Mistaking the jungle they have landed in for the surface of a normal planet, the Tardis crew find they are actually inside a gigantic spaceship. The miniaturised population of earth are being taken to Refusis to start a new population there with the Guardians monitoring their safety, while the reptilian Monoids act as their servants. Dodo's cold starts to infect them all, and the travellers are put on trial but the Doctor soon puts this right, and they depart, only to materialise on the Space Ark again, hundreds of years in the future when the Monoids now rule, and the humans are their slaves...

Episode One - THE STEEL SKY (05/03/66) (5.5m)
Episode Two - THE PLAGUE (12/03/66) (6.9m)
Episode Three - THE RETURN (19/03/66) (6.2m)
Episode Four - THE BOMB (26/03/66) (7.4m)

Commander . . . . Eric Elliott
Zentos . . . . Inigo Jackson
Manyak . . . . Roy Spencer
Rhos . . . . Michael Sheard
Maharis . . . . Terence Woodfield
Dassuk . . . . Brian Wright
Monoid . . . . Edmund Coulter
Monoid . . . . Frank George
Director . . . . Michael Imison
Designer (& Vis Fx) . . . . Barry Newbery
Costume Design . . . . Daphne Dare

THE CELESTIAL TOYMAKER (Serial Y)
(Episode four exists)
Written by Brian Hayles (4 Episodes)
Uncredited Rewrite by Gerry Davis
The Doctor is turned invisible, and realises that the Tardis has become trapped in the domain of a being known as the Toymaker. He is separated from Steven and Dodo, who have to complete a series of tests to win the Tardis back, while the Doctor plays the Trilogic Game. If any of the Travellers fail to win, they will become the Toymakers play things for all eternity...

Episode One - THE CELESTIAL TOYROOM (02/04/66) (8.0m)

Episode Two - THE HALL OF DOLLS (09/04/66) (8.0m)
Episode Three - THE DANCING FLOOR (16/04/66) (7.8m)
Episode Four - THE FINAL TEST (23/04/66) (7.8m)

The Toymaker. . . . . Michael Gough
Clown . . . . Campbell Singer (plus other characters)
Clown . . . . Carmen Silvera (plus other characters)
Cyril . . . . Peter Stephens (Plus One of The Hearts)
Heart . . . . Reg Lever
Director . . . . Bill Sellars
Designer (& Vis Fx). . . . . John Wood
Costume Design . . . . Daphne Dare

THE GUNFIGHTERS (Serial Z)
Written by Donald Cotton (4 Episodes)
The search for a dentist to cure the Doctor's bad toothache takes the Tardis to Tombstone in the wild west, and the only physician in the area happens to be Doc Holliday, fore whom the Doctor is mistaken. With Steven and Dodo working as entertainers to avoid being executed as outlaws, the Doctor has to get them away from the town before the legendary gunfight at the OK Corral takes place...

Episode One - A HOLIDAY FOR THE DOCTOR (30/04/66) (6.5m)
Episode Two - DON'T SHOOT THE PIANIST (07/05/66) (6.6m)
Episode Three - JOHNNY RINGO (14/05/66) (6.2m)
Episode Four - THE OK CORRAL (21/05/66) (5.7m)

Ike Clanton. . . . . William Hurndall
Phineas Clanton . . . . Maurice Good
Billy Clanton . . . . David Cole
Seth Harper. . . . . Shane Rimmer
Wyatt Earp. . . . . John Alderson
Doc Holliday . . . . Anthony Jacobs
Bat Masterson. . . . . Richard Beale
Pa Clanton . . . . Reed de Rouen
Johnny Ringo . . . . Laurence Payne
Director. . . . . Rex Tucker
Designer (& Vis Fx) . . . . Barry Newbery
Costume Design . . . . Daphne Dare

THE SAVAGES (Serial AA) (No episodes exist)
Written by Ian Stuart Black (4 Episodes)
Returning to a planet he has been to once before, the Doctor finds a sinister situation has arisen since his last visit. The Elders are experimenting on the primitives of their race, and draining their lifeforce to prolong their own lifespans. After the Doctor finds a way to stop this taking place, Steven decides to stay behind on the planet to try and bring the two races together...

Episode One – (28/05/66) (4.8m)
Episode Two – (04/06/66) (5.6m)
Episode Three – (11/06/66) (5.0m)
Episode Four – (18/06/66) (4.5m)

Chal. . . . . Ewan Solon
Tor Patrick Godfrey
Captain Edal . . . . Peter Thomas
Exorse . . . . Geoffrey Frederick
Jano . . . . Frederick Jaeger
Nanina . . . . Clare Jenkins
Senta . . . . Norman Henry
Wylda. . . . . Edward Caddick
Director. . . . . Christopher Barry
Designer (& Vis Fx) . . . . Stuart Walker
Costume Design . . . . Daphne Dare

THE WAR MACHINES (Serial BB)
Written by Ian Stuart Black (4 Episodes)
Finally arriving back in modern London, the Doctor is intrigued by the recently completed GPO Tower, and senses something is wrong. Investigating further, he finds that an artificial intelligence computer, called WOTAN, has been built within. Dodo is put under the machine's control, and after the Doctor has recovered from an attempt to take over his mind, he finds that WOTAN has unleashed a number of tank-like machines throughout central London. Helped by a sailor, Ben Jackson, and a secretary, Polly, the Doctor manages to defeat WOTAN, and sets off for the Tardis alone, as Dodo has decided to stay behind, but Ben and Polly soon join him...

Episode One – (25/06/66) (5.4m)
Episode Two – (02/07/66) (4.7m)
Episode Three – (09/07/66) (5.3m)
Episode Four – (16/07/66) (5.5m)

Professor Brett . . . . John Harvey
Major Green . . . . Alan Curtis
Polly . . . . Anneke Wills
Ben Jackson . . . . Michael Craze
Sir Charles Summer . . . . . . William Mervyn
Professor Krimpton . . . . John Cater
Kitty . . . . Sandra Bryant
Newsreader . . . . Kenneth Kendall
Director . . . . Michael Ferguson
Designer (& Vis Fx). . . . . Raymond London
Costumer Design. . . . . Daphne Dare

Season Four

Regular Cast
The Doctor. (Serial CC-DD) William Hartnell
The Doctor . . . . (Serial EE onwards) Patrick Troughton
Polly . . . . (Serial CC-KK) Anneke Wills
Ben Jackson . . (Serial CC-KK) Michael Craze
Jamie . . . . (Serial FF Onwards) Frazer Hines
Victoria . . . . (Serial LL Onwards) Deborah Watling

Regular Production Team
Innes Lloyd . . . . Producer
Gerry Davis. . . . . Script Editor
Peter Bryant. . . . . Script Editor (From Serial LL/Episode 4)

THE SMUGGLERS (Serial CC)
(No episodes exist)
Written by Brian Hayles (4 Episodes)
Arriving on the Cornish Coast in the 17th Century, a seemingly harmless message from a Church warden leads the Tardis crew into a confrontation with some Pirates. The Doctor has to persuade Customs and Excise Officers to help him defeat Captain Pike, who is in league with the local Squire, before sentence is passed on Ben and Polly, who have been framed for the murder of the now dead Church warden...

Episode One – (10/09/66) (4.3m)
Episode Two – (17/09/66) (4.9m)
Episode Three – (24/09/66) (4.2m)
Episode Four – (01/10/66) (4.5m)

Cherub . . . . George A. Cooper
Squire . . . . Paul Whitsun-Jones
Captain Pike . . . . Michael Godfrey
Blake . . . . John Ringham
Jacob Kewper . . . . David Blake Kelly
Tom . . . . Mike Lucas
Director. . . . . Julia Smith
Designer (& Vis Fx) . . . . Richard Hunt
Costume Design . . . . Daphne Dare

THE TENTH PLANET (Serial DD) (Episodes 1-3 exist)
Written by Kit Pedlar with Gerry Davis (for episodes three and four)
At a tracking station on the South Pole, radars pick up signals from a new planet heading into orbit, which drains the energy from a space shuttle, and then starts to do the same to the Earth. It's inhabitants are revealed to be the Cybermen, who need the energy to carry out their plan to turn humans into their own kind. A first inva-

sion force is defeated, and after the Doctor manages to overcome a second, Mondas (Earth's long-lost twin world) is blown up. The experience seems to age the Doctor, and on returning to the Tardis, Ben and Polly can only watch as he collapses and starts to regenerate...

Episode One - (08/10/66) (5.5m)
Episode Two - (15/10/66) (6.4m)
Episode Three - (22/10/66) (7.6m)
Episode Four - (29/10/66) (7.5m)

General Cutler. . . . . Robert Beatty
Dyson . . . . Dudley Jones
Barclay . . . . David Dodimead
Radar Technician . . . Christopher Matthews
Winger . . . . Steve Plytas
Cybermen Voices by Roy Skelton & Peter Hawkins
Director . . . . Derek Martinus
Designer (& Vis Fx). . . . . Peter Kindred
Costume Designer. . . . . Sandra Reid

THE POWER OF THE DALEKS (Serial EE)
(no episodes exist)
Written by David Whitaker (6 Episodes)
With Uncredited rewrites by Dennis Spooner
Still suspicious of the stranger claiming to be the Doctor, Ben and Polly keep a careful eye on him as the Tardis arrives on Vulcan, where the Doctor is mistaken for being the Earth Examiner. Nobody takes heed of his warnings as he realises the implications of three Daleks being reactivated, after being found in a capsule in a Mercury swamp. Sure enough, a Dalek production line is quickly up and running, with the creatures attempting to over-run the colony before the Doctor can defeat them...

Episode One - (05/11/66) (7.9m)
Episode Two - (12/11/66) (7.8m)
Episode Three - (19/11/66) (7.5m)
Episode Four - (26/11/66) (7.8m)
Episode Five - (03/12/66) (8.0m)
Episode Six - (10/12/66) (7.8m)

Quinn. . . . . Nicholas Hawtrey
Bragen . . . . Bernard Archard
Lesterson. . . . . Robert James
Janley . . . . Pamela Ann Davy
Hensell. . . . . Peter Bathurst
Valmar. . . . . Richard Kane
Kebble . . . . Steven Scott
Dalek Voices by Peter Hawkins
Director. . . . . Christopher Barry
Designer (& Vis Fx) . . . . Derek Dodd
Costume Design . . . . Sandra Reid

THE HIGHLANDERS (Serial FF)
(No episodes exist)
Written by Elwyn Jones with additional material by Gerry Davis (4 Episodes)
The Tardis lands in Scotland during the Battle of Culloden in 1746, and the Doctor and his companions become involved with a group of slave traders. The Doctor sets about freeing the men and arming them, whilst revealing to the English Redcoats the identity of the man behind the operation, a solicitor called Grey. With everything resolved, the Tardis leaves with an extra occupant, the piper Jamie McCrimmon...

Episode One - (17/11/66) (6.7m)
Episode Two - (24/12/66) (6.8m)
Episode Three - (31/12/66) (7.4m)
Episode Four - (07/01/67) (7.3m)

Lieutenant Algernon Ffinch . Michael Elwyn
Laird. . . . . Donald Bisset
Kirsty . . . . Hannah Gordon
Solicitor Grey. . . . . David Garth
Perkins . . . . Sydney Arnold
Trask . . . . Dallas Cavell
Sergeant . . . . Peter Welch
Director. . . . . Hugh David
Designer (& Vis Fx) . . . . Geoff Kirkland
Costume Design . . . . Sandra Reid

THE UNDERWATER MENACE (Serial GG)
(Episode 3 exists)
Written by Geoffrey Orme (4 Episodes)
Materialising on an apparently uninhabited extinct volcano on Earth, the Tardis crew are captured by primitive Atlanteans and taken below ground, where they find they are entering the lost city of Atlantis. They are saved from being sacrificed by Professor Zaroff, an insane scientist intent on destroying the world, who has made a false promise to the Atlanteans that he will raise their city from the ocean floor. The Doctor has to convince city's slaves and workers that Zaroff has to be stopped...

Episode One - (14/01/67) (8.3m)
Episode Two - (21/01/67) (7.5m)
Episode Three - (28/01/67) (7.1m)
Episode Four - (04/02/67) (7.0m)

Zaroff . . . . Joseph Furst
Lolem. . . . . Peter Stephens
Ramo . . . . Tom Watson
Ara Catherine Howe
Damon . . . . Colin Jeavons
Jacko . . . . Paul Anil
Sean. . . . . P.G. Stephens
Director. . . . . Julia Smith
Designer (& Vis Fx). . . . . Jack Robinson
Costume Design . . . . Sandra Reid & Juanita Robinson

THE MOONBASE (Serial HH) (Episodes 2 & 4 exist)
Written by Kit Pedlar with Additional Material by Gerry Davis (4 Episodes)
The year is 2070, and the Earth's weather is being controlled by a machine called the Gravitron, housed on the moon. Exploring the lunar surface, the Tardis crew head towards the moonbase when Jamie is injured. They find the staff on the moonbase under siege from a mysterious illness and sabotage. The Cybermen are revealed to be behind it, with a plan to use the Gravitron to help render the Earth powerless to an invasion attempt. The Doctor has very little time to stop them...

Episode One - (11/02/67) (8.1m)
Episode Two - (18/02.67) (8.9m)
Episode Three - (25/02/67) (8.2m)
Episode Four - (04/03/67) (8.1m)

Hobson . . . . Patrick Barr
Benoit . . . . Andre Maranne
Nils . . . . Michael Wolf
Sam . . . . John Rolfe
Doctor Evans. . . . . Alan Rowe
Ralph. Mark Heath
Cybermen Voices by Peter Hawkins
Director . . . . Morris Barry
Designer (& Vis Fx). . . . . Colin Shaw
Costume Design . . . . Daphne Dare & Mary Woods

THE MACRA TERROR (Serial JJ)
(No episodes exist)
Written by Ian Stuart Black (4 Episodes)
On a planet where an Earth colony is run like a holiday camp, the Doctor begins to suspect that something is wrong when the Tardis lands there. The colonists are under the control of the Macra, giant crab-like creatures, who use them to mine for the gas which is vital for the creatures' survival. With the Doctor imprisoned and Ben under the power of the Macra, Jamie and Polly have to try and save them both, before they too succumb to the Macra......

Episode One - (11/03/67) (8.0m)
Episode Two - (18/03/67) (7.9m)
Episode Three - (25/03/67) (8.5m)
Episode Four - (01/04/67) (8.4m)

Pilot . . . . Peter Jeffrey
Ola . . . . Gertan Klauber
Medok . . . . Terence Lodge
Controller. . . . . Graham Leaman
Sunnaa . . . . Jane Enshawe
Control Voice . . . . Denis Goacher
Director. . . . . John Davies
Designer (& Vis Fx) . . . . Kenneth Sharp
Costume Design . . . . Daphne Dare

THE FACELESS ONES (Serial KK) (Episode 1 & 3 exist)
Written by David Ellis & Malcolm Hulke (6 Episodes)
The Tardis arrives in 1966, and lands on the runway of Gatwick Airport. The Doctor becomes suspicious of one of the tour groups, and it's revealed that Chameleon Tours is run by a group of aliens who have no identity, and they're using charter flights to kidnap both airline staff and passengers to steal their likenesses. Realising they're back on Earth on the day they left on their first trip in the Tardis, Ben and Polly elect to stay behind, and as the Doctor and Jamie return to the time machine, they see it being driven away on the back of a lorry...

Episode One - (08/04/67) (8.0m)
Episode Two - (15/04/67) (6.4m)
Episode Three - (22/04/67) (7.9m)
Episode Four - (29/04/67) (6.9m)
Episode Five - (06/05/67) (7.1m)
Episode Six - (13/05/67) (8.0m)

Meadows . . . . George Selway
Commandant . . . . Colin Gordon
Jean Rock . . . . Wanda Ventham
Blade . . . . Donald Pickering
Spencer . . . . Victor Winding
Jenkins . . . . Christopher Tranchell
Samantha Briggs . . . . Pauline Collins
Crossland . . . . Bernard Kay
Ann Davidson . . . . Gilly Fraser
Director . . . . Gerry Mill
Designer (& Vis Fx) . . . . Geoff Kirkland
Costume Design . . . . Daphne Dare & Sandra Reid

THE EVIL OF THE DALEKS (Serial LL) (Episode 2 exists)
Written by David Whitaker (7 Episodes)
Trying to trace the Tardis eventually leads Jamie and the Doctor to Edward Waterfield, an antique dealer with items that are just too good. Both of them are then kidnapped and taken back to 1866, where it is revealed that Waterfield and his associate, Theodore Maxtible, are in league with the Daleks, who are holding his daughter, Victoria Waterfield, as a hostage to ensure he complies with their plans. Their plan is to distil the 'Human Factor' and destroy it, and use the Doctor, once he has the 'Dalek Factor' installed in him, to conquer both time and space. Taken to Skaro, where the Doctor confronts the Emperor Dalek, the situation is saved by Waterfield, who sacrifices himself to end the evil. With her Father dead, the Doctor promises to take care of Victoria, and she joins the Tardis crew...

Episode One - (20/05/67) (8.1m)
Episode Two - (27/05/67) (7.5m)
Episode Three - (03/06/67) (6.1m)
Episode Four - (10/06/67) (5.3m)
Episode Five - (17/06/67) (5.1m)
Episode Six - (24/06/67) (6.8m)
Episode Seven - (01/07/67) (6.1m)

Edward Waterfield . . . . John Bailey
Theodore Maxtible . . . . Marius Goring
Mollie Dawson . . . . Jo Rowbottom
Ruth Maxtible . . . . Brigit Forsyth
Toby . . . . Windsor Davies
Kemel . . . . Sonny Caldinez
Dalek Voice by Peter Hawkins & Roy Skelton
Dalek Emperor Voice by Roy Skelton
Director . . . . Derek Martinus
Designer . . . . Chris Thompson
Special Effects . . . . Michael John Harris
Costume Design . . . . Sandra Reid

Season Five

Regular Cast

The Doctor . . . . Patrick Troughton
Jamie . . . . Frazer Hines
Victoria . . (Serial MM-RR) Deborah Watling
Zoe. . . (Serial SS onwards) Wendy Padbury

Regular Production Team

Innes Lloyd . . . . . . Producer (Serial NN-PP)
Peter Bryant . . . Script Editor (Serial NN-PP)
Producer (Serial MM & QQ-SS)
Victor Pemberton . Script Editor (Serial MM)
Derrick Sherwin . . Script Editor (Serial QQ-SS)

THE TOMB OF THE CYBERMEN (Serial MM)
Written by Gerry Davis & Kit Pedler (4 Episodes)
An earth expedition is trying to excavate the tombs of the Cybermen on the planet Telos, and when the Tardis crew arrive, they are immediately suspected as a rival party. One of the expedition, Klieg, deliberately reactivates the Cybermen, thinking that he can control them, but they attack the humans using the rodent-like Cybermats, which home in on brain waves. The Doctor has to overcome Klieg's schemes, and the ruthless Cybercontroller, and reseal the tombs before the Tardis can leave the planet...

Episode One - (02/09/67) (6.0m)
Episode Two - (09/09/67) (6.4m)
Episode Three - (16/09/67) (7.2m)
Episode Four - (23/09/67) (7.4m)

Professor Parry . . . . Aubrey Richards
John Viner. . . . . Cyril Shaps
Eric Klieg . . . . George Pastell
Kaftan . . . . Shirley Cooklin
Toberman . . . . Roy Stewart
Captain Hooper . . . . George Roubicek
Jim Callum. . . . . Clive Merrison
Cybercontroller . . . . Michael Kilgarriff
Cybermen voices by Peter Hawkins
Director . . . . Morris Barry
Designer. . . . . Martin Johnson
Special Effects . . . . . Michael John Harris & Peter Day
Costume Design . . . . Sandra Reid & Dorothea Wallace

THE ABOMINABLE SNOWMEN (Serial NN) (Episode 2 exists)
Written by Mervyn Haisman & Henry Lincoln (6 Episodes)
The Doctor and his companions arrive in Tibet in the mid-1930s, where he plans to return a holy relic to the Det-sen monastery, having been asked to look after it by Phadmasambhava decades previously. Travers, one of the members of an expedition attacked by Yetis, accuses the Doctor of murdering his partner. The Doctor is shocked to learn that Phadmasambhava is still alive; he is possessed by the 'Great Intelligence', who has used him to construct the robot Yetis roaming the wilderness and plans to take over the Earth. The Doctor must outwit the 'Intelligence' and free his old friend from his torment...

Episode One - (30/09/67) (6.3m)
Episode Two - (07/10/67) (6.0m)
Episode Three - (14/10/67) (7.1m)
Episode Four - (21/10.67) (7.1m)
Episode Five - (28/10/67) (7.2m)
Episode Six - (04/11/67) (7.4m)

Professor Travers. . . . . Jack Watling
Khrisong . . . . Norman Jones
Thonmi . . . . David Spencer
Rinchen . . . . David Grey
Sapan . . . . Raymond Llewellyn
Songsten. . . . . Charles Morgan
Ralpachan . . . . David Baron
Padmasambhava . . . . Wolfe Morris
Director . . . . Gerald Blake
Designer . . . . Malcolm Middleton
Visual Effects . Ron Oates & Ulrich Grossner
Costumer Design . . . . Martin Baugh

THE ICE WARRIORS (Serial 00) (Episode 1 & 4-6 exist)
Written by Brian Hayles (6 Episodes)
During the second ice age in the Earth's

future, a computer is used at the Brittanicus Base, to keep the ice flows at bay. A towering alien warrior is excavated from the snow, thought to be long dead, but it slowly comes back to life. Varga's ship crashlanded in the ice centuries ago, and he is determined to revive his men, who are still frozen. He kidnaps Victoria when the Tardis arrives, and the Doctor has to outwit him to get her back and stop Leader Clent at Brittanicus from using an ioniser to destroy the Martian ship...

Episode One - (11/11/67) (6.7m)
Episode Two - (18/11/67) (7.1m)
Episode Three - (25/11/67) (7.4m)
Episode Four - (02/12/67) (7.3m)
Episode Five - (09/12/67) (8.0m)
Episode Six - (16/11/67) (7.5m)

Leader Clent . . . . Peter Barkworth
Miss Garrett . . . . Wendy Gifford
Penley. Peter Sallis
Arden . . . . George Waring
Walters . . . . Malcolm Taylor
Storr. . . . . Angus Lennie
Varga . . . . Bernard Bresslaw
Director . . . . Derek Martinus
Designer . . . . Jeremy Davies
Special Effects . . Bernard Wilkie & Ron Oates
Costume Design . . . . Martin Baugh

THE ENEMY OF THE WORLD (Serial PP) (Episode 3 exists)

Written by David Whitaker (6 Episodes)

After being attacked and rescued by a helicopter pilot called Astrid on an Australian beach, her boss, Giles Kent, reveals that the Doctor is a doppleganger for the corrupt political leader, Salamander. The Doctor tries to expose Salamander for what he really is, and in a final confrontation on board the Tardis the dictator gets ejected into space.....

Episode One - (23/12/67) (6.8m)
Episode Two - (30/12/67) (7.6m)
Episode Three - (06/01/68) (7.1m)
Episode Four - (13/01/68) (7.8m)
Episode Five - (20/01/68) (6.9m)
Episode Six - (27/01/68) (8.3m)

Giles Kent . . . . Bill Kerr
Astrid . . . . Mary Peach
Donald Bruce . . . . Colin Douglas
Swann . . . . Christopher Burgess
Benik . . . . Milton Johns
Salamander. . . . . Patrick Troughton
Colin . . . . Adam Verney
Mary . . . . Margaret Hickey
Director. . . . . Barry Letts
Designer . . . . Christopher Pemsel
Special Effects. . . . . (N/A)
Costume Design . . . . Martin Baugh

THE WEB OF FEAR (Serial QQ) (Episode 1 exists)

Written by Mervyn Haisman & Henry Lincoln (6 Episodes)

Attacked by a mysterious web-like substance in space, the Tardis has to materialise on Earth to escape and lands in a London underground station. The Doctor and his two companions meet up with Professor Travers, who explains that the web has caused London to be evacuated, after it started killing people on the Underground system, where Yetis have been sighted. The 'Great Intelligence' is once again on the planet, and the Doctor is assisted in defeating it by Colonel Lethbridge-Stewart, without either of them realising how much they would come to rely on each other in the future.....

Episode One - (03/02/68) (7.2m)
Episode Two - (10/02/68) (6.8m)
Episode Three - (17/02/68) (7.0m)
Episode Four - (24/02/68) (8.4m)
Episode Five - (02/03/68) (8.3m)
Episode Six - (20/04/68) (6.9m)

Professor Travers. . . . . Jack Watling
Anne Travers . . . . Tina Packer
Corporal Lane. . . . . Rod Beacham
Corporal Blake . . . . Richardson Morgan
Captain Knight . . . . Ralph Watson
Staff Sergeant Arnold. . . . . . . Jack Woolgar
Colonel Lethbridge-Stewart . . . . . Nicholas Courtney
Harold Chorley . . . . Jon Rollason
Director . . . . Douglas Camfield
Designer . . . . . . David Myerscough-Jones
Visual Effects . . . . Ron Oates
Costume Design . . . . Martin Baugh

FURY FROM THE DEEP (Serial RR) (No episodes exist)

Written by Victor Pemberton (6 Episodes)

At a refinery off the North Sea, the Doctor is blamed by its boss, Robson, for the disappearance of several staff members and for sabotaging the pipes. Others believe that there is something mysterious in the pipes, and whatever it is seems to control the mysterious Mr Quill and Mr Oak. They are the human agents for a lethal, mutant sea weed creature, which is trying to expand its race by taking over humans. The amplified sounds of Victoria's screams kill it, and when it comes to leaving, she opts to stay behind on the Earth.....

Episode One - (16/03/68) (8.2m)
Episode Two - (23/03/68) (7.9m)
Episode Three - (30/03/68) (7.7m)
Episode Four - (06/04/68) (6.6m)
Episode Five - (13/04/68) (5.9m)

Robson . . . . Victor Maddern
Harris . . . . Roy Spencer
Price. . . . . Graham Leaman
Maggie Harris . . . . June Murphy
Van Lutyens . . . . John Abineri
Mr Quill . . . . Bill Burridge
Mr Oak . . . . John Gill
Chief Engineer . . . . Hubert Rees
Director . . . . Hugh David.
Designer. . . . . Peter Kindred
Visual Effects. . . . . Peter Day & Len Hutton
Costume Design . . . . Martin Baugh

THE WHEEL IN SPACE (Serial SS) (Episode 3 & 6 exist)

Written by David Whitaker (6 Episodes)

From A Storyline by Kit Pedler

The Tardis materialises on an abandoned rocket, where the Doctor is attacked and knocked out by a Servo Robot. On arriving at a giant space station, where the Doctor receives medical treatment and recovers, both he and Jamie are alarmed by the rumours that metal rodents are on board. They soon find out they're Cybermats, and that the Cybermen are planning to use the station as part of an invasion attempt on the Earth. The Doctor defeats them and as he and Jamie leave, they find they have a stowaway in the form of Zoe Herriott. The Doctor shows her a mental projection of the kind of situations she'll face if she joins the crew (leading into a repeat of THE EVIL OF THE DALEKS for the next seven weeks).....

Episode One - (27/04/68) (7.2m)
Episode Two - (04/05/68) (6.9m)
Episode Three - (11/05/68) (7.5m)
Episode Four - (18/95/68) (8.6m)
Episode Five - (25/05/68) (6.8m)
Episode Six - (01/06/68) (6.5m)

Leo Ryan. . . . . Eric Flynn
Doctor Gemma Corwyn . . . . . Anne Ridler
Tanya Lernov . . . . Clare Jenkins
Enrico Casali . . . . Donald Sumpter
Jarvis Bennett . . . . Michael Turner
Armand Vallance . . . . Derrick Gilbert
Sean Flannigan. . . . . James Mellor
Director . . . . Tristan de Vere Cole
Designer. . . . . Derek Dodd
Visual Effects . . . . . Bill King & Trading Post
Costume Design . . . . Martin Baugh

Season Six

Regular Cast
The Doctor . . . . Patrick Troughton
Jamie . . . . Frazer Hines
Zoe. . . . . Wendy Padbury

Regular Production Team
Peter Bryant . . . . . . Producer (Serial TT-YY)
Derrick Sherwin . . . . Script Editor (Serial TT-UU & YY) Producer (Serial ZZ)
Terrance Dicks. . . . . Script Editor (Serial VV-XX & ZZ)

THE DOMINATORS (Serial TT)
Written by Norman Ashby (5 Episodes) (Mervyn Haisman & Henry Lincoln's false name)
The Dominators have taken over the planet of Dulkis with their robotic Quarks, with a plan to detonate a vast nuclear device in the planet's core which would turn the world into nothing more than radioactive waste. This would then be used to power the Dominators' fleet of spacecraft. The Dulcians are natural pacifists, and so the Doctor must find a way to stop the Dominators' scheme.....

Episode One - (10/08/68) (6.1m)
Episode Two - (17/08/68) (5.9m)
Episode Three - (24/08/68) (5.4m)
Episode Four - (31/08/68) (7.5m)
Episode Five - (07/09/68) (5.9m)

Rago . . . . Ronald Allen
Toba . . . . Kenneth Ives
Cully. . . . . Arthur Cox
Kando . . . . Felicity Gibson
Balan . . . . Johnson Bayly
Teel . . . . Giles Block
Senex . . . . Walter Fitzgerald
Director . . . . Morris Barry
Designer. . . . . Barry Newbery
Visual Effects . . . . Ron Oates
Costume Design . . . . Martin Baugh

THE MIND ROBBER (Serial UU)
Written by Peter Ling (5 Episodes) & Derrick Sherwin (uncredited as writer of part one)
To escape a lava rush from a volcano, the Doctor uses an emergency take-off, and the Tardis lands in a white void. As they try to escape, the Tardis disintegrates and the three travellers find they are now in the Land of Fiction. The Doctor has to defeat the Master of the Land, who is capable of creating characters out of nothing by simply thinking them into reality, by taking him on in the same way and calling up all the characters from literature he can think of. If he fails, the Tardis crew will become absorbed into fiction, and the Doctor's mind will be absorbed...

Episode One - (14/09/68) (6.6m)
Episode Two - (21/09/68) (6.5m)
Episode Three - (28/09/68) (7.2m)
Episode Four - (05/10/68) (7.3m)
Episode Five - (12/10/68) (6.7m)

The Master . . . . Emrys Jones
A Stranger (Gulliver) . . . . . Bernard Horsfall
Rapunzel. . . . . Christine Pirie
The Karkus . . . . Christopher Robbie
The Medusa . . . . Sue Pulford
The Other Jamie . . . . Hamish Wilson
D'Artagnan & Sir Lancelot . . . . John Greenwood
Director . . . . David Maloney
Designer . . . . Evan Hercules
Visual Effects . . . . . Bill King & Trading Post
Costume Design . . . . Martin Baugh & Susan Wheel

THE INVASION (Serial VV) (Episodes 2-3 & 5-8 Exist)
Written by Derrick Sherwin (8 Episodes)
Based on an idea by Kit Pedler
On the Tardis scanner, the Doctor and his companions see a vast fleet of ships hidden behind the dark side of the Earth's moon. Materialising on the planet, the crew try and find Professor Travers, whom they discover has leant his home to a colleague, Professor Watkins, while he and Anne are away. The Doctor learns from Watkins' niece, Isobel, that Watkins is working for magnate Tobias Vaughn, who is in reality using the scientist's work to make a device that can induce emotions in Cybermen. Vaughn is helping the aliens orchestrate an invasion of Earth, with their battle fleet waiting behind the moon, and wants the Cerebraton Mentor as a fail-safe to control them. As the Doctor tries to prevent his plans, he once again meets Lethbridge-Stewart, now a Brigadier, who has set up the United Nations Intelligence Taskforce (UNIT) to counter attack such threats. The two join forces to try and save mankind.....

Episode One - (02/11/68) (7.3m)
Episode Two - (09/11/68) (7.1m)
Episode Three - (16/11/68) (7.1m)
Episode Four - (23/11/68) (6.4m)
Episode Five - (30/11/68) (6.7m)
Episode Six - (07/11/68) (6.5m)
Episode Seven - (14/11/68) (7.2m)
Episode Eight - (21/11/68) (7.0m)

Professor Watkins . . . . . . Edward Burnham
Isobel Watkins . . . . Sally Faulkner
Tobis Vaughn. . . . . Kevin Stoney
Packer . . . . Peter Halliday
Brigadier Lethbridge-Stewart . . . . Nicholas Courtney
Sergeant Walters . . . . James Thornhill
Captain Turner . . . . Robert Sidaway
Benton . . . . John Levene
Cyber Voices by Peter Halliday
Director . . . . Douglas Camfield
Designer . . . . Richard Hunt
Visual Effects . . . . . Bill King & Trading Post
Costume Design . . . . Bobi Bartlett

THE KROTONS (Serial WW)
Written by Robert Holmes (4 Episodes)
The Gonds are all controlled by the Krotons, and each year, the brightest male and female students of their race are selected and sent into the Kroton's machine to work with them, or so they are led to believe. The Doctor discovers that they are actually being mentally absorbed, with their bodies then being vaporised. The Doctor has to fight to defeat them, before any other Gonds are destroyed...

Episode One - (28/12/68) (9.0m)
Episode Two - (4/1/69) (8.4m)
Episode Three - (11/1/69) (7.5m)
Episode Four - (18/1/94) (7.1m)

Selris. . . . . James Copeland
Varna . . . . Madeleine Mills
Thara . . . . Gilbert Wynne
Eelek . . . . Philip Madoc
Axus . . . . Richard Ireson
Beta . . . . James Cairmcross
Kroton voices by Roy Skelton & Patrick Tull
Director . . . . David Maloney
Designer . . . . Ray London
Visual Effects . . . . . Bill King & Trading Post
Costume Design . . . . Bobbi Bartlett

THE SEEDS OF DEATH (Serial XX)
Written by Brian Hayles (6 Episodes)
A T-Mat station on the moon seems to have broken down, when in reality it's been invaded by Ice Warriors, under the command of their Ice Lord, Slaar. The T-Mat system transports anything to any point in an instant, and the breakdown has stopped food supplies being moved around world wide. The Ice Warriors use the system to send deadly seed pods to various points around the globe, with the resulting fungus quickly sucking all the oxygen out of the atmosphere. The Tardis lands in a museum, and the Doctor has to

pilot one of it's old rockets to the moon to be able to defeat the Martians.....

Episode One - (25/01/69) (6.6m)
Episode Two - (01/02/69) (6.8m)
Episode Three - (08/02/69) (7.5m)
Episode Four - (15/02/69) (7.1m)
Episode Five - (22/02/69) (7.6m)
Episode Six - (01/03/69) (7.7m)

Gia Kelly . . . . Louise Pajo
Commander Radnor . . . Ronald Leigh-Hunt
Brent. Ric Felgate
Fewsham . . . . Terry Scully
Eldred. Philip Ray
Slaar . . . . Alan Bennion
Phipps. . . . . Christopher Coll
Director . . . . Michael Ferguson
Designer . . . . Paul Allen
Visual Effects . . . . . Bill King & Trading Post
Costume Design . . . . Bobi Bartlett

THE SPACE PIRATES (Serial YY) (Episode 2 Exists)
Written by Robert Holmes (6 Episodes)
The Tardis and the travellers become separated when they land in a space beacon, and an eccentric old miner is their only means of help. The International Space Corps are on his trail, wrongly believing Milo Clancey to have stolen one of the beacons. The Doctor has to travel to the planet Ta, where the true culprits, the Space Pirates led by the murderous Craven.....

Episode One - (08/03/69) (5.8m)
Episode Two - (15/03/68) (6.8m)
Episode Three - (22/03/69) (6.4m)
Episode Four - (29/03/69) (5.8m)
Episode Five - (05/04/69) (5.4m)
Episode Six - (12/04/69) (5.3m)

General Hermack . . . . Jack May
Craven . . . . Dudley Foster
Milo Clancey . . . . Gordon Gostelow
Dervish . . . . Brian Peck
Major Ian Warne . . . . Donald Gee
Technician Penn . . . . George Layton
Madeleine Issigri . . . . Lisa Daniely
Dom Issigri. . . . . Esmond Knight
Lieutenant Sorba . . . . Nick Zaven
Director . . . . Michael Hart
Designer. . . . . Ian Watson
Visual Effects . . . . John Wood
Costume Design. . . . . Nicholas Bullen

THE WAR GAMES (Serial ZZ)
Written by Terrance Dicks & Malcolm Hulke (10 Episodes)
Materialising in No Man's Land during the First World War, the Tardis crew are captured and General Smythe insists that they

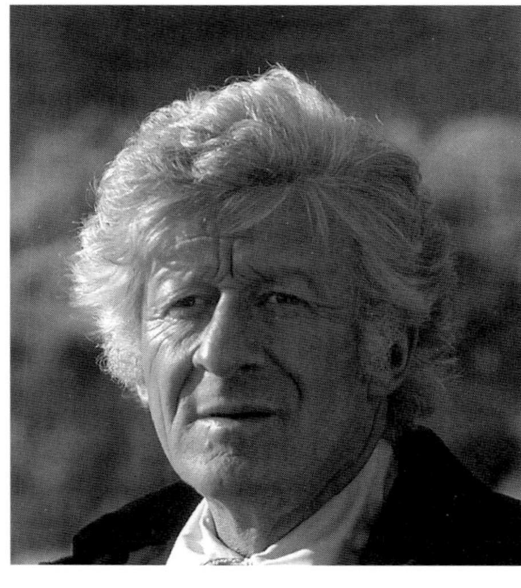

are executed, but the Doctor and his companions manage to escape. Moving through a strange area of mist, they suddenly find themselves entering Roman times. The Doctor uncovers the fact that they are in the middle of a vast war game being played out by aliens, using captured soldiers from various periods in Earth's history. The whole thing is masterminded by a renegade from the Doctor's own race, known as the War Chief, who answers to the War Lord. When he arrives, the Doctor realises he can't win, and calls for help from his people, the Time Lords, but tries to get away from the planet before they arrive. There is no escape, and they force his Tardis to land back on his home planet, where he is put on trial for 'interference', the greatest crime a Time Lord can commit. Jamie and Zoe are returned to their own times, with their memories wiped of all bar their first adventure with the Doctor, who is exiled to earth, with a forced regeneration.....

Episode One - (19/04/69) (5.5m)
Episode Two - (26/04/69) (6.3m)
Episode Three - (03/05/69) (5.1m)
Episode Four - (10/05/69) (5.7m)
Episode Five - (17/05/69) (5.1m)
Episode Six - (24/05/69) (4.2m)
Episode Seven - (31/05/69) (4.9m)
Episode Eight - (07/06/69) (3.5m)
Episode Nine - (14/06/69) (4.1m)
Episode Ten - (21/06/69) (5.0m)

Lady Jennifer Buckingham . . . Jane Sherwin
Lieutenant Carstairs . . . . David Saville
General Smythe . . . . Noel Coleman
General Von Weich . . . . David Garfield
War Chief. . . . . Edward Brayshaw
Security Chief . . . . James Bree
War Lord. . . . . Philip Madoc
Scientist . . . . Vernon Dobtcheff
Russell . . . . Graham Weston
Moor . . . . David Troughton
Time Lord . . . . Bernard Horsfall
Time Lord . . . . Clyde Pollitt
Time Lord . . . . Trevor Martin
Director . . . . David Maloney
Designer . . . . Roger Cheveley
Visual Effects . . . . Michael John Harris
Costume Design. . . . . Nicholas Bullen

Season Seven

Regular Cast
The Doctor . . . . Jon Pertwee
Liz Shaw . . . . Caroline John
Brigadier Lethbridge-Stewart . . . . Nicholas Courtney
Sergeant Benton (Serial CCC on) . . . . John Levene

Regular Production Team
Derrick Sherwin . . . . Producer (Serial AAA)
Barry Letts . . . . Producer (Serial BBB Onwards)
Terrance Dicks. . . . . Script Editor

SPEARHEAD FROM SPACE (Serial AAA)
Written by Robert Holmes (4 Episodes)
A swarm of Nestene meteorites lands in Oxley Woods, as does the newly regenerated Doctor, who collapses outside the Tardis and is taken to a nearby hospital. The Brigadier is not convinced that the man who claims to be the Doctor is the same one that he knew. The Nestenes, who are able to control and bring plastic to life, have taken over a plastics factory and are mass-producing Autons. Disguised as shop-window dummies, the Autons start to slaughter the general public. The Doctor has to prevent the octopus-like Nestene consciousness from wiping out mankind....

Episode One - (03/01/70) (8.4m)
Episode Two - (10/01/70) (8.1m)
Episode Three - (17/01/70) (8.3m)
Episode Four - (24/01/70) (8.1m)

Sam Seeley . . . . Neil Wilson
Captain Munro. . . . . John Breslin
Channing . . . . Hugh Burden
Hibbert. . . . . John Woodnutt
Major General Scobie . . . . . Hamilton Dyce
Ransome. . . . . Derek Smee
Director . . . . Derek Martinus
Designer . . . . Paul Allen
Visual Effects. . . . . John Horton
Costume Design . . . . Christine Rawlins

DOCTOR WHO AND THE SILURIANS
(Serial BBB)
Written by Malcolm Hulke (7 Episodes)
At a power station on Wenley Moor, energy from the generators is being siphoned off, with the help of Doctor Quinn, into the Silurian base deep in the rocks below, where the creatures are slowly being revived. They were the original dominant race on earth, but went into hibernation when they saw a satellite heading towards their world, thinking it would land and cause mass destruction. The satellite became the moon, and their machines never woke them. The Doctor makes contact and one of the older creatures is keen for their race to live in peace with the humans, but a younger Silurian and a Silurian scientist plot against this and release a lethal plague to rid the planet of what they see as an intruding race. The Doctor has to find a cure and bring peace to the situation, but the Brigadier has other plans for the fate of the reptiles.....

Episode One - (31/01/70) (8.8m)
Episode Two - (07/02/70) (7.3m)
Episode Three - (14/02/70) (7.5m)
Episode Four - (21/02/70) (8.2m)
Episode Five - (28/02/70) (7.5m)
Episode Six - (07/03/70) (7.2m)
Episode Seven - (14/03/70) (7.5m)

Doctor Lawrence . . . . Peter Miles
Major Baker . . . . Norman Jones
Doctor Quinn . . . . Fulton Mackay
Miss Dawson . . . . Thomasine Heiner
Masters. . . . . Geoffrey Palmer
Captain Hawkins . . . . Paul Darrow
Silurian Voices by Peter Halliday
Director. . . . . Timothy Combe
Designer. . . . . Barry Newbery
Visual Effects . . . . Jim Ward
Costume Design . . . . Christine Rawlins

THE AMBASSADORS OF DEATH (Serial CCC)
Written by David Whitaker (7 Episodes)
With Uncredited Rewrites by Malcolm Hulke
Space Control are deeply worried about the fact that there has been radio silence from the Mars Probe Seven ship since it started the return journey to Earth seven months earlier. A recovery ship makes contact, but its radio also goes dead. The Doctor discovers that there are signals, but they're being rerouted to a warehouse, and the UNIT troops storm it. The Recovery Seven lands, but all three astronauts are kidnapped by General Carrington's men. They are in reality aliens, who have replaced the Earth astronauts, and Carrington plans to discredit them and bring in a policy that all aliens should be destroyed. The Doctor travels to the aliens' ship, finds the humans are safe, and manages to negotiate a peaceful swap with the aliens to get the crew back, but Carrington has other ideas.....

Episode One - (21/03/70) (7.1m)
Episode Two - (28/03/70 (7.6m)
Episode Three - (04/04/70) (8.0m)
Episode Four - (11/04/70) (7.1m)
Episode Five - (18/04/70) (7.1m)
Episode Six - (25/04/70) (6.9m)
Episode Seven - (02/05/70) (5.4m)

General Carrington . . . . John Abineri
Ralph Cornish. . . . . Ronald Allen
Van Lyden. . . . . Ric Felgate
Quinlan . . . . Dallas Cavell
Taltalian . . . . Robert Cawdron
Reegan . . . . William Dysart
Astronaut . . . . Steve Peters
Astronaut . . . . Neville Simons
Director . . . . Michael Ferguson
Designer . . . . David Myerscough-Jones
Visual Effects. . . . . Peter Day
Costume Design . . . . Christine Rawlins

INFERNO (Serial DDD)
Written by Don Houghton (7 Episodes)
A potential energy source has been discovered at the Earth's core and Professor Stahlman has a drilling operation underway to release it, but a strange green slime is being brought up the mine shaft which induces extreme personality changes when it comes into contact with flesh. Skin turns green and anything the victims touch becomes red hot. The Doctor is using the drilling plant's energy banks to try and get the Tardis console working again and is accidentally projected into a parallel universe, where he meets the fascist counterparts of both the Brigadier and Liz. The drilling there has nearly been completed, and the slime has turned people into rampaging creatures. The Doctor realises the Earth is doomed on that time line, and only just manages to escape. He has to stop Stahlman causing the destruction of the planet in his own time stream.....

Episode One - (09/05/70) (5.7m)
Episode Two - (16/05/70) (5.9m)
Episode Three - (23/05/70) (4.8m)
Episode Four - (30/05/70) (6.0m)
Episode Five - (06/06/70) (5.4m)
Episode Six - (13/06/70) (5.7m)
Episode Seven - (20/06/70) (5.5m)

Professor Stahlman. . . . . Olaf Pooley
Greg Sutton . . . . Derek Newark
Petra Williams . . . . Sheila Dunn
Sir Keith Gold . . . . . . Christopher Benjamin
Bromley . . . . Ian Fairbairn
Director . . . . Douglas Camfield
Uncredited work on studio recording . . Barry Letts
Designer . . . . Jeremy Davies
Visual Effects . . . . Len Hutton
Costume Design . . . . Christine Rawlins

Season Eight

Regular Cast

The Doctor . . . . Jon Pertwee
Jo Grant . . . . Katy Manning
Brigadier Lethbridge-Stewart . . . . Nicholas Courtney
Captain Mike Yates . . . . . . Richard Franklin
(All serials bar HHH)
Sergeant Benton . . . . John Levene
(All serials bar HHH)
The Master . . . . Roger Delgado

Regular Production Team

Barry Letts . . . . Producer
Terrance Dicks. . . . . Script Editor

TERROR OF THE AUTONS (Serial EEE)
Written by Robert Holmes (4 Episodes)
A renegade Time Lord called the Master arrives on Earth with a plan to use new Autons to instigate a second Nestene invasion attempt. The Doctor, working alongside his new assistant, Jo Grant, has to contend with all manor of Nestene devices, ranging from lethal plastic daffodils to animated troll dolls, before stopping the Master from allowing the Nestene consciousness to land on Earth.....

Episode One - (02/01/71) (7.3m)
Episode Two - (09/01/71) (8.0m)
Episode Three - (16/01/71) (8.1m)
Episode Four - (23/01/71) (8.4m)

Rossini . . . . John Baskcomb
Professor Philips . . . . . Christopher Burgess
Rex Farrel. . . . . Michael Wisher
McDermott . . . . Harry Towb
Mrs. Farrel . . . . Barbara Leake
Auton Police Constable . . . . . . Terry Walsh
Auton Leader . . . . Pat Gorman
Director. . . . . Barry Letts
Designer. . . . . Ian Watson
Visual Effects . . . . Michael John Harris
Costume Design . . . . Ken Trew

THE MIND OF EVIL (Serial FFF)
Written by Don Houghton (6 Episodes)
The Keller Machine extracts all evil impulses from the human mind and the Doctor and Jo visit a prison to watch the tests being carried out on convicts. A series of bizarre deaths at the prison follow, and the Doctor realises that the machine is using people's worst fears to frighten them to death. The creator of the machine is in reality the Master, who plans to kidnap a thunderbolt missile, which UNIT are escorting, and use it to threaten and then blackmail a world peace conference. The Keller Machine contains a mind parasite, which is quickly growing too powerful to control. Somehow, the Doctor has to destroy the machine and stop the Master.....

Episode One - (30/01/71) (9.2m)
Episode Two - (06/02/71) (8.8m)
Episode Three - (13/02/71) (7.5m)
Episode Four - (20/02/71) (7.4m)
Episode Five - (27/02/71) (7.3m)
Episode Six - (06/03/71) (7.3m)

Doctor Summers . . . . Michael Sheard
Barnham . . . . Neil McCarthy
Mailer . . . . William Marlowe
Vosper . . . . Haydn Jones
Captain Chin Lee . . . . Pik-Sen Lim
Prison Governor . . . . . . Raymond Westwell
Corporal Bell . . . . Fernando Marlowe
Director . . . . Timothy Combe
Designer . . . . Ray London
Visual Effects . . . . Jim Ward
Costume Design . . . . Bobi Bartlett

THE CLAWS OF AXOS (Serial GGG)
Written by Bob Baker & Dave Martin (4 Episodes)
The organic Axon spaceship, with its beautiful gold-skinned crew, lands near a power station and asks for help to restore its depleted power supply. It offers Axonite, which has the properties to make living matter grow, as an exchange for energy. The Master is trapped on the ship and has lead the creatures to Earth, because behind the facade, they are really a power absorbing parasitic organism and they plan to drain the planet dry. The Doctor has to join forces with the Master to try and trap Axos in a time loop, but can their combined efforts succeed?

Episode One - (13/03/71) (7.3m)
Episode Two - (20/03/71) (8.0m)
Episode Three - (27/03/71) (6.4m)
Episode Four - (03/04/71) (7.8m)

Chinn . . . . Peter Bathurst
Bill Filer . . . . Paul Grist
Winser . . . . David Saville
Captain Harker . . . . Tim Pigott-Smith
Sir George Hardiman . . . . . Donald Hewlett
Corporal Bell . . . . Fernando Marlowe
Minister . . . . Kenneth Benda
Axon Man . . . . Bernard Holley
Director . . . . Michael Ferguson
Designer . . . . Kenneth Sharp
Visual Effects . . . . John Horton
Costume Design . . . . Barbara Lane

COLONY IN SPACE (Serial HHH)
Written by Malcolm Hulke (6 Episodes)
The Doomsday Weapon is one of the most powerful in existence, and the Master has discovered where it is. The Time Lords dispatch the Doctor, with Jo Grant, to the world of Exarius, where they find the earth colonists being killed off by giant lizards, or so they think. The Interplanetary Mining Corporation want to get rid of the settlers and exploit the minerals of the planet. They use a mining robot to commit the murders, using vast reptilian claws, to try and scare them away. The war between the factions has to be settled and an Earth adjudicator arrives – The Master in disguise. The Doctor has to stop him reaching the weapon at all costs.....

Episode One - (10/04/71) (7.6m)
Episode Two - (17/04/71) (8.5m)
Episode Three - (24/04/71) (9.5m)
Episode Four - (01/05/71) (8.1m)
Episode Five - (08/05/71) (8.8m)
Episode Six - (15/05/71) (8.7m)

Ashe . . . . John Ringham
Mary Ashe . . . . Helen Worth
Winton . . . . Nicholas Pennell
Norton . . . . Roy Skelton
Caldwell . . . . Bernard Kay
Dent . . . . Morris Perry
Morgan . . . . Tony Caunter
Primative . . . . Pat Gorman
The Guardian . . . . Norman Atkyns
Director . . . . Michael E. Briant
Designer . . . . Tim Gleeson
Visual Effects . . . . Bernard Wilkie
Costume Design . . . . Michael Burdle

THE DAEMONS (Serial JJJ)
Written by Guy Leopold (5 Episodes)
Pen Name for Robert Sloman & Barry Letts
The Devil's Hump barrow is due to be opened by an archaeologist live on BBC3, and as a result, psionic alien forces are unleashed and the village of Devil's End becomes trapped inside a vast forcefield dome, much to the delight of the new vicar, Reverend Magister, in reality the Master. He is trying to summon up Azal, last of the Daemons, to claim the right to inherit his powers, by using a black magic coven in the Church's crypt. With the creature being more than capable of destroying the world, the Doctor has to try and stop the Master.....

Episode One - (22/05/71) (9.2m)
Episode Two - (29/05/71) (8.0m)
Episode Three - (05/06/71) (8.1m)
Episode Four - (12/06/71) (8.1m)
Episode Five - (19/06/71) (8.3m)

Miss Hawthorne . . . . Damaris Hayman
Doctor Reeves . . . . Eric Hillyard
Winstanley . . . . Rollo Gamble
Tom Girton . . . . Jon Croft
Bert . . . . Don McKillop
Bok . . . . Stanley Mason
Azal . . . . Stephen Thorne
Director . . . . Christopher Barry
Designer . . . . Roger Ford
Visual Effects . . . . Peter Day
Costume Design . . . . Barbara Lane

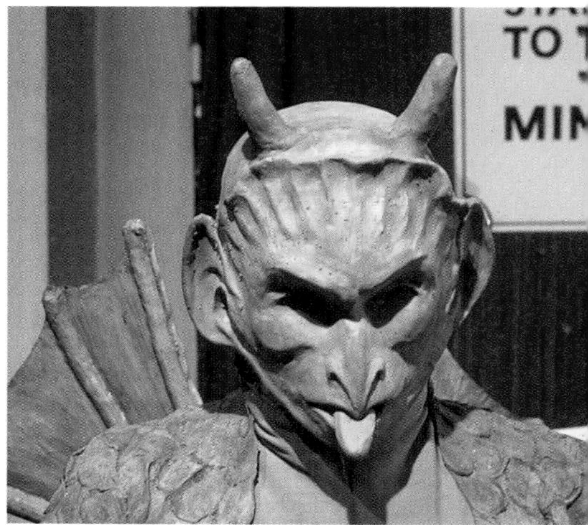

Season Nine

Regular Cast
The Doctor . . . . Jon Pertwee
Jo Grant . . . . Katy Manning
Brigadier Lethbridge-Stewart . . . . Nicholas Courtney
(Serial KKK & OOO Only)
Captain Mike Yates . . . . . . Richard Franklin
(Serial KKK & OOO Only)
Sergeant Benton . . . . John Levene
(Serial KKK & OOO Only)
The Master . . . . Roger Delgado

Regular Production Team
Barry Letts . . . . Producer
Terrance Dicks . . . . Script Editor

DAY OF THE DALEKS (Serial KKK)
Written by Louis Marks (4 Episodes)
With Sir Reginald Styles, a major diplomat at the World Peace Conference due to be held at Auderley House, attacked by what he describes as a ghost, the Doctor and Jo decide to spend a night there to see if it returns. It does, and in force, as a team of rebels from the 22nd century arrive, and say Styles is responsible for a war that will take place allowing the Daleks to take over the Earth. The Doctor travels to the future, joining the freedom fighters to try and defeat the Daleks, but the aliens travel back to the 20th century intent on mass destruction.....

Episode One - (01/01/72) (9.8m)
Episode Two - (08/01/72) (10.4m)
Episode Three - (15/01/72) (9.1m)
Episode Four - (22/01/72) (9.1m)

Sir Reginald Styles . . . . Wilfrid Carter
Controller . . . . Aubrey Woods
Anat . . . . Anna Barry
Shura . . . . Jimmy Winston
Boaz . . . . Scott Fredericks
Monia . . . . Valentine Palmer
Dalek Voices by Oliver Gilbert & Peter Messaline
Director . . . . Paul Bernard
Designer . . . . David Myerscough-Jones
Visual Effects . . . . Jim Ward
Costume Design . . . . Mary Husband

THE CURSE OF PELADON (Serial MMM)
Written by Brian Hayles (4 Episodes)
Arriving on the planet Peladon, the Doctor is quickly mistaken as the Earth delegate of the Galactic Federation and Jo is thought to be a Princess. With two Ice Warriors present, the Doctor is immediately suspicious, thinking they are behind the various sabotage attempts to destroy Peladon's credibility and chances of joining the federation, but he has to look within the ranks of Peladon's high-ranking officials to find the real villain.....

Episode One - (29/01/72) (10.3m)
Episode Two - (05/02/72) (11.0m)
Episode Three - (12/02/72) (7.8m)
Episode Four - (19/02/72) (8.4m)

King Peladon . . . . David Troughton
Hepesh . . . . Geoffrey Toone
Izlyr . . . . Alan Bennion
Ssorg . . . . Sonny Caldinez
Alpha Centuri . . . . Stuart Fell
(Voice by Ysanne Churchman)
Arcturus . . . . Murphy Grumbar
(Voice by Terry Bale)
Grun . . . . Gordon St. Clair
Aggedor . . . . Nick Hobbs
Director . . . . Lennie Mayne
Designer . . . . Gloria Clayton
Visual Effects . . . . Ian Scoones
Costume Design . . . . Barbara Lane

THE SEA DEVILS (Serial LLL)
Written by Malcolm Hulke (6 Episodes)
The Doctor and Jo visit the Master on his remote island prison, where the Governor, Colonel Trenchard, says he's now a changed man. The Doctor investigates reports that shipping in the area has been attacked, and uncovers the fact that the Sea Devils, distant aquatic cousins of the Silurians, have been woken in their sea bed base. The Master is communicating with them, trying to persuade them to destroy mankind. Trenchard has been conned by the Master, believing his lies that agents are destroying the submarines and ships, so he has been compliant and helped him with his plans. The Doctor has to stop the Sea Devils when a series of depth charges convince them mankind should be eradicated.....

Episode One - (26/02/72) (6.4m)
Episode Two - (04/03/72) (9.7m)
Episode Three - (11/03/72) (8.3m)
Episode Four - (18/03/72) (7.8m)
Episode Five - (25/03/72) (8.3m)
Episode Six - (01/04/72) (8.5m)

Colonel Trenchard . . . . Clive Morton
Captain Hart . . . . Edwin Richfield
Third Officer Jane Blythe . . . . . June Murphy
Commander Ridgeway . . . Donald Sumpter
Lieutenant Commander . . . Mitchell.David Griffin
Ldg Telegraphist Bowman . . . . Alec Wallis
Chief Sea Devil . . . . Peter Forbes-Robertson
Director . . . . Michael E. Briant
Designer . . . . Tony Snoaden
Visual Effects . . . . Peter Day
Costume Design . . . . Maggie Fletcher

THE MUTANTS (Serial NNN)
Written by Bob Baker & Dave Martin (6 Episodes)
Armed with a container from the Time Lords, which will only open for one special person, the Doctor and Jo are taken in the Tardis to a space station orbiting the planet Solos. The planet is meant to have its independence, but the evil Marshal is not willing to give up his control of the natives so easily. The Solonians are going through a bizarre period of mutations, genetically reshaping into giant insects, and the Marshal plans to wipe them out using a bomb to purify the atmosphere. The container turns out to be for the rebel leader, Ky. The Doctor has to stop the Marshal, and allow the mutants to evolve into their next stage of existence....

Episode One - (08/04/72) (9.1m)
Episode Two - (15/04/72) (7.8m)
Episode Three - (22/04/72) (7.9m)
Episode Four - (29/04/72) (7.5m)
Episode Five - (06/05/72) (7.9m)
Episode Six - (13/05/72) (6.5m)

The Marshal . . . . Paul Whitsun-Jones
Stubbs . . . . Christopher Coll
Cotton . . . . Rick James
Varan . . . . James Mellor
Ky . . . . Garrick Hagan
Sondergard . . . . John Hollis
Jaeger . . . . George Pravda
Administrator . . . . Geoffrey Palmer
Director . . . . Christopher Barry
Designer . . . . Jeremy Bear
Visual Effects . . . . John Horton
Costume Design . . . . James Acheson

THE TIME MONSTER (Serial OOO)
Written by Robert Sloman (6 Episodes)
The Master uses the Transmission of Matter Through Interstitial Time machine (TOMTIT), to try and ensnare the power of the Chronovore, Kronos, a creature that feeds off time. To be able to complete his power, the Master heads back to Atlantis where he plots with Queen Gallaia. When the Doctor arrives to try and stop him, the inevitable destruction of Atlantis is brought about in the ensuing confrontation.....

Episode One - (20/05/72) (7.6m)
Episode Two - (27/05/72) (7.4m)
Episode Three - (03/06/72) (8.1m)
Episode Four - (10/06/72) (7.6m)
Episode Five - (17/06/72) (6.0m)
Episode Six - (24/06/72) (7.6m)

Doctor Ruth Ingram . . . . Wanda Moore
Stuart Hyde . . . . Ian Collier
Krasis . . . . Donald Eccles
Hippias . . . . Aidan Murphy
Kronos . . . . Marc Boyle
Dalios . . . . George Cormack
Galleia . . . . Ingrid Pitt
Lakis . . . . Susan Penhaligon
Minotaur . . . . Dave Prowse
Director . . . . Paul Bernard
Designer . . . . Tim Gleeson
Visual Effects . . . . . . Michael John Harris & Peter Pegrum
Costume Design . . . . Barbara Lane

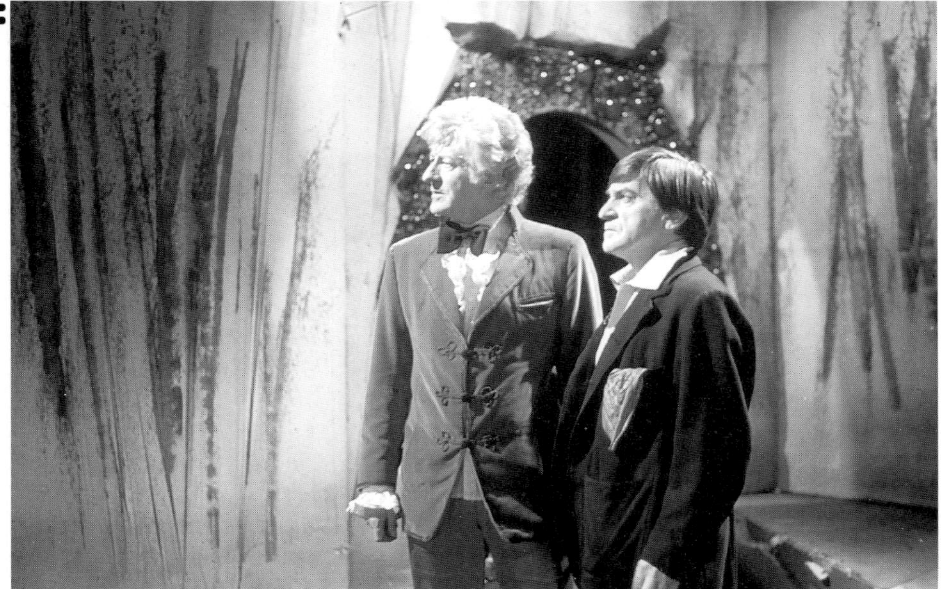

Season Ten

Regular Cast
The Doctor . . . . Jon Pertwee
Jo Grant . . . . Katy Manning
Brigadier Lethbridge-Stewart . . . . Nicholas Courtney (Serial RRR & TTT Only)
Captain Mike Yates . . . . . . Richard Franklin (Serial TTT Only)
Sergeant Benton . . . . John Levene (Serial RRR & TTT Only)
The Master . . . . Roger Delgado (Serial QQQ Only)

Regular Production Team
Barry Letts . . . . Producer
Terrance Dicks. . . . . Script Editor

THE THREE DOCTORS (Serial RRR)
Written by Bob Baker & Dave Martin (4 Episodes)
The Time Lords are under siege, with their power being drained into a world of anti-matter where the embittered galactic engineer, Omega, who discovered the energy source in the first place, is absorbing it and planning his revenge. The UNIT Headquarters comes under attack from Omega's shapeless guards, as they hunt the Doctor down and trap him inside the Tardis. His second incarnation is sent by the Time Lords to help, but their personalities clash, and the first Doctor acts as a mediator, trapped in a time bubble and only able to advise from a monitor screen. They travel to Omega's domain, where they have to combine their wits to try and stop him.....

Episode One - (30/12/72) (9.6m)
Episode Two - (06/01/73) (10.8m)
Episode Three - (13/01/73) (8.8m)
Episode Four - (20/01/73) (11.9m)

The Doctor . . . . Patrick Troughton
The Doctor . . . . William Hartnell
Doctor Tyler . . . . Rex Robinson
Omega . . . . Stephen Thorne
President Of The Council. . . . . . Roy Purcell
Chancellor. . . . . Clyde Pollitt
Time Lord. . . . . Graham Leaman
Arthur Ollis . . . . Laurie Webb
Director. . . . . Lennie Mayne
Designer . . . . Roger Liminton
Visual Effects . . . . . . Michael John Harris & Len Hutton
Costume Design. . . . . James Acheson

CARNIVAL OF MONSTERS (Serial PPP)
Written by Robert Holmes (4 Episodes)
With the Doctor's exile on Earth now lifted, he takes Jo on a test flight in the Tardis, and they land on a cargo ship in 1926, but the crew keep going through the same set of motions again and again, with history repeating itself. They are trapped in a miniscope, on the planet Inter Minor, and have become part of a peepshow. One of the politicians sees his chance to seize power by releasing the deadly Drashigs from the machine, which run riot through the capitol. The Doctor has to fight to stop the carnage.....

Episode One - (27/01/73) (9.5m)
Episode Two - (03/02/73) (9.0m)
Episode Three - (10/02/73) (9.0m)
Episode Four - (17/02/73) (9.2m)

Vorg . . . . Leslie Dwyer
Shirna . . . . Cheryl Hall
Major Daly . . . . Tenniel Evans
Claire Daly. . . . . Jenny McCracken
Captain Andrews . . . . Ian Marter
Kalik . . . . Michael Wisher
Pletrac . . . . Peter Halliday
Orum . . . . Terence Lodge
Director. . . . . Barry Letts
Designer . . . . Roger Liminton
Visual Effects. . . . . John Horton
Costume Design. . . . . James Acheson

FRONTIER IN SPACE (Serial QQQ)
Written by Malcolm Hulke (6 Episodes)
To avoid a crash, the Tardis materialises on a craft which is attacked by Ogrons, though a strange sound makes the crew see them as being reptilian Draconians, a race whose relationship with the Earth is worsening. With the Tardis stolen by the Ogrons, the Doctor and Jo are taken to Earth, where their story falls on disbelieving ears. The Doctor is taken to a prison colony, while Jo is rescued by the Master, who then frees the Doctor. He is working for a 'Third Party', with his task being to start a war between the humans and Draconians, but the Doctor manages to arbitrate and, with representatives of both sides, he heads to the Ogron's planet, where the Master reveals the 'Third Party' are the Daleks.....

Episode One - (24/02/73) (9.1m)
Episode Two - (03/03/73) (7.8m)
Episode Three - (10/03/73) (7.5m)
Episode Four - (17/03/73) (7.1m)
Episode Five - (24/03/73) (7.7m)
Episode Six - (31/03/73) (8.9m)

General Williams . . . . Michael Hawkins
President of Earth . . . . Vera Fusek
Professor Dale . . . . Harold Goldblatt
Gardiner . . . . Ray Lonnen
Draconian Prince. . . . . Peter Birrel
Draconian Emperor. . . . . . . John Woodnutt
Draconian Captain. . . . . Bill Wilde
Dalek Voices by Michael Wisher
Director . . . . Paul Bernard
Designer . . . . Cynthia Kljuco
Visual Effects . . . . Bernard Wilkie & Ian Scoones
Costume Design. . . . . Barbara Kidd

PLANET OF THE DALEKS (Serial SSS)
Written by Terry Nation (6 Episodes)
Tracking the Daleks to the jungle world of Spiridon, the Doctor and Jo meet a party of Thals on a suicide mission to destroy the small number of Daleks there. With the help of Wester, one of the invisible Spiridons, Jo and the others discover the

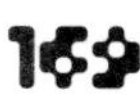

fact that there are tens of thousands of Daleks in hibernation beneath their base, waiting to be reactivated with their plan being to conquer space. The Doctor realises the answer might lie in activating an ice volcano.....

Episode One - (07/04/73) (11.0m)
Episode Two - (14/04/73) (10.7m)
Episode Three (21/04/73) (10.1m)
Episode Four - (28/04/73) (8.3m)
Episode Five - (05/05/73) (9.7m)
Episode Six - (12/05/73) (8.5m)

Taron . . . . Bernard Horsfall
Vaber . . . . Prentis Hancock
Codal . . . . Tim Preece
Rebec . . . . Jane How
Latep. Alan Tucker
Marat . . . . Hilary Minister
Wester . . . . Roy Skelton
Dalek Voices by Michael Wisher & Roy Skelton
Director . . . . David Maloney
Designer . . . . John Hurst
Visual Effects . . . . Cliff Culley
Costume Design. . . . . Hazel Pethig

<u>THE GREEN DEATH</u> (Serial TTT)
Written by Robert Sloman (6 Episodes)
In Wales, a community of miners becomes suspicious when one of their number dies from an infection that turns his skin bright green. They blame Global Chemicals for dumping waste in the mines, and Jo joins the group protesting against their continual pollution, led by Professor Jones. The Doctor and the Brigadier discover that the waste is causing mutations, with giant maggots and flies slowly starting to infest the mines. Captain Yates is sent undercover into the company, but is hypnotised by the computer running it, BOSS. The Doctor manages to overcome it, after defeating Yates' attempts to kill him on BOSS's orders. Everything returns to normal with all of the maggots now destroyed. Jo decides that she and the Professor are going to get married, and that it's time to leave UNIT and the Doctor.....

Episode One - (19/05/73) (9.2m)
Episode Two - (26/05/73) (7.2m)
Episode Three - (02/06/73) (7.8m)
Episode Four - (09/06/73) (6.8m)
Episode Five - (16/06/73) (8.3m)
Episode Six - (23/06/73) (7.0m)

Professor Clifford Jones . . . . Stewart Bevan
Stevens . . . . Jerome Willis
Hinks . . . . Ben Howard
Elgin. Tony Adams
Dave. . . . . Talfryn Thomas
Nancy . . . . Mitzi McKenzie
Voice of BOSS by John Dearth
Director . . . . Michael E. Briant
Designer . . . . John Borrowes
Visual Effects . . . Ron Oates, Colin Mapson & Richard Conway
Costume Design. . . . . Barbara Kidd

Season Eleven

Regular Cast
The Doctor . . . . Jon Pertwee
Sarah Jane Smith. . . . . Elisabeth Sladen
Brigadier Lethbridge-Stewart . . . . Nicholas Courtney (Serial UUU-WWW &ZZZ)
Captain Mike Yates . . . . . . Richard Franklin (Serial WWW & ZZZ)
Sergeant Benton. . . . . John Levene (Serial WWW & ZZZ)

Regular Production Team
Barry Letts . . . . Producer
Terrance Dicks. . . . . Script Editor

<u>THE TIME WARRIOR</u> (Serial UUU)
Written by Robert Holmes (4 Episodes)
A Sontaran (Linx) crash lands in 12th century England, and starts kidnapping scientists from the late 20th century to help with repairs to his ship. The Doctor, with a stowaway in the form of reporter Sarah Jane Smith, tracks Linx to the Castle of local warlord Irongron in his Tardis. The Sontaran would rather use the Doctor's mind than co-operate peacefully, and Sarah joins the rival castle owned by the nobility to try and defeat Irongron. Not only does the Doctor have to stop Linx, he also has to convince Sarah that he's not the villain!

Episode One - (15/12/73) (8.7m)
Episode Two - (22/12/73) (7.0m)
Episode Three - (29/12/73) (6.6m)
Episode Four - (05/01/74) (10.6m)

Irongron . . . . David Daker
Bloodaxe . . . . John J. Carney
Linx . . . . Kevin Lindsay
Professor Rubeish . . . . Donald Pelmear
Meg . . . . Sheila Fay
Eleanor . . . . June Brown
Edward of Wessex . . . . Alex Rowe
Hal . . . . Jeremy Bulloch
Director . . . . Alan Bromly
Designer. . . . . Keith Cheetham
Visual Effects . . . . Jim Ward
Costume Design. . . . . James Acheson

<u>INVASION OF THE DINOSAURS</u> (Serial WWW)
Written by Malcolm Hulke (6 Episodes)
Returning to an apparently deserted London, the Doctor and Sara Jane are arrested as looters and put on trial, but they escape from the vehicle transporting them when it's attacked by a Tyrannosaurus Rex. On finding the Brigadier, he explains that the evacuation took place when dinosaurs started to appear on the streets, although they soon vanish without trace. The whole thing is part of a plot by Sir Charles Grover and a group of scientists to revert the Earth to a time before technology corrupted society, and it's up to the Doctor to try and defeat their Operation Golden Age.....

Episode One - (12/01/74) (11.0m)
Episode Two - (19/01/74) (10.1m)
Episode Three - (26/01/74) (11.0m)
Episode Four - (02/02/74) (9.0m)
Episode Five - (09/02/74) (9.0m)
Episode Six - (16/02/74) (7.5m)

Sir Charles Grover . . . . Noel Johnson
Professor Whitaker . . . . Peter Miles
Butler . . . . Martin Jarvis
General Finch . . . . John Bennett
Mark. . . . . Terence Wilton
Adam . . . . Brian Badcoe
Director . . . . Paddy Russell
Designer . . . . Richard Morris
Visual Effects . . . . Cliff Culley
Costume Design. . . . . Barbara Kidd

<u>DEATH TO THE DALEKS</u> (Serial XXX)
Written by Terry Nation (4 Episodes)
All of the Tardis power banks are drained, and it has to land on the planet Exxilon, where a vast city absorbs all of the energy of passing spacecraft, forcing them down on the rocky terrain. The Doctor and Sarah meet a stranded Earth expedition, who are trying to find Parranium, the only known cure to a deadly space plague. When the Daleks arrive, unable to use their guns due to the power drain, an unholy alliance between them and the humans occurs, but can the Daleks be trusted?

Episode One - (23/02/74) (8.1m)
Episode Two - (02/03/74) (9.5m)
Episode Three - (09/03/74) (10.5m)
Episode Four - (16/03/74) (9.5m)

Lieutenant Dan Galloway. . Duncan Lamont
Lieutenant Peter Hamilton. . . . . . Julian Fox
Captain Richard Railton . . . . . . John Abineri
Jill Tarrant . . . . Joy Harrison
Bellal. . . . . Arnold Yarrow
Astronaut . . . . Terry Walsh

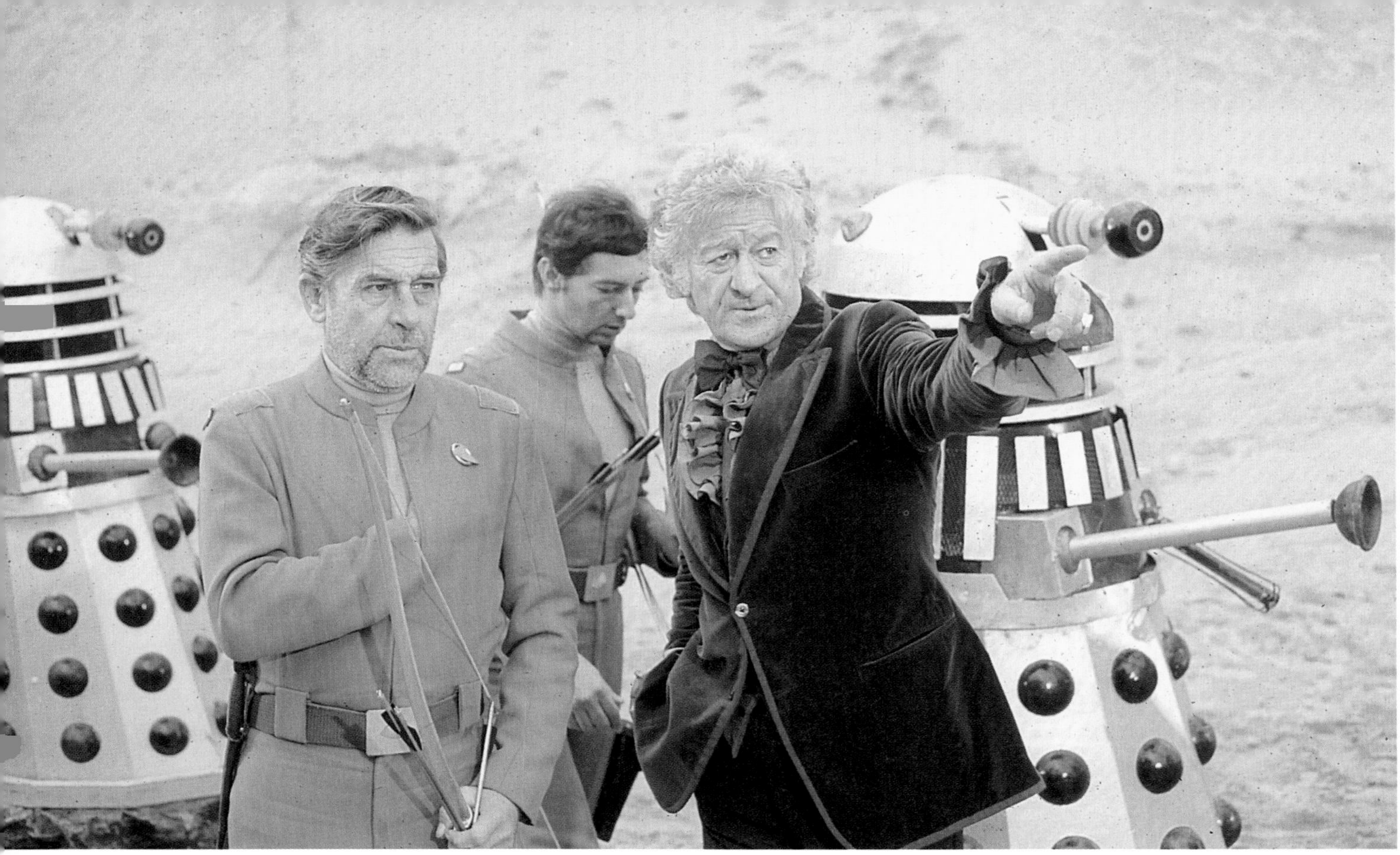

Dalek Voices by Michael Wisher
Director . . . . *Michael E. Briant*
Designer . . . . *Colin Green*
Visual Effects . . . . *Jim Ward*
Costume Design . . . . . . *L. Rowland Warne*

<u>THE MONSTER OF PELADON</u> (Serial YYY)
Written by Brian Hayles (6 Episodes)
The Tardis lands on Peladon, fifty years after the Doctor's last visit. Queen Tharila, a direct descendant of King Peladon, is trying to control the miners of the planet, who are rebelling against using Federation equipment, as it offends Aggador's spirit, which appears and kills anyone who operates the machines. The Doctor uncovers a conspiracy by enemy agents, led by Eckersley and a group of Ice Warriors, led by Azaxyr. The Doctor has to try and defeat them and return peace to Peladon.....

Episode One - (23/03/74) (9.2m)
Episode Two - (30/03/74) (6.8m)
Episode Three - (06/04/74) (7.4m)
Episode Four - (13/04/74) (7.2m)
Episode Five - (20/04/74) (7.5m)
Episode Six - (27/04/74) (8.1m)

Queen Thalira . . . . Nina Thomas
Eckersley . . . . Donald Gee
Ettis . . . . Ralph Watson
Ortron . . . . Frank Gatliff
Azaxyr . . . . Alan Bennion
Sskel . . . . Sonny Caldinez
Gebek . . . . Rex Robinson
Alpha Centuri . . . . Stuart Fell
(Voice by Ysanne Churchman)
Aggedor . . . . Nick Hobbs
Director . . . . *Lennie Mayne*
Designer . . . . *Gloria Clayton*
Visual Effects . . . . *Peter Day*
Costume Design . . . . *Barbara Kidd*

<u>PLANET OF THE SPIDERS</u> (Serial ZZZ)
Written by Robert Sloman (6 Episodes)
Jo Grant sends the blue crystal from Metabilis Three that the Doctor gave to her as a wedding present back to him. A giant spider from that planet materialises at a meditation centre, and takes over Lupton, commanding him to retrieve the said gem. The Doctor, Sarah and Lupton end up on

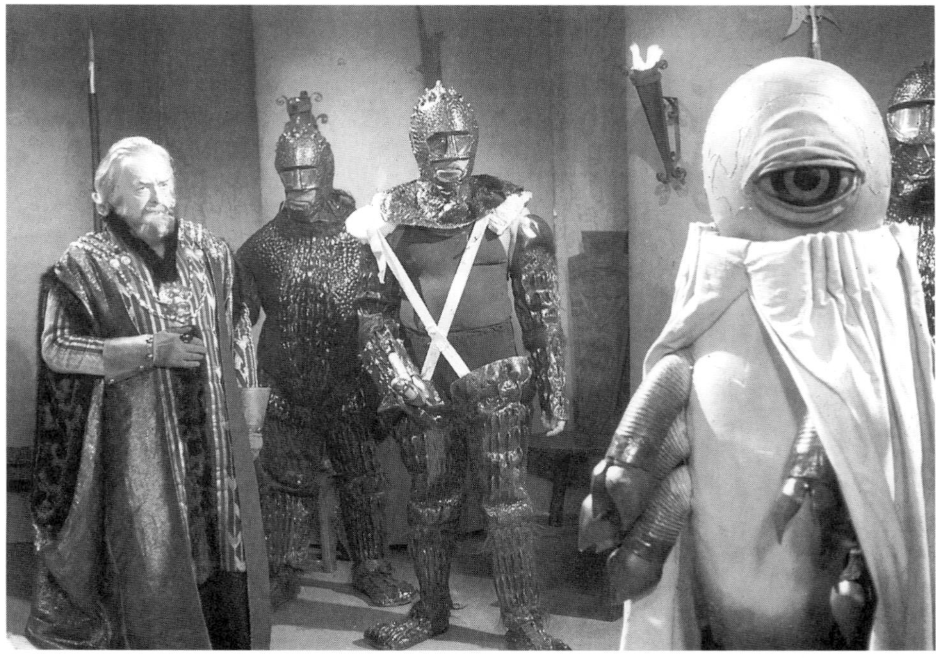

the planet where the Spiders rule, and their powerful queen, 'The Great One', needs the missing crystal to complete a giant one which will give it immense power. The Doctor confronts it, and the radiation from its cave destroys his body. The Tardis manages to get him back to the UNIT lab, where the Brigadier and Sarah watch in amazement as he collapses and regenerates.....

Episode One - (04/05/74) (10.1m)
Episode Two - (11/05/74) (8.9m)
Episode Three - (18/05/74) (8.8m)
Episode Four - (25/05/74) (8.2m)
Episode Five - (01/06/74) (9.2m)
Episode Six - (08/06/74) (8.9m)

Lupton . . . . John Dearth
Moss . . . . Terence Lodge
Keaver. . . . . Andrew Staines
Barnes . . . . Christopher Burgess
Land . . . . Carl Forgoine
Cho-je . . . . Kevin Lindsay
Tommy . . . . John Kane
Tuar. . . . . Ralph Arliss
Arak . . . . Gareth Hunt
Voice of Lupton's Spider by Ysanne Churchman
Voice of Queen Spider by Kismet Delgado
Voice of The Great One by Maureen Morris
Director. . . . . Barry Letts
Designer. . . . . Rochelle Selwyn
Visual Effects . . . . Bernard Wilkie
Costume Design . . . . . . L. Rowland Warne

Season Twelve

Regular Cast

The Doctor . . . . Tom Baker
Sarah Jane Smith. . . . . Elisabeth Sladen
Harry Sullivan . . . . Ian Marter
Brigadier Lethbridge-Stewart . . . . Nicholas Courtney (Serial 4A)
Sergeant Benton. . . John Levene(Serial 4A)

Regular Production Team

Barry Letts . . . . Producer (Serial 4A)
Philip Hinchcliffe . . . . Producer (Serial 4B Onwards)
Robert Holmes . . . . Script Editor

<u>ROBOT</u> (Serial 4A)
Written by Terrance Dicks (4 Episodes)
Some powerful creature is stealing all the components to build a disintegrator gun, and the newly regenerated Doctor deduces that it must be something big. The KI Robot Sarah is investigating fits the bill. The Robot is being used by a group of elitist scientists who want to a new ruling order of only the highest intelligences. When the robot's creator, Professor Kettlewell, is killed, it goes on the rampage. The Doctor has to take on the vast creature, when the Brigadier unwittingly causes it to grow to gigantic proportions.....

Episode One - (28/12/74) (10.8m)
Episode Two - (04/01/75) (10.7m)
Episode Three - (11/01/75) (10.1m)
Episode Four - (18/01/75) (9.0m)

Professor Kettlewell. . . . . Edward Burnham
Miss Winters . . . . Patricia Maynard
Jellicoe . . . . Alec Linstead
The Robot . . . . Michael Kilgarriff
Security Guard. . . . . Pat Gorman
Director. . . . . Christopher Barry
Designer . . . . Ian Rawnsley
Visual Effects . . . . Cliff Culley
Costume Design. . . . . Barbara Kidd

<u>THE ARK IN SPACE</u> (Serial 4C)
Written by Robert Holmes (4 Episodes)
The test flight for the new Doctor in the Tardis lands him, along with Sarah and Harry, on the space station Nerva, in the distant future. The Earth has been laid to waste by solar flares and the Nerva holds an enormous cryogenic store of all the survivors, waiting to be revived when enough time has passed for the planet to be habitable again. An alien parasitic insect, the Wirrn, invaded the station and laid its eggs in one of the sleeping humans. The Doctor has to race to stop the creatures from using the rest of the humans as incubators for their larvae.....

Episode One - (21/01/75) (9.4m)
Episode Two - (01/02/75) (13.6m)
Episode Three - (08/02/75) (11.2m)
Episode Four - (15/02/75) (10.2m)

Vira . . . . Wendy Williams
Noah. . . . . Kenton Moore
Rogan . . . . Richardson Morgan
Libri . . . . Christopher Masters
Voices by Gladys Spencer & Peter Tuddenham
Director. . . . . Rodney Bennett
Designer. . . . . Roger Murray-Leach
Visual Effects. . . . . John Friedlander & Tony Oxley
Costume Design. . . . . Barbara Kidd

<u>THE SONTARAN EXPERIMENT</u> (Serial 4B)
Written by Bob Baker & Dave Martin (2 Episodes)
Sent to Earth to try and repair the Nerva's transmat beam, they find it a wasteland of weeds, but habitable and seemingly

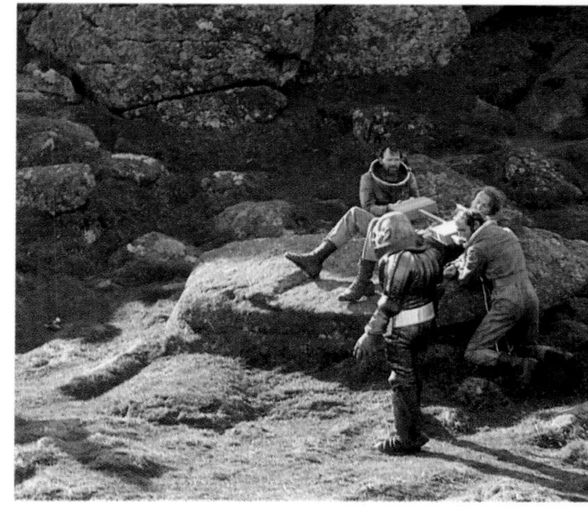

deserted. The Doctor and his two companions soon discover that there is a group of Glasec colonists stranded there, and that one by one they're being captured and tortured by a Sontaran, Styre, who's carrying out experiments to assess whether humans would be a threat to a Sontaran invasion force. The Doctor has to take the warrior on in combat to try and defeat him.....

Episode One - (22/02/75) (11.0m)
Episode Two - (01/03/75) (10.5m)

Field Major Styre . . . . Kevin Lindsay
Erak. Peter Walshe
Krans. . . . . Glyn Jones
Roth . . . . Peter Rutherford
Vural . . . . Donald Douglas
The Marshal . . . . Kevin Lindsay
Director. . . . . Rodney Bennett
Designer. . . . . Roger Murray-Leach
Visual Effects. . . . . John Friedlander & Tony Oxley
Costume Design. . . . . Barbara Kidd

<u>GENESIS OF THE DALEKS</u> (Serial 4E)
Written by Terry Nation (6 Episodes)
Diverted from the transmat beam taking them back to the Nerva, the Doctor, Sarah and Harry find themselves on Skaro. The Time Lords have given the Doctor a mission to stop or at least hinder the creation of the Daleks, and in the Kaled bunker, he witnesses the crippled scientist Davros proudly showing off his new Mark Three travel machine, housing the genetically mutated body of a Kaled – primitive, but it's undoubtedly a Dalek. As Davros betrays his own race, and then wipes out the Thals, the Doctor has to try and find it within himself to commit genocide and wipe out the Daleks forever.....

Episode One - (08/03/75) (10.7m)
Episode Two - (15/03/75) (10.5m)
Episode Three - (22/03/75) (8.5m)

Episode Four - (29/03/75) (8.8m)
Episode Five - (05/04/75) (9.8m)
Episode Six - (12/04/75) (9.1m)

Davros . . . . Michael Wisher
Nyder. Peter Miles
Gharman . . . . Dennis Chinnery
Ronson. . . . . James Garbutt
Kavell . . . . Tom Georgeson
Bettan . . . . Harriet Philpin
Sevrin. . . . . Stephen Yardley
Dalek Voices by Roy Skelton &
(Uncredited) Michael Wisher
Director . . . . David Maloney
Designer . . . . David Spode
Visual Effects. . . . . Peter Day
Costume Design. . . . . Barbara Kidd

REVENGE OF THE CYBERMEN (Serial 4D)
Written by Gerry Davis (4 Episodes)

The Time Ring given to the travellers by the Time Lord when they arrived on Skaro returns them to Nerva, but it's in an earlier time period when the station was still a beacon. A plague has killed off a large percentage of the crew, with only four survivors, one of whom is the treacherous Kellman. He is working for the Vogans, using Cybermats to kill off the humans, whilst laying a trap for the Cybermen, who want to destroy Voga, the planet of gold – the only substance that can kill them. The Cybermen arrive, and send the Doctor down to Voga with two of the beacon's crew as living bombs. He has to overcome that situation, and save Sarah and Harry, who are still on the beacon, before the Cybermen find out.....

Episode One - (19/04/75) (9.5m)
Episode Two - (26/04/75) (8.3m)
Episode Three - (03/04/75) (8.9m)
Episode Four - (10/04/75) (9.4m)

Commander Stevenson . . Ronald Leigh-Hunt
Kellman . . . . Jeremy Wilkin
Lester . . . . William Marlowe
Vorus. . . . . David Collings
Magrik . . . . Michael Wisher
Tyrum . . . . Kevin Stoney
Sheprah. . . . . Brian Grellis
Cyberleader . . . . Christopher Robbie
Director . . . . Michael E. Briant
Designer. . . . . Roger Murray-Leach
Visual Effects . . . . Jim Ward
Costume Design . . . . Prue Handley

Season Thirteen

Regular Cast

The Doctor . . . . Tom Baker
Sarah Jane Smith. . . . . Elisabeth Sladen
Harry Sullivan . . . . Ian Marter (Serial 4F & 4J Only)
Brigadier Lethbridge-Stewart . . . . Nicholas Courtney (Serial 4F)
RSM Benton . . . . John Levene (Serial 4F & 4J Only)

Regular Production Team

Philip Hinchcliffe . . . . Producer
Robert Holmes . . . . Script Editor

TERROR OF THE ZYGONS (Serial 4F)
Written by Robert Banks-Stewart (4 Episodes)

Arriving back on Earth, following a mayday call from the Brigadier, the Tardis lands near Loch Ness. Oil Rigs are apparently being destroyed by the famous 'Nessie', and the Doctor's investigations reveal some startling facts; the creature is actually a vast Cyborg, under the control of the Zygons, whose spacecraft is at the bottom of the Loch. They have a shapeshifting ability, which they use to full advantage to take over positions of authority, and the Doctor has to thwart their plans to take over the Earth for colonisation. Rather than travel back to UNIT Headquarters in the Tardis, Harry decides to head back to London with the Brigadier on a train, leaving the Doctor and Sarah to take off on their own.

Episode One - (30/08/75) (8.4m)
Episode Two - (06/09/75) (6.1m)
Episode Three - (13/09/75) (8.2m)
Episode Four - (20/09/75) (7.2m)

The Duke of Forgill & Broton . . . . John Woodnutt
The Caber. . . . . Robert Russell
Sister Lamont . . . . Lillias Walker
Angus . . . . Angus Lennie
Zygon . . . . Ronald Gough
Zygon . . . . Keith Ashley
Director . . . . Douglas Camfield
Designer . . . . Nigel Curzon
Visual Effects. . . . . John Horton
Costume Design. . . . . James Acheson

PLANET OF EVIL (Serial 4H)
Written by Louis Marks (4 Episodes)

The Doctor answers a distress call from the edge of the universe, and the Tardis lands on Zeta Minor, where a scientific expedition has been picked off one by one by an alien force. When a rescue ship arrives from Morestra, the Doctor and Sarah are immediately accused of being guilty of the murders. When the ship tries to take-off, it's dragged back to the planet's surface, because the only survivor of the expedition, Professor Sorenson, has taken samples of anti-matter – the planet acts as a gateway between worlds of anti-matter and matter – and a powerful creature from the other universe wants them back. The Doctor has to persuade the Morestrans to hand back the anti-matter, and overcome Sorenson, now mutating through exposure to anti-matter.....

Episode One - (27/09/75) (10.4m)
Episode Two - (04/10/75) (9.9m)
Episode Three - (11/10/75) (9.1m)
Episode Four - (18/10/75) (10.1m)

Professor Sorenson . . . . . . Frederick Jaeger
Vishinsky . . . . Ewan Solon
Salamar. . . . . Prentis Hancock
De Haan . . . . Graham Weston
Morelli . . . . Michael Wisher

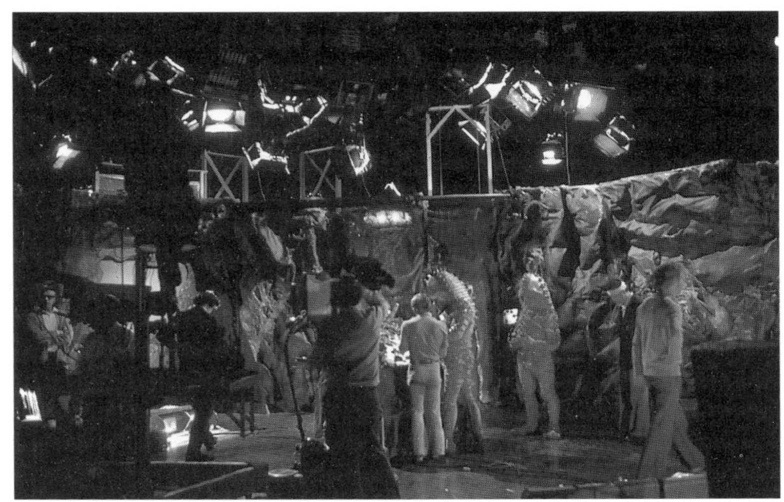

Reig . . . . Melvyn Bedford
Director . . . . David Maloney
Designer. . . . . Roger Murray-Leach
Visual Effects . . . . Dave Havard
Costume Design . . . . Andrew Rose

<u>PYRAMIDS OF MARS</u> (Serial 4G)
Written by Stephen Harris (4 Episodes)
Uncredited Rewrite by Robert Holmes
From The Original Scripts by Lewis Greifer
The Tardis finally returns to the UNIT Headquarters, but it's 1911, and the Doctor and Sarah are in the old priory that the building was later built over. Lawrence Scarman and his associate, Doctor Warlock, are protesting to Namin, an uncivil Egyptian, over his apparent take-over of the priory in the absence of its owner, Lawrence's brother, Marcus Scarman. Namin worships the evil God, Sutekh, whom he manages to summon and is promptly killed for his trouble. Sutekh uses the body of Marcus Scarman, captured when he broke into his tomb in Egypt, as the creature is actually an Osirian who was imprisoned in the tomb by his own race. Capturing the Doctor, Sutekh forces him to take the Tardis to Mars, where a series of traps have to be solved to free him from his prison. Unfortunately, if he does escape, it will mean the end of the universe.....

Episode One - (25/10/75) (10.5m)
Episode Two - (01/11/75) (11.3m)
Episode Three - (08/11/75) (9.4m)
Episode Four - (15/11/75) (11.7m)

Marcus Scarman . . . . Bernard Archard
Doctor Warlock . . . . Peter Copley
Laurence Scarman . . . . Michael Sheard
Namin. . . . . Peter Maycock
Sutekh . . . . Gabriel Woolf
Director . . . . Paddy Russell
Designer. . . . . Christine Ruscoe
Visual Effects . . . . Ian Scoones
Costume Design. . . . . Barbara Kidd

<u>THE ANDROID INVASION</u> (Serial 4J)
Written by Terry Nation (4 Episodes)
The Tardis lands in the picturesque village of Devesham, which has a space defence centre stationed nearby. The Doctor soon realises something is wrong with the behaviour of the local people, and discovers that they are all android duplicates, and that they're not on Earth at all. The Kraals of the planet Oseidon have laid their own world to waste, and are planning to stage an invasion of Earth, spearheading the way with the androids, which include Benton and Harry. The Doctor has to stop them when they arrive on Earth, before a lethal plague can be unleashed, which will eradicate mankind.....

Episode One - (22/11/75) (11.9m)
Episode Two - (29/11/75) (11.3m)
Episode Three - (06/12/75) (12.1m)
Episode Four - (13/12/75) (11.4m)

Corporal Adams . . . . Max Faulkner
Morgan. . . . . Peter Welch
Guy Crayford . . . . Milton Johns
Styggron. . . . . Martin Friend
Colonel Faraday . . . . Patrick Newell
Kraal . . . . Roy Skelton
Kraal. . . . . Stuart Fell
Director. . . . . Barry Letts
Designer. . . . . Philip Lindley
Visual Effects . . . . Len Hutton
Costume Design . . . . Barbara Lane

<u>THE BRAIN OF MORBIUS</u> (Serial 4K)
Written by Robin Bland (4 Episodes)
Original Script by Terrance Dicks
Rewritten by Robert Holmes
On the planet Karn, the brilliant Surgeon Mehendri Solon is searching for a suitable head to house the brain of Morbius, a renegade Time Lord executed on the planet years before with Solon retrieving the only surviving organ before the rest of the body was atomised. When the Doctor and Sarah arrive, Solon sees the perfect cranium for Morbius on the Time Lord. The Doctor has to contend with the Sisterhood of Karn, suspicious of his motives for visiting their world, thinking the Time Lords have sent him to steal their elixir of life, and then the mobile form of Morbius, when Solon puts the brain in a container fixed to a body constructed out of many parts retrieved from the wreckage of space crashes on the planet's surface......

Episode One - (03/01/76) (9.5m)
Episode Two - (10/01/76) (9.3m)
Episode Three - (17/01.76) (10.1m)
Episode Four - (24/01.76 (10.2m)

Solon. . . . . Philip Madoc
Condo . . . . Colin Fay
Chica . . . . Gilly Brown
Maren . . . . Cynthia Grenville
Voice of Morbius by Michael Spice
Director. . . . . Christopher Barry
Designer. . . . . Barry Newbery
Visual Effects. . . . . John Horton
Costume Design . . . . . . L. Rowland Warne

<u>THE SEEDS OF DOOM</u> (Serial 4L)
Written by Robert Banks-Stewart (6 Episodes)
Sent to the antarctic by the World Ecology Bureau, the Doctor and Sarah find that a Krynoid pod has been excavated from the ice. Once unleashed, its spores infect flesh and take over, mutating into sentient vegetable life. With the potential disaster averted there, the Doctor traces a second pod to Harrison Chase, a multi-millionaire in England, who is obsessed by all forms of plant life. He lets the pod infect another man, who mutates until he becomes a full Krynoid and starts to manipulate vegetation, using it to kill humans. The Doctor has to destroy the creature before its infection spreads world-wide.....

Episode One - (31/01/76) (11.4m)
Episode Two - (07/02/76) (11.4m)
Episode Three - (14/02/76) (10.3m)
Episode Four - (21/02/76) (11.1m)
Episode Five - (28/02/76) (9.9m)
Episode Six - (06/03/78) (11.5m)

Harrison Chase . . . . Tony Beckley
Scorby . . . . John Challis
Richard Dunbar . . . . Kenneth Gilbert
Hargreaves . . . . Seymour Green
Sir Colin Thackery . . . . . Michael Barrington
Amelia Ducat . . . . Sylvia Coleridge
Arnold Keeler. . . . . Mark Jones
Krynoid Voice by Mark Jones
Director . . . . Douglas Camfield
Designer. . . . . Roger Murray-Leach
(Episodes 1-2 Only) Jeremy Bear
Visual Effects. . . . . Richard Conway
Costume Design . . . . Barbara Lane

Season Fourteen

Regular Cast
The Doctor . . . . Tom Baker
Sarah Jane Smith. . . . . Elisabeth Sladen
(Serial 4M & 4N Only)
Leela . . . . Louise Jameson
(Serial 4Q Onwards)

Regular Production Team
Philip Hinchcliffe . . . . Producer
Robert Holmes . . . . Script Editor

<u>THE MASQUE OF MANDRAGORA</u>
(Serial 4M)
Written by Louis Marks (4 Episodes)
Part of the malevolent Mandragora Helix energy gets on board the Tardis, and the Doctor accidentally transports it to Italy in the fifteenth century, where it uses the

ancient cult of Demnos to instigate plans to take over the Earth. A celebration by the local nobility will see a party where all the guests will be the great thinkers and artists of the period. The Doctor has to stop the Mandragora energy before it can kill them all, and as a result, some of the greatest inventions will never be made, and the Earth will remain in the dark ages for eternity.....

Episode One - (04/09/76) (8.3m)
Episode Two - (11/09/76) (9.8m)
Episode Three - (18/09/76) (9.2m)
Episode Four - (25/09/76) (10.6m)

Count Frederico .... Jon Laurimore
Captain Rossini .... Anthony Carrick
Giuliano .... Gareth Armstrong
Hieronymous .... Norman Jones
Marco .... Tim Pigott-Smith
High Priest............... Robert James
Brother .... Brian Ellis
Director............... Rodney Bennett
Designer............... Barry Newbery
Visual Effects.............. Ian Scoones
Costume Design......... James Acheson

THE HAND OF FEAR (Serial 4N)
Written by Bob Baker & Dave Martin (4 Episodes)
The Tardis land in a quarry on Earth as several large explosions take place, and Sarah gets buried under rubble. She grips a fossilised hand, which the detonation unearthed, and it starts to control her mind, making her take it to a nuclear reactor. Feeding on the radiation, the hand grows a new body, in the shape of Eldred, a Kastrian criminal, who demands that the Doctor takes her back to her home planet so she can exact her revenge on her race, for executing her in the first place. Kastria is, however, a dead world, but a series of traps set in case Eldred ever returned lead to the creature's demise. The Doctor is summoned back to Gallifrey, and leaves Sarah on Earth, unable to take her with him.....

Episode One - (02/10/76) (10.5m)
Episode Two - (09/10/76) (10.2m)
Episode Three - (16/10/76) (11.1m)
Episode Four - (23/10/76) (12.0m)

Professor Watson .... Glyn Houston
Doctor Carter .... Rex Robinson
Miss Jackson........... Frances Pidgeon
Eldred.................... Judith Paris
Driscoll .... Roy Boyd
Eldred (Male Incarnation). . Stephen Thorne
Director................ Lennie Mayne
Designer .... Christine Roscoe
Visual Effects .... Colin Mapson
Costume Design .... Barbara Lane

THE DEADLY ASSASSIN (Serial 4P)
Written by Robert Holmes (4 Episodes)
The Doctor has a premonition that someone is about to assassinate the President on Gallifrey, so he tries to find the murderer before he can carry out his plan. The assassination, however, goes ahead and the Doctor is framed so that he is caught with the gun in his hand. The Doctor buys time before his inevitable execution for the crime, by declaring himself as a candidate for Presidential election, and then finds that the Master is behind the whole set-up. The Doctor has to stop the Master from absorbing a new cycle of bodily regenerations from the Eye of Harmony, and stop him from destroying Gallifrey......

Episode One - (30/10/76) (11.8m)
Episode Two - (06/11/76) (12.1m)
Episode Three - (13/11/76) (13.0m)
Episode Four - (20/11/76) (11.8m)

Chancellor Goth .... Bernard Horsfall
Castellan Spandrell .... George Pravda
Cardinal Borusa.......... Angus Mackay
Co-Ordinator Engin .... Erik Chitty
Commander Hildred .... Derek Seaton
Commentator Runcible..... Hugh Walters
The President of Gallifrey. . . Llewellyn Rees
The Master................. Peter Pratt
Director .... David Maloney
Designer........... Roger Murray-Leach
Visual Effects..... Len Hutton & Peter Day
Costume Design....... James Acheson & Joan Ellacott

THE FACE OF EVIL (Serial 4Q)
Written by Chris Boucher (4 Episodes)
On a primitive world, the tribe of the Sevateem fear the mighty God, Xoanon, while the Tesh work for it. The Doctor has been there before, when he helped repair a vast computer by giving it his personality, but it's now totally schizoid and trying to create the perfect species. The Doctor repairs the machine, and bridges the gap between the tribes so they can live in peace. One of the Sevateem, Leela, joins him to travel on the Tardis.....

Episode One - (01/01/77) (10.7m)
Episode Two - (08/01/77) (11.1m)
Episode Three - (15/01/77) (11.3m)
Episode Four - (22/01/77) (11.7m)

Neeva .... David Garfield
Tomas .... Brendan Price
Calib .... Leslie Schofield
Jabel .... Leon Eagles
Gentek.................... Mike Elles
Director .... Pennant Roberts
Designer................ Austin Ruddy
Visual Effects .... Mat Irvine
Costume Design .... John Bloomfield

THE ROBOTS OF DEATH (Serial 4R)
Written by Chris Boucher (4 Episodes)
The decadent crew of the vast sandminer, ploughing across an alien wasteland mining for minerals, are served by a series of robots, with varying degrees of intelligence; the Dums are basic labourers, the Vocs have a certain amount of intelligence, while the Super-Vocs actually co-ordinate the whole mining operation. As the Tardis arrives, the Doctor and Leela become immediate suspects for the murders that are taking place amongst the crew. None of them will believe the Doctor's theory that some of the robots have been reprogrammed to kill their masters, or the possibility that it's one of the crew that's doing it.....

Episode One - (29/01.77) (12.8m)
Episode Two - (05/02/77) (12.4m)
Episode Three - (12/02/77) (13.1m)
Episode Four - (19/02/77) (12.6m)

Commander Uvanov ...... Russell Hunter
Toos.................. Pamela Salem
Poul.................. David Collings
Dask .... David Ballie
Borg .... Brian Croucher
SV7 .... Miles Fothergill

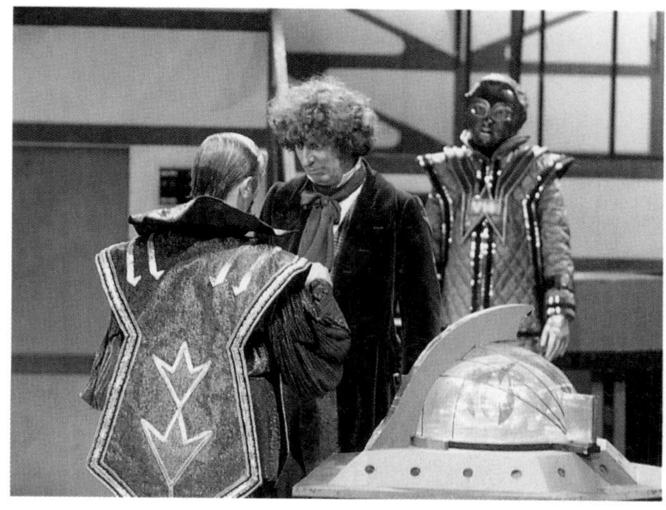

D84 . . . . Gregory de Polney
Director . . . . Michael E. Briant
Designer . . . . Kenneth Sharp
Visual Effects . . . . Richard Conway
Costume Design . . . . Elizabeth Waller

THE TALONS OF WENG-CHIANG (Serial 4S)
Written by Robert Holmes (6 Episodes)
In Victorian England, the Doctor starts to investigate the background to a number of disappearances by young girls and a murder. Working with a pathologist, Professor Lightfoot, and a theatre manager, Henry Jago, they discover that the oriental magician Li H'sen Chang is part of a tong cult worshipping the ancient God, Weng Chiang. Magnus Greel, a war criminal from the future, who was terribly mutated by the journey he made into the past in a primitive time machine, is posing as the God and he is behind the disappearing girls, whose lifeforce he drains to keep him alive. The Doctor has to stop him from endangering countless lives as he tries to get back to the future. . . .

Episode One - (26/02/77)(11.3m)
Episode Two - (05/03/77)(9.8m)
Episode Three - (12/03/77)(10.2m)
Episode Four - (19/03/77)(11.4m)
Episode Five - (26/03/77)(10.1m)
Episode Six - (02/04/77)(9.3m)

Professor Lightfoot . . . . Trevor Baxter
Henry Litefoot . . . . . Christopher Benjamin
Li H'sen Chang . . . . John Bennett
Weng-Chiang/Magnus Greel . . Michael Spice
Mister Sin . . . . Deep Roy
Casey . . . . Chris Gannon
Lee Tony Then
Director . . . . David Maloney
Designer. . . . . Roger Murray-Leach
Visual Effects . . . . Michael John-Harris
Costume Design . . . . John Bloomfield

Season Fifteen

Regular Cast
The Doctor . . . . Tom Baker
Leela . . . . Louise Jameson

Regular Production Team
Graham Williams . . . . Producer
Robert Holmes . . . . Script Editor (Serial 4V-4W)
Anthony Read . . . . Scrip Editor (Serial 4Y Onwards)

HORROR OF FANG ROCK (Serial 4V)
Written by Terrance Dicks (4 Episodes)
Still travelling at the turn of the century, the Tardis lands on the rocks outside a lighthouse and, along with the survivors of a shipwreck, they find themselves being murdered one by one. The murderer is a Rutan, one of the shape-changing creatures locked in a never-ending war with the Sontarans. The Doctor has to stop its murderous rampage before it can send a signal to its mothership for Earth to be colonised.

Episode One - (03/09/77)(6.8m)
Episode Two - (10/09/77)(7.1m)
Episode Three - (17/09/77)(9.8m)
Episode Four - (24/09/77)(9.9m)

Reuben. . . . . Colin Douglas
Vince . . . . John Abbott
Skinsdale . . . . Alan Rowe
Lord Palmerdale . . . . Sean Caffrey
Adelaide. . . . . Annette Woollett
Director . . . . Paddy Russell
Designer . . . . Paul Allen
Visual Effects. . . . . Peter Pegrum
Costume Design . . . . Joyce Hawkins

THE INVISIBLE ENEMY (Serial 4V)
Written by Bob Baker & Dave Martin (4 Episodes)
An intelligent space virus infects the crew of a space station and then attacks the Doctor, implanting itself in his brain. With the help of Professor Marius, the Doctor and Leela are cloned, miniaturised and injected into the Doctor's blood stream to try and find the creature in his brain. The Nucleus escapes and starts to multiply its swarm so it can take over the medical centre, and then the universe now that it has a physical form. After destroying the creature, the Doctor is asked to look after Marinus's robot dog, K9, so the Tardis leaves with a new passenger. . . .

Episode One - (01/01/77)(8.6m)
Episode Two - (08/10/77)(7.3m)
Episode Three - (15/10/77)(7.5m)
Episode Four - (22/10/77)(8.3m)

Professor Marius . . . . Frederick Jaeger
Lowe . . . . Michael Sheard
Safran . . . . Brian Grellis
Opthalmologist . . . . Jim McManus
Technician . . . . Pat Gorman
Voice of the Nucleus & K9 by John Leeson
Director . . . . Derrick Goodwin
Designer. . . . . Barry Newbery
Visual Effects . . Ian Scoone & Tony Harding
Costume Design . . . . Raymond Design

IMAGE OF THE FENDAHL (Serial 4X)
Written by Chris Boucher (4 Episodes)
Time experiments around an ancient skull, led by Doctor Fendelman with his team of scientists based at Fetch Priory, unwittingly release the power of the Fendahl, an energy force that drains the energy of life itself from humans. As the slug-like Fendahleens start to materialise, and Thea Ransome becomes possessed by the power which turns her into a human manifestation of its evil, the Doctor uses science and the folklore magic of old Martha Tyler to overcome the threat. . . .

Episode One - (29/10/77)(6.7m)
Episode Two - (05/11/77)(7.5m)
Episode Three - (12/11/77)(7.9m)
Episode Four - (19/11/77)(9.1m)

Doctor Fendelman . . . . Denis Lill
Thea Ransome . . . . Wanda Ventham
Maximillian Stael . . . . Scott Fredericks
Adam Colby . . . . Edward Arthur

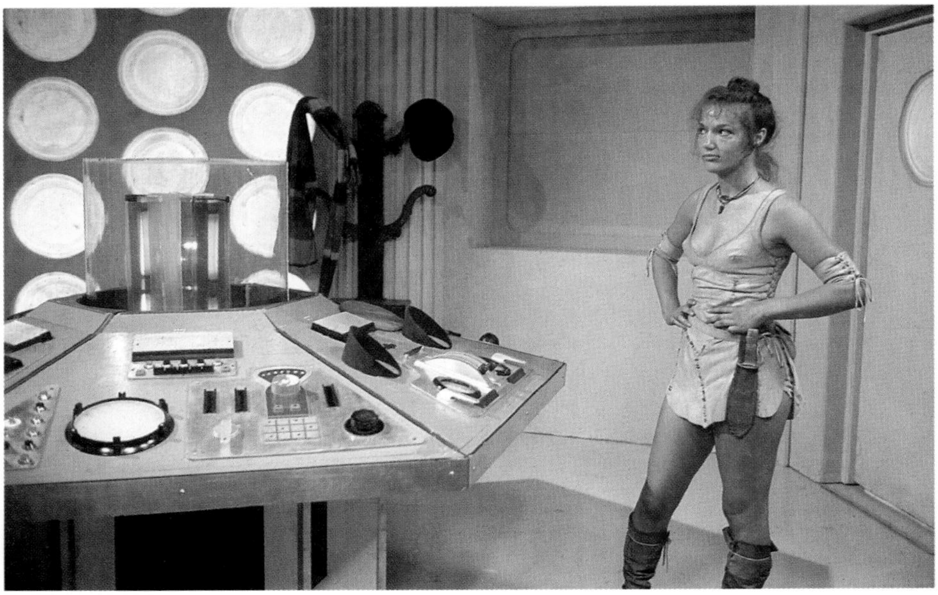

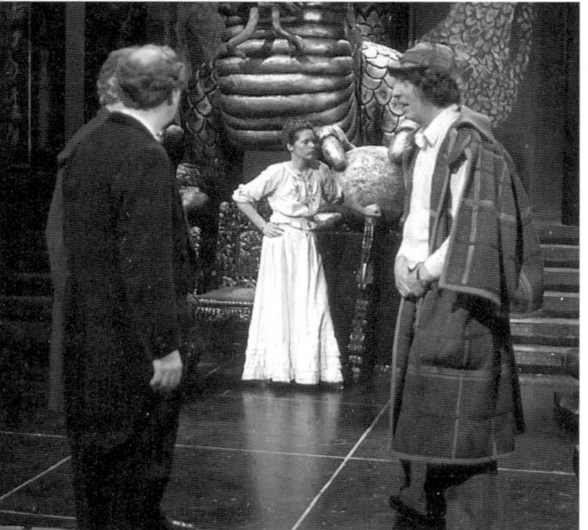

Ted Moss . . . . Edward Evans
David Mitchell . . . . Derek Martin
Martha Tyler . . . . Daphne Heard
Jack Tyler. . . . . Geoffrey Hinsliff
Director . . . . George Spenton Foster
Designer. . . . . Anne Ridley
Visual Effects . . . . Colin Mapson
Costume Design . . . . Amy Roberts

THE SUN MAKERS (Serial 4W)
Written by Robert Holmes(4 Episodes)
The Usurians' lives seems to revolve around money, and the economy of Megropolis Pluto has an astronomical tax rate that has reduced the workers to poverty, while the Gatherer of Taxes leads an opulent lifestyle, and answers only to the wheelchair bound Collector, who is obsessed with profit, no matter what the cost on human lives. The Doctor and Leela join forces with the rebels in the city, and manage to defeat the Collector, who reverts to his natural form, which appears to be nothing more than a lump of seaweed. . . .

Episode One - (26/11/77)(8.5m)
Episode Two - (03/12/77)(9.5m)
Episode Three - (10/12/77)(8.9m)
Episode Four - (17/12/77)(8.4m)

Gatherer Hade . . . . Richard Leech
The Collector . . . . Henry Woolf
Cordo . . . . Roy Macready
Mandrel. . . . . William Simons
Goudry . . . . Michael Keating
Marn . . . . Jonina Scott
Veet. . . . . Adrienne Burgess
Bisham . . . . David Rowlands
Synge . . . . Derek Crewe
Director . . . . Pennant Roberts
Designer . . . . Tony Snoaden
Visual Effects . . . . Peter Day & Peter Logan
Costume Design . . . . . . Christine Rawlins

UNDERWORLD (Serial 4Y)
Written by Bob Baker & Dave Martin
The race banks of the Minyans went missing centuries ago on a ship called the P7E, and the Tardis materialises on another Minyan ship carrying out an epic search for it. The P7E is at the heart of a planet, which has formed around it and the descendants of the original crew are now either its slaves or cybernetic seers, working to the orders of the Oracle, the ship's computer which is now worshipped and runs their lives. The Doctor helps the Minyans in the fight to retrieve the race banks from the computer's control room.

Episode One - (07/01/78)(8.9m)
Episode Two - (14/01/78)(9.1m)
Episode Three - (21/01/78)(8.9m)
Episode Four - (28/01/78)(11.7m)

Jackson. . . . . James Maxwell
Tala . . . . Imogen Bickford-Smith
Herrick . . . . Alan Lake
Orfe . . . . Johnathan Newth
Idmon . . . . Jimmy Gardner
Idas . . . . Norman Tipton
Tarn. . . . . Godfrey James
Rask . . . . James Marcus
Director . . . . Norman Stewart
Designer . . . . Dick Coles
Visual Effects. . . . . Richard Conway
Costume Design. . . . . Rupert Jarvis

THE INVASION OF TIME (Serial 4Z)
Written by David Agnew (6 Episodes)
False Name for Graham Williams & Anthony Read
The Doctor returns to Gallifrey, with his behaviour becoming more and more erratic, and claims his rightful place as the President of Gallifrey, then promptly betrays his own race by letting an invasion force of Vardans land on Gallifrey. A rebellion is started by one of the guard commanders, Andred, to try and depose the Doctor, and Leela is banished to the wastelands of the planet, but the Doctor is setting a trap for the Vardans. When he succeeds in defeating them, everything seems as though it will go back to normal but, while the defence barriers around Gallifrey were down, an invasion force of Sontarans landed, and they try and take over the power of the Time Lords. The Doctor has to use a D-Mat gun to stop them, and as he goes to leave, both Leela, who is in love with Andred, and K9 decide to stay on Gallifrey. As the Tardis takes off, the Doctor pulls out a box, containing all the components he needs to build a K9 Mark II. . . .

Episode One - (04/02/78)(11.2m)
Episode Two - (11/02/78)(11.4m)
Episode Three - (18/02/78)(9.5m)
Episode Four - (25/02/78)(10.9m)
Episode Five - (04/03/78)(10.3m)
Episode Six - (11/03/78)(9.8m)

Cardinal Borusa . . . . John Arnatt
Castellan Kelner . . . . Milton Johns
Commander Andred . . . . . . Chris Tranchell
Rodan . . . . Hilary Ryan
Nesbin . . . . Max Faulkener
Presta . . . . Gai Smith
Vardan Leader . . . . Stan McGowan
Stor . . . . Derek Deadman
Sontaran. . . . . Stuart Fell
Director . . . . Gerald Blake
Designer. . . . . Barbara Gosnold
Visual Effects. . . . . Richard Conway & Colin Mapson
Costume Design . . . . Dee Kelly

Season Sixteen

Regular Cast
The Doctor . . . . Tom Baker
Romana. . . . . Mary Tamm
Voice of K9 by John Leeson (Except Serial 5E)

Regular Production Team
Graham Williams . . . . Producer
Anthony Read. . . . . Script Editor

THE RIBOS OPERATION (Serial 5A)
Written by Robert Holmes (4 Episodes)
The Doctor is sent on a quest by the White Guardian, a being of immense power who exists outside the dimensions of space and time, to collect the six segments of the Key to Time, which have been scattered throughout the universe. He has a new assistant, in the shape of the Time Lady, Romana, and a new model of K9. The first segment is found on the planet Ribos, in the form of a lump of Jethrik, a precious stone that Garron and Unstoffe are using to help try and con the Graff Vynda-K into buying the planet, by making him believe that there are Jethrik mines throughout the world . . .

Episode One - (02/09/78)(8.3m)
Episode Two - (09/09/78)(8.1m)
Episode Three - (16/09/78)(7.9m)
Episode Four - (23/09/78)(8.2m)

The White Guardian . . . . Cyril Luckham
Garron . . . . Iain Cuthbertson
Unstoffe. . . . . Nigel Plaskitt
Graff Vynda-K . . . . Paul Seed
Sholakh. . . . . Robert Keegan

Captain . . . . Prentis Hancock
Director . . . . George Spenton Foster
Designer. . . . . Ken Ledsham
Visual Effects . . . . Dave Havard
Costume Design . . . . June Hudson

THE PIRATE PLANET (Serial 5B)
Written by Douglas Adams (4 Episodes)
The second segment is the entire planet of Calufrax, but the Doctor and Romana are mystified when they find the planet of Zanak in its place. The Captain, a blustering figure with a partially cybernised head and left arm, rules from his headquarters, assisted by Mr Fibuli and his ever present Nurse. The Doctor discovers that Zanak is a vast hollow ship, which materialises around planets, and then absorbs all their natural energy, until all that's left is a small lump of rock. The Doctor has to defeat the Captain and find the second segment, while K9 has to battle the Polyphase Avatron, the Captain's deadly metal parrot.

Episode One - (30/09/78)(9.1m)
Episode Two - (07/10/78)(7.4m)
Episode Three - (14/10/78)(8.2m)
Episode Four - (21/10/78)(8.4m)

The Captain . . . . Bruce Purchase
Mister Fibuli . . . . Andrew Robertson
Pralix . . . . David Sibley
Mula . . . . Primi Townsend
Kimus. . . . . David Warwick
Mentiad . . . . Bernard Finch
Queen Xanxia . . . . Rosalind Lloyd
Director . . . . Pennant Roberts
Designer. . . . . Jon Pusey
Visual Effects . . . . Colin Mapson
Costume Design . . . . Rowland Warne

THE STONES OF BLOOD (Serial 5C)
Written by David Fisher (4 Episodes)
Professor Amelia Rumford is working around the stone circle, known as the Nine Travellers, with her assistant Vivien Fay, when the Doctor and Romana arrive on the scene. Local devil worship has activated some of the stones with blood sacrifices, as they are in reality the Ogri, who need to absorb nutrients from haemoglobin to live. The Doctor discovers that there is a spaceship hovering over the circle in hyperspace, thus making it invisible to people in this dimension. On board, the fact becomes clear that one of the prisoners, Cessair of Dilpos has escaped, and the Megara, shapeless justice machines, accuse the Doctor of aiding her and sentence him to death. Cessair is really Vivien Fay, and the Doctor has to convince the Megara that this is her true identity to save his life. . . .

Episode One - (28/10/78)(8.6m)
Episode Two - (04/11/78)(6.6m)
Episode Three - (11/11/78)(9.3m)
Episode Four - (18/11/78)(7.6m)

Professor Amelia Rumford . . Beatrix Lehmann
Vivien Fay . . . . Susan Engel
Doctor Vries . . . . Nicholas McArdle
Martha . . . . Elaine Ives-Cameron
Megara Justice Machine Voices by Gerald Cross & David McAlister
Director. . . . . Darrol Blake
Designer . . . . John Stout
Visual Effects . . . . Mat Irvine
Costume Design. . . . . Rupert Jarvis

THE ANDROIDS OF TARA (Serial 5D)
Written by David Fisher (4 Episodes)
The planet of Tara holds the fourth segment of the Key as a statue, and the Doctor becomes involved in the feud that exists between Count Grendel and Prince Reynart. Grendel has kidnapped Reynart in an attempt to seize the throne, but the Prince's followers have substituted an android in his place so that the coronation can go ahead. Grendel manages to sabotage the device. Reynart's true love is Princess Strella, whom Grendel also holds captive and much to his surprise, he finds that Romana is a doppleganger for her when they meet. The Doctor has to defeat Grendel and ensure the Prince inherits his rightful title, as well as rescuing Romana, before he can leave to search for the fifth segment. . . .

Episode One - (25/11/78)(8.5m)
Episode Two - (02/12/78)(10.1m)
Episode Three - (09/12/78)(8.9m)
Episode Four - (16/12/78)(9.0m)

Count Grendel. . . . . Peter Jeffrey
Prince Reynart . . . . Neville Jason
Zadek . . . . Simon Lack
Farrah. Paul Lavers
Till Declan Mulholland
Larnia . . . . Lois Baxter
Archimandrite. . . . . Cyril Shaps
Kurster . . . . Martin Matthews
Director. . . . . Michael Hayes
Designer . . . . Valerie Warrender
Visual Effects . . . . Len Hutton
Costume Design. . . . . Doreen James

THE POWER OF KROLL (Serial 5E)
Written by Robert Holmes (4 Episodes)
On one of the moons of Delta Magna, a primitive tribe called the Swampies worship the monstrous Kroll, and they are opposed to all forms of alien technology, which makes life awkward for an earth refinery set up there. A human gun runner called Rohm-Dutt is supplying the Swampies with all the weapons they need to overthrow the humans, who mistake the Doctor for being Dutt when the Tardis lands in the middle of the swamp lands. Kroll rises from the depths, and the Doctor has to somehow get the key tracer near it to revert it to its natural form. The creature is only that big due to the fact that it swallowed the fifth segment centuries before.

Episode One - (23/12/78)(6.5m)
Episode Two - (30/12/78)(12.4m)
Episode Three - (06/01/79)(8.9m)
Episode Four - (13/01/79)(9.9m)

Rohm-Dutt . . . . Glyn Owen
Fenner . . . . Philip Madoc
Thawn . . . . Neil McCarthy
Dugeen. . . . . John Leeson
Varlik . . . . Carl Rigg
Ranquin . . . . John Abineri
Skart. . . . . Frank Jarvis
Director . . . . Norman Stewart
Designer. . . . . Don Giles
Visual Effects. . . . . Tony Harding
Costume Design . . . . Colin Lavers

THE ARMAGEDDON FACTOR (Serial 5F)
Written by Bob Baker & Dave Martin
The planet of Atrios had been fighting its direct neighbour, Zeos, for years. When the Tardis arrives, the Doctor is lured onto Zeos, where he finds that a computer K9 is able to communicate with is actually what the Atrians are fighting – a strategic planner. The war is kept going by the Shadow, a malevolent agent of the Black Guardian, and the Doctor is able to overthrow him with the help of another Time Lord, Drax. The Shadow reveals that the sixth segment is Princess Astra, and she is converted into the crystal. With everything settled between the planets, the Doctor leaves and puts the key together, and the White Guardian appears on the scanner screen. When it becomes clear that he was the Black Guardian all along, the Doctor disperses the key through space once again, and the evil guardian swears revenge. . . .

Episode One - (20/01/79)(7.5m)
Episode Two - (27/01/79)(8.8m)
Episode Three - (03/02/79)(7.8m)
Episode Four - (10/02/79)(8.6m)
Episode Five - (17/02/79)(8.6m)
Episode Six - (24/02/79)(9.6m)

The Marshal . . . . John Woodvine
Merak . . . . Ian Saynor

Princess Astra . . . . Lalla Ward
Shapp . . . . Davyd Harries
Drax . . . . Barry Jackson
The Shadow . . . . William Squire
The Black Guardian . . . . Valentine Dyall
Director. . . . . Michael Hayes
Designer . . . . Richard McManan-Smith
Visual Effects . . . Jim Francis, John Horton & Steve Lucas
Costume Design . . . . Michael Burdle

Season Seventeen

Regular Cast
The Doctor . . . . Tom Baker
Romana. . . . . Lalla Ward
Voice of K9 by David Brierley (Serial 5G-5M)

Regular Production Team
Graham Williams . . . . Producer
Douglas Adams . . . . Script Editor

DESTINY OF THE DALEKS (Serial 5J)
Written by Terry Nation (4 Episodes)
With the Tardis now fitted with a Randomiser, so that the Black Guardian will not be able to trace their flight paths, the first landing the Doctor makes is on Skaro. They explore and eventually become separated, with the Doctor meeting the Movellans, and Romana becoming the prisoner of the Daleks. The Daleks are trying to excavate the bunker where Davros was buried as they are at war with the Movellans, and their battle computers have reached stalemate. Both factions have realised that human intuitions would give one side an advantage, and Davros is the ideal scientist to induce this in either of the robotic races. The Doctor has to try and stop them finding Davros, but time is running out. . . .

Episode One - (01/09/79)(13.0m)
Episode Two - (08/09/79)(12.7m)
Episode Three - (15/09/79)(13.8m)
Episode Four - (22/09/79)(14.4m)

Tyssan . . . . Tim Barlow
Commander Sharrel . . . . Peter Straker
Agella . . . . Suzanne Danielle
Davros . . . . David Gooderson
Lan Tony Osoba
Veldan . . . . David Yip
Jall Penny Casdagli
Dalek Voices by Roy Skelton
Director . . . . Ken Grieve
Designer. . . . . Ken Ledsham
Visual Effects . . . . Peter Logan
Costume Design . . . . June Hudson

CITY OF DEATH (Serial 5H)
Written by David Agnew (4 Episodes)
Based on the Premise by David Fisher
Rewritten Uncredited by Graham Williams & Douglas Adams
A plot set up by Count Scarlioni to steal the Mona Lisa from the Louvre Gallery in Paris leads the Doctor to his home, where he discovers that time experiments are being carried out in the Count's cellar by Professor Kerensky. The Count is really Scaroth, one of twelve splinters of a Jagaroth pilot scattered throughout earth's history when his ship exploded in prehistoric times. He is financing the experiments by selling duplicate Mona Lisas he had Leonardo da Vinci bash out, but he can only do this if he owns the one in the Louvre, otherwise the buyers will suspect. He wants to go back in time and stop his ship from being destroyed, but as the explosion triggered the creation of life on Earth, the Doctor has to stop him at all costs. . . .

Episode One - (29/09/79)(12.4m)
Episode Two - (06/10/79)(14.1m)
Episode Three - (13/10/79)(15.4m)
Episode Four - (20/10/79)(16.1m)

Count Scarlioni & Scaroth. . . . Julian Glover
Duggan . . . . Tom Chadbon
Countess Scarlioni . . . . Catherine Schell
Professor Kerensky. . . . . David Graham
Hermann . . . . Kevin Flood
Guard Captain . . . . Peter Halliday
Art Gallery Critic . . . . John Cleese
Art Gallery Critic. . . . . Eleanor Bron
Director. . . . . Michael Hayes
Designer . . . . Richard McManan-Smith
Visual Effects . . . . Ian Scoones
Costume Design. . . . . Doreen James

THE CREATURE FROM THE PIT (Serial 5G)
Written by David Fisher (4 Episodes)
Metal is practically priceless on the planet Chloris, as it is such a rare object, and when the Tythonian Ambassador arrived wishing to swap metal ore for vegetation, Lady Adastra had it thrown down a pit fearing that such trading would threaten her hold on the population. The Doctor finds a way to communicate with the creature, who explains that there has been such a protracted silence from him communicating with his race, that they have sent a neutron star towards Chloris to destroy it. The Doctor has to join forces with the creature to save the planet. . . .

Episode One - (27/10/79)(9.3m)
Episode Two - (03/11/79)(10.8m)
Episode Three - (10/11/79)(10.2m)
Episode Four - (17/11/79)(9.6m)

Lady Adastra. . . . . Myra Frances
Karela. . . . . Eileen Way
Torvin . . . . John Bryans
Edu. . . . . Edward Kelsey
Organon . . . . Geoffrey Bayldon
Ainu . . . . Tim Munro
Director. . . . . Christopher Barry
Designer . . . . Valerie Warrender
Visual Effects . . . . Mat Irvine
Costume Design . . . . June Hudson

NIGHTMARE OF EDEN (Serial 5K)
Written by Bob Baker (4 Episodes)
Emerging from Hyperspace at the same moment, a star liner and a freighter crash in space and fuse. The Tardis lands on board, and the Doctor and Romana find that huge creatures called Madrels have escaped from a Continuous Event Transmitter, and are roaming the ship killing the passengers. Mandrels disintegrate into a powder when they die, which is also a highly addictive drug called Vraxoin. The Doctor determines to smash the drug ring which is smuggling the live creatures. . . .

Episode One - (24/11/79)(6.0m)
Episode Two - (01/12/79)(8.8m)
Episode Three - (08/12/79)(9.6m)
Episode Four - (15/12/79)(9.4m)

Professor Tryst . . . . Lewis Flander
Figg . . . . David Daker
Dymond. . . . . Geoffrey Bateman
Stott . . . . Barry Andrews

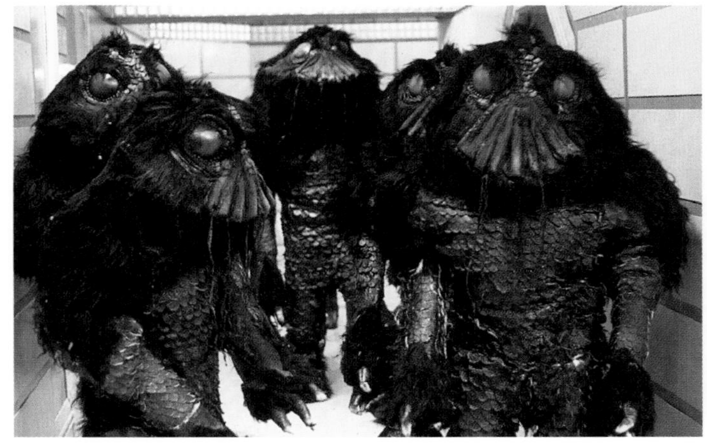

Della . . . . Jennifer Lonsdale
Fisk Geoffrey Hinsliff
Costa . . . . Peter Craze
Director . . . . Alan Bromly
Uncredited additional work by Graham Williams
Designer . . . . Roger Cann
Visual Effects . . . . Colin Mapson
Costume Design. . . . . Rupert Jarvis

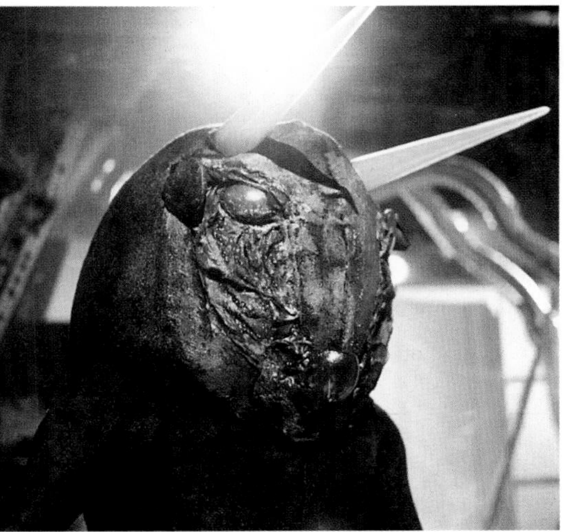

THE HORNS OF NIMON (Serial 5L)
Written by David Fisher (4 Episodes)
Regular freighter loads of sacrificial offerings are being taken from the planet Anneth to Skonnos, where the high-priest, Soldeed, sends them into the lair of the Nimon, bull-like creatures whom he believes to be Gods. The Doctor proves they are planning to invade Skonnos, and Romana makes a trip to the last planet they laid to waste, where she learns of their only weakness, which must be exploited to destroy them. . . .

Episode One - (22/12/79)(6.0m)
Episode Two - (29/12/79)(8.8m)
Episode Three - (05/01/80)(9.8m)
Episode Four - (12/01/80)(10.4m)

Soldeed . . . . Graham Crowden
Sorak. . . . . Michael Osborne
Seth. . . . . Simon Gipps-Kent
Teka . . . . Janet Ellis
Co-Pilot. . . . . Malcolm Terris
Voice of the Nimon by Clifford Norgate
Director. . . . . Kenny McBain
Designer. . . . . Graeme Story
Visual Effects. . . . . Peter Pegrum
Costume Design . . . . June Hudson

SHADA (Serial 5M) (Story not completed)
Written by Douglas Adams (6 Episodes)
The Doctor and Romana visit a Time Lord called Professor Chronotis, now living in retirement as a Cambridge College lecturer. He asks them to take back a powerful book to his home planet called 'The Ancient Law of Gallifrey', and the Doctor is horrified when he finds out it ever left the planet in the first place. Skagra, a malevolent mind-thief, wants to use the book to travel to Shada, a prison planet where he will free the legendary Salyavin, a rogue Time Lord. Chronotis is in reality Salyavin, who now just wants to live out the rest of his years in peace, and the Doctor has to follow Skagra to Shada to try and stop his scheme. . . .

Broadcast Details – N/A

Professor Chronotis . . . . Denis Carey
Skagra . . . . Christopher Neame
Clare Keightley. . . . . Victoria Burgoyne
Chris Parsons . . . . Daniel Hill
Director . . . . Pennant Roberts
Designer . . . . Victor Meredith
Visual Effects . . . . Dave Havard
Costume Design. . . . . Rupert Jarvis

Season Eighteen

Regular Cast
The Doctor . . . . Tom Baker
Romana . . . . . . Lalla Ward (Serial 5N – 5S)
Voice of K9 . . John Leeson (Serial 5N – 5S)
Adric . . . . Matthew Waterhouse (Serial 5R Onwards)
Nyssa . . . . Sara Sutton (Serial 5T Onwards)
Tegan . . Janet Fielding (Serial 5V Onwards)

Regular Production Team
John Nathan-Turner . . . . Producer
Christopher H. Bidmead . . . . . Script Editor
Barry Letts . . . . Executive Producer

THE LEISURE HIVE (Serial 5N)
Written by David Fisher (4 Episodes)
After a disappointing holiday attempt in Brighton, with K9 getting waterlogged in the sea, the Doctor and Romana head for the planet Argolis, famed for its leisure complex. The Argolins are being forced to sell out to the Foamasi, an enemy of the race for generations, and Pangol uses the Argolin Generator to mass-clone himself as an army to wage war against the creatures. The Doctor, who has accidentally been aged five hundred years, has to race to stop Pangol, and uncover the Foamasi agent in their midst. . . .

Episode One - (30/09/80)(5.9m)
Episode Two - (06/09/80)(5.0m)
Episode Three - (13/09/80)(5.0m)
Episode Four - (20/09/80)(4.5m)

Mena . . . . Adrienne Corri
Brock . . . . John Collin
Vargos . . . . Martin Fisk
Pangol . . . . David Haig
Hardin . . . . Nigel Lambert
Klout . . . . Ian Talbot
Director . . . . Lovett Bickford
Designer. . . . . Tom Yardley-Jones
Visual Effects . . . . Andrew Lazell
Costume Design . . . . June Hudson

MEGLOS (Serial 5Q)
Written by John Flanagan & Andrew McCulloch (4 Episodes)
Gigantic screens dominate the wasteland of Zolpha-Thura, and a group of Gaztec mercenaries take a kidnapped human there, where Meglos, a cactus-like creature, uses the man's form as a blueprint for a new body. With the Tardis trapped, Meglos takes on the Doctor's form and heads for Tigella, where he steals the Dodechahedron, the Tigellans main power source. With it, he plans to rule the universe, whilst the Doctor has to convince the Tigellans that it was not really him who stole it. . . .

Episode One - (27/09/80)(5.0m)
Episode Two - (04/10/80)(4.2m)
Episode Three - (11/10/80)(4.7m)
Episode Four - (18/10/80)(4.7m)

General Grugger . . . . Bill Fraser
Lieutenant Brotadac . . . . . Frederick Treves
Zastor. . . . . Edward Underdown
Caris . . . . Colette Gleeson
Deedrix. . . . . Crawford Logan
Lexa . . . . Jacqueline Hill
Earthling . . . . Christopher Owen
Director. . . . . Terence Dudley
Designer. . . . . Philip Lindley
Visual Effects . . . . Steven Drewett
Costume Design . . . . June Hudson

FULL CIRCLE (Serial 5R)
Written by Andrew Smith (4 Episodes)
The Tardis is trapped in an alternate universe called E-Space, and lands on the planet Alzarius, where the populace live on board the Starliner, a vast spaceship that crashed on the planet centuries before. Ruled by the Deciders, the passive race retreat into the ship as Mistfall approaches, and the Marshmen rise from the swamps. The Doctor deduces that the humanoids are actually mutations from the Marshmen, in part of a lifecycle unique to the planet. The Deciders have known all along and are also hiding the fact that the Starliner could take off at any time. The Doctor helps them

to leave the planet, and dematerialises unaware that he has a stowaway on board – a young Alzarian Maths student called Adric. . . .

Episode One - (25/10/80)(5.9m)
Episode Two - (01/11/80)(m3.7)
Episode Three - (08/11/80)(5.9m)
Episode Four - (15/11/80)(5.5m)

Login . . . . George Baker
Tylos . . . . Bernard Padden
Varsh . . . . Richard Willis
Nefred . . . . James Bree
Keara . . . . June Page
Garif . . . . Alan Rowe
Omril . . . . Andrew Forbes
Dexeter . . . . Tony Calvin
Director . . . . Peter Grimwade
Designer . . . . Janet Budden
Visual Effects . . . . John Brace
Costume Design . . . . Amy Roberts

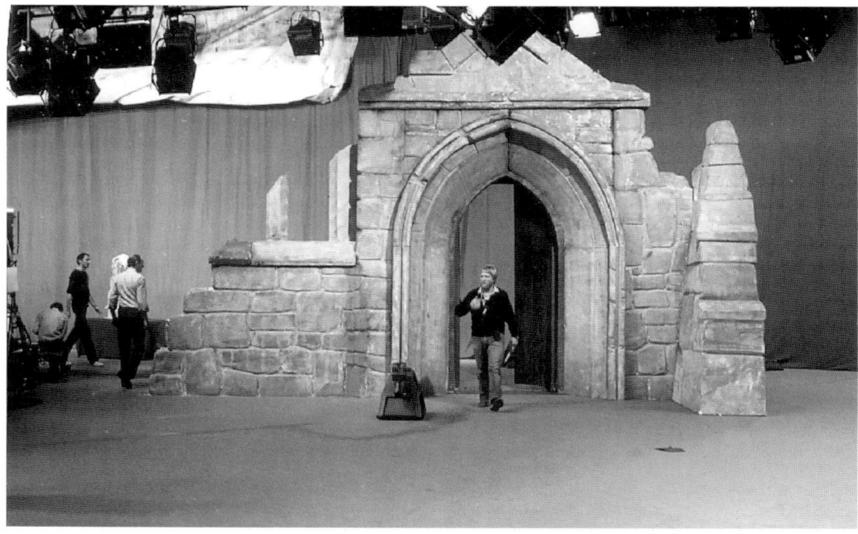

STATE OF DECAY (Serial 4P)
Written by Terrance Dicks (4 Episodes)
The Tardis lands on a mediaeval world, where the local peasants are terrified of their masters, the Three Who Rule, to whom they must sacrifice their young to join them in their castle as guards . . . but some are never heard of again. The Castle is really the remains of a spaceship, drawn into E-Space centuries before, and the three lords are the original pilots, under the control of the Great Vampire, buried way below ground. The creature is beginning to stir, and the Doctor has to stop one of the greatest threats the galaxy would ever face from breaking free from the ground. . . .

Episode One - (22/11/80)(5.8m)
Episode Two - (29/11/80)(5.3m)
Episode Three - (06/12/80)(4.4m)
Episode Four - (13/12/80)(5.4m)

Aukon . . . . Emrys James
Zargo . . . . William Lindsay
Camilla . . . . Rachel Davies
Ivo . . . . Clinton Greyn
Veros . . . . Stacy Davies
Tarak . . . . Thane Bettany
Kalmar . . . . Arthur Hewlett
Director . . . . Peter Moffatt
Designer. . . . . Christine Ruscoe
Visual Effects. . . . . Tony Harding
Costume Design . . . . Amy Roberts

WARRIOR'S GATE (Serial 5S)
Written by Steve Gallagher (4 Episodes)
The Tardis arrives at the gateway between E-Space and N-Space, and encounters a group of Privateers, brutally using a cargo of time sensitive Tharils to try to locate precisely the gateway. The Doctor encounters the Tharil empire at its height, by travelling through time mirrors, and sees how they were slaughtered by Gundan Robots, built by their human slaves to kill their captors. The Tharils are now a peaceful race, and the Doctor realises he has to try and save the last of their kind, who are being held captive on the Privateers' ship, but its Captain is going to try and get back to N-Space by blasting through the mirrors with their engines, and this destroys their ship. Romana and K9 stay with the Tharils, while the Doctor and Adric leave in the Tardis. . .

Episode One -(03/01/81)(7.1m)
Episode Two - (10/01/81)(6.7m)
Episode Three - (17/01/81)(8.3m)
Episode Four - (24/01/81)(7.8m)

Captain Rorvik . . . . Clifford Rose
Packard . . . . Kenneth Cope
Royce . . . . Harry Waters
Aldo . . . . Freddie Earlle
Sagan . . . . Vincent Pickering
Lane. . . . . David Kincaid
Lazlo . . . . Jeremy Gittins
Biroc . . . . David Weston
Director . . . . Paul Joyce
Designer. . . . . Graeme Story
Visual Effects . . . . Mat Irvine
Costume Design . . . . June Hudson

THE KEEPER OF TRAKEN (Serial 5T)
Written by Johnny Byrne (4 Episodes)
The Keeper of Traken materialises inside the Tardis, asking the Doctor for help as he believes the harmony of his world is in danger. The threat is the Melkur, an alien who turned to stone, calcifying when he landed on the planet as he was unable to cope with the inherent goodness of the race. On Traken, with a new Keeper soon due to take over, the Doctor uncovers a plot by Kassia to manoeuvre the Melkur to take over the Keeper's power. Melkur is actually housing the Master's Tardis. He is still in his decaying form and, although defeated at the end, manages to escape and meld into the body of Tremas, thus taking on a new physical form. . . .

Episode One - (31/01/81)(7.6m)
Episode Two - (07/02/81)(6.1m)
Episode Three - (14/02/81)(5.2m)
Episode Four - (21/02/81)(6.1m)

(Nyssa, introduced in this story, joins Tardis crew in LOGOPOLIS)

The Keeper . . . . Denis Carey
Consul Tremas. . . . . Anthony Ainley
Consul Kassia. . . . . Sheila Ruskin
Seron . . . . John Woodnutt
Luvic. Robin Soans
Katura . . . . Margot Van der Burgh
Neman . . . . Roland Oliver
The Master . . . . Geoffrey Beevers
Voice of the Melkur by Geoffrey Beevers
Director . . . . John Black
Designer. . . . . Tony Burrough
Visual Effects. . . . . Peter Logan
Costume Design . . . . Amy Roberts

LOGOPOLIS (Serial 5V)
Written by Christopher H. Bidmead (4 Episodes)
In order to repair the Tardis chameleon circuit, the Doctor goes to Logopolis, where the Logopolitans puremaths is used to create matter. Measuring a Police Box on Earth to get the dimensions exactly right, the Tardis materialises around the Master's, which is disguised as the blue box in question. The Doctor seems to be followed by a mysterious white figure, the Watcher, and no matter how often Adric asks who he is,

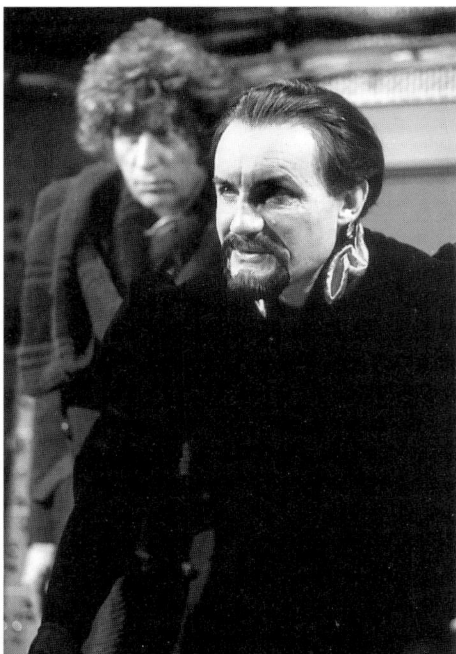

the Doctor never answers, although it's clear he knows. Air stewardess Tegan Jovenka's car breaks down near where the Tardis is, and her aunt is murdered by the Master – a crime which the Doctor is accused of committing. He escapes to Logopolis, unwittingly taking both the Master and Tegan with him. The Master starts destroying the planet, and begins to cause the universe to collapse, as the combined forces of the Logopolitans is keeping entropy at bay, so the Doctor has to use a beam projected from the Pharos Project radar dish on earth to slow the effect down. As the Doctor tries to stop the Master hijacking the equipment to hold the universe to ransom, he falls from the tower. The Watcher, a future projection of the Time Lord, merges with him, and Tegan, Nyssa and Adric watch in amazement as the Doctor regenerates. . . .

Episode One - (28/02/81)(7.1m)
Episode Two - (07/03/81)(7.7m)
Episode Three - (14/03/81)(5.8m)
Episode Four - (21/03/81)(6.1m)

The Master . . . . Anthony Ainley
Aunt Vanessa . . . . Delores Whiteman
Detective Inspector . . . . . . Tom Georgeson
The Monitor . . . . John Fraser
Security Guard . . . . Christopher Hurst
Director . . . . Peter Grimwade
Designer . . . . Malcolm Thornton
Visual Effects . . . . John Horton
Costume Design . . . . June Hudson

Season Nineteen

Regular Cast

The Doctor . . . . Peter Davison
Adric . . . . Matthew Waterhouse (Until Serial 6B)
Tegan . . . . Janet Fielding
Nyssa . . . . Sarah Sutton

Regular Production Team

John Nathan-Turner . . . . Producer
Anthony Root . . . . Script Editor (Serials 5W, 5X & 6B)
Eric Saward . . . . Script Editor (Serials 5Z, 5Y, 6A & 6C)

CASTROVALVA (Serial 5Z)
Written by Christopher H. Bidmead (4 Episodes)

Tegan and Nyssa help the newly regenerated Doctor back to the Tardis, but Adric is kidnapped by the Master, who uses the boy's mental abilities to project a fake Adric on board and programme the Doctor's time machine to head back to the Hydrogen inrush that created the universe, which will destroy the craft. The Doctor starts to recover, and tells Tegan how to escape. When the Tardis lands on Castrovalva, the local inhabitants are all too happy to help with the Doctor's recovery but he realises something is wrong. The whole city is another one of Adric's projections. . . .

Episode One - (04/01/82)(10.1m)
Episode Two - (05/01/82)(8.7m)
Episode Three - (11/01/82)(10.4m)
Episode Four - (12/01/82)(10.5m)

The Master & The Portreeve . . . . . Anthony Ainley
Shardovan . . . . Derek Waring
Mergrave . . . . Michael Sheard
Ruther . . . . Frank Wylie
Head of Security at Pharos Project . . Dallas Cavell
Director . . . . Fiona Cumming
Designer . . . . Janet Budden
Visual Effects . . . . Simon MacDonald
Costume Design. . . . . Odile Dicks-Mireaux

FOUR TO DOOMSDAY (Serial 5W)
Written by Terence Dudley (4 Episodes)

Monarch, leader of the Urbankans, is heading towards the Earth in a vast spaceship with his assistants Enlightenment and Persuasion. When the Tardis arrives, the Doctor and his companions find the vessel populated with android replicants of the original humans Monarch kidnapped throughout history on his previous visits to the planet. Their original personalities are stored on a micro-circuit inside their bodies. Although Monarch is convincing with his explanations that his is a peaceful mission, the Doctor discovers that he intends to colonise the Earth with the frog-like Urbankans, after wiping out mankind with a deadly poison. . . .

Episode One - (18/01/82)(8.6m)
Episode Two - (19/01/82)(8.8m)
Episode Three - (25/01/82)(9.1m)
Episode Four - (26/01/82)(9.6m)

Monarch . . . . Stratford Johns
Enlightenment . . . . Annie Lambert
Persuasion. . . . . Paul Shelley
Bigon . . . . Philip Locke
Lin Fitu . . . . Burt Kwouk
Kurkutji . . . . Illario Bisi Pedro
Villagra . . . . Nadia Hamman
Director . . . . John Black
Designer . . . . Tony Burrough
Visual Effects . . . . Mickey Edwards
Costume Design . . . . Colin Lavers

KINDA (Serial 5Y)
Written by Christopher Bailey (4 Episodes)

After collapsing in the console room, Nyssa remains on board the Tardis, while the Doctor explores the jungle world of Deva Loka with Tegan and Adric. Sleeping in a forest clearing, Tegan's mind is invaded by an evil force called the Mara. The Doctor and Adric become trapped in an earth colony base, where one of the crew has become power crazed and dangerous, and when they escape with the base's scientist, Todd, they meet Panna, a prophet, who speaks of the Mara's return. Tegan passes the Mara on to a young member of the primitive, but peaceful Kinda tribe, who tries to lead them in a rebellion. The Doctor manages to defeat the power, which manifests itself as a vast snake butTegan is fearful that some element of the force may still be in her mind. . . .

Episode One - (01/02/82)(8.5m)
Episode Two - (02/02/82)(9.5m)
Episode Three - (08/02/82)(8.7m)
Episode Four - (09/02/82)(9.1m)

Sanders . . . . Richard Todd
Todd . . . . Nerys Hughes
Hindle . . . . Simon Rouse
Panna . . . . Mary Morris
Karunna . . . . Sarah Prince
Anatta . . . . Anna Wing
Dukkha . . . . Jeffrey Stewart
Director . . . . Peter Grimwade

Designer . . . . *Malcolm Thornton*
Visual Effects . . . . *Peter Logan*
Costume Design . . . . *Barbara Kidd*

THE VISITATION (Serial 5X)
Written by Eric Saward (4 Episodes)
In the 17th Century, the Tardis lands in a woodland, where they meet out-of-work actor and highwayman, Richard Mace, who explains that England is in the grip of a plague. A party of three Terileptil convicts, on the run from the tnclavic mines of the planet Raaga, have crashed nearby, and they are using the peasants to help prepare an escape attempt from the Earth. The Doctor traces them to Pudding Lane in London, where a confrontation leads to the creatures' demise, and the start of a certain fire that would be remembered throughout English history. . . .

Episode One - (15/02/82)(9.3m)
Episode Two - (16/02/82)(9.5m)
Episode Three - (22/02/82)(10.1m)
Episode Four - (23/02/82)(10.2m)

Richard Mace . . . . Michael Robbins
Squire John . . . . John Savident
Charles . . . . Anthony Calf
Elizabeth . . . . Valerie Fyfer
Ralph . . . . John Baker
Android . . . . Peter Van Dissel
Terileptil Leader . . . . Michael Melia
Director . . . . *Peter Moffatt*
Designer . . . . *Ken Starkey*
Visual Effects . . . . *Peter Wragg*
Costume Design . . . . . *Odile Dicks-Mireaux*

BLACK ORCHID (Serial 6A)
Written by Terence Dudley (2 Episodes)
The Tardis arrives in the 1920s, materialising at a railway station, where a case of mistaken identity leads the Doctor and his companions to being the guests of the Cranleigh family, with the Time Lord indulging in his passion for the game of cricket for an afternoon. However, the Cranleighs are hiding a dark secret in their mansion, with a hideously deformed relative locked in a back room, who escapes and mistakes Nyssa for Ann Talbot, her doppelganger and his old love. The Doctor has to try and persuade him to bring her down off the blazing rooftop. . . .

Episode One - (01/03/82)(9.1m)
Episode Two - (02/03/82)(9.2m)

Charles Cranleigh . . . . . . Michael Cochrane
Lady Cranleigh . . . . Barbara Murray
Ann Talbot . . . . Sarah Sutton
Sir Robert Muir . . . . Moray Watson
Latoni . . . . Ahmed Khalil
George Cranleigh/The Unknown . . . Gareth Milne
Sergeant Markham . . . . Ivor Salter
Director . . . . *Ron Jones*
Designer . . . . *Tony Burrough*
Visual Effects . . . . *Tony Auger*
Costume Design . . . . *Rosalind Ebbutt*

EARTHSHOCK (Serial 6B)
Written by Eric Saward (4 Episodes)
An archaeological expedition into a cave region has been slaughtered one by one, with a pair of featureless androids stalking through the shadows. A military investigation starts to meet the same fate, until the Tardis arrives and the Doctor finds that the robots are protecting a powerful bomb, which the Doctor defuses and traces the signals being sent to it from a vast space freighter. On board, he encounters the Cybermen, who turn the freighter into a bomb, intent on crashing it into the Earth, but Adric's tampering with the guidance systems sends the ship back in time where it is destroyed in the Earth's outer atmosphere, and it in turn wipes out the dinosaurs, as it has gone back to prehistoric times. Adric was on board, and to the Doctor, Tegan and Nyssa's horror, they are unable to save him. . . .

Episode One - (08/03/94)(9.3m)
Episode Two - (09/03/94)(9.0m)
Episode Three - (15/03/94)(9.9m)
Episode Four - (16/03/94)(9.1m)

Professor Kyle . . . . Clare Clifford
Lieutenant Scott . . . . James Warwick
Briggs . . . . Beryl Reid
Ringway . . . . Alec Sabin
Berger . . . . June Bland
Cyberlead . . . . David Banks
Cyberlieutenent . . . . Mark Hardy
Director . . . . *Peter Grimwade*
Designer . . . . *Bernard Lloyd*
Visual Effects . . . . *Steve Bowman*
Costume Design . . . . *Dinah Collins*

TIME-FLIGHT (Serial 6C)
Written by Peter Grimwade (4 Episodes)
The Tardis arrives at Heathrow, and the Doctor becomes involved in investigating the mysterious disappearance of a Concorde. Using the Tardis to follow a time trail, the plane is found in prehistoric times, where the Master is using the passengers and flight crew as slaves to try and utilise the powers of the Xeraphin to rebuild his Tardis engines. The Doctor manages to defeat him and banish him to Xeriphas, and get everyone back to modern day Heathrow, where Tegan is accidentally left behind when the Tardis takes off. . . .

Episode One - (22/03/82)(10.1m)
Episode Two - (23/03/82)(8.5m)
Episode Three - (29/03/82)(9.1m)
Episode Four - (30/03/82)(8.3m)

The Master & Kalid . . . . . . Anthony Ainley
Professor Hayter . . . . Nigel Stock
Captain Stapley . . . . Richard Easton
First Officer Bilton . . . . . . Michael Cashman
Flight Engineer Scobie . . . . . . Keith Drinkel
Angela Clifford . . . . Judith Byfield
Anithon . . . . Hugh Hayes
Director . . . . *Ron Jones*
Designer . . . . *Richard McManan-Smith*
Visual Effects . . . . *Peter Logan*
Costume Design . . . . *Amy Roberts*

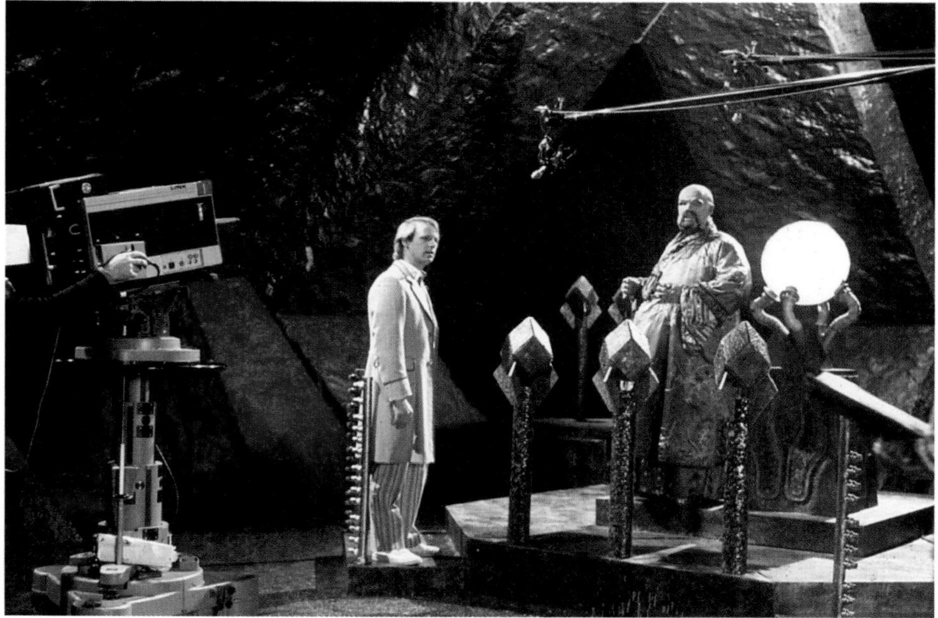

Season Twenty

Regular Cast

The Doctor . . . . Peter Davison
Tegan . . . . Janet Fielding
Nyssa. . . . . Sarah Sutton (Seriel 6E-6G)
Turlough . . . . Mark Strickson (Serial 6F Onwards)

Regular Production Team

John Nathan Turner . . . . Producer
Eric Saward. . . . . Script Editor

ARC OF INFINITY (Serial 6E)
Written by Johnny Byrne (4 Episodes)
On Gallifrey, Councillor Hedin is helping the long-thought dead Omega to return via the arc of infinity, but he needs a body print to give him a physical form, so he 'bonds' with the Doctor, and retreats to a hideout on the Earth in Amsterdam. The Doctor is brought back to his home world, where he is sentenced to death to try and stop Omega passing over from his universe of anti-matter by using his bio-scan. The Doctor escapes, and tracks Omega down on Earth, with the help of Tegan, whom he and Nyssa meet up with. With the renegade Time Lord defeated, Tegan rejoins the Tardis crew. . . .

Episode One - (04/01/83)(7.2m)
Episode Two - (05/01/83)(7.3m)
Episode Three - (11/01/83)(6.9m)
Episode Four - (12/01/83)(7.2m)

President Borusa . . . . Leonard Sachs
Councillor Hedin . . . . Michael Gough
Castellan. . . . . Paul Jerricho
Chancellor Thalia . . . . Elspet Gray
Commander Maxil . . . . Colin Baker
Omega. Ian Collier
Ergon . . . . Malcolm Harvey
Director . . . . Ron Jones
Designer. . . . . Marjorie Pratt
Visual Effects . . . . Chris Lawson
Costume Design . . . . Dee Robson

SNAKEDANCE (Serial 6D)
Written by Christopher Bailey (4 Episodes)
The Mara takes possession of Tegan's mind once again as the Tardis arrives on Mannusa, the Mara's homeworld, where the power plans to re-emerge and take over the planet during a madri-gras. Assisted by the hermit Dojjen, the Doctor prepares himself for a final confrontation as the giant snake materialises for a second time. In the aftermath, it becomes clear that Tegan is now free of its influence forever. . . .

Episode One - (18/01/83)(6.7m)
Episode Two - (19/01/83)(7.7m)
Episode Three - (25/01/83)(6.6m)
Episode Four - (26/01/83)(7.4m)

Lon . . . . Martin Clunes
Tahna . . . . Colette O'Neill
Ambril. John Carson
Dojjen. . . . . Preston Lockwood
Chela. . . . . Jonathan Morris
Dugdale. . . . . Brian Miller
Director. . . . . Fiona Cumming
Designer. . . . . Jan Spoczynski
Visual Effects . . . . Andy Lazell
Costume Design . . . . Ken Trew

MAWDRYN UNDEAD (Serial 6F)
Written by Peter Grimwade (4 Episodes)
Visitor Turlough, who appears to be nothing more than a schoolboy, is actually an alien stranded on Earth, whom the Black Guardian starts to manipulate in a plan to get revenge against the Doctor. Arriving at the school, the Doctor meets the Brigadier, who is now a maths teacher there. He's investigating a transmat beacon, which a mysterious, seemingly abandoned spaceship comes into focus with once every seven years. Separated in time, Tegan and Nyssa find an occupant in the capsule in 1977, and mistake him for the Doctor, thinking that he's been badly injured, and they seek help from the Brigadier of that period. The creature is actually Mawdryn, part of a race banished by the Time Lords on the spaceship, for their meddling with time experiments. The Doctor has to help the creatures find a way to die, and keep the two Brigadiers apart, because if they met, the resulting collision of Time Energy could be deadly. As everything is resolved, Turlough accepts the Doctor's offer to join the Tardis crew. . . .

Episode One - (01/02/83)(6.5m)
Episode Two - (02/02/83)(7.5m)
Episode Three - (08/02/83)(7.4m)
Episode Four - (09/02/83)(7.7m)

Brigadier Lethbridge-Stewart . . . . Nicholas Courtney
Mawdryn. . . . . David Collings
Ibbotson . . . . Stephen Garlick
Doctor Runciman Roger Hammond
Headmaster . . . . Angus MacKay
Matron . . . . Sheila Gill
The Black Guardian . . . . Valentine Dyall
Director . . . . Peter Moffatt
Designer . . . . Stephen Scott
Visual Effects . . . . Stuart Brisdon
Costume Design . . . . Amy Roberts

TERMINUS (Serial 6G)
Written by Steve Gallagher (4 Episodes)
Still under the influence of the Black Guardian, Turlough follows his instructions on sabotaging the Tardis, which causes the ship to start to break up and lock onto the side of another vessel. Nyssa becomes lost on the other craft, and the Doctor and his remaining companions start to search for her on board. When the Doctor finds her, they become the captives of two space pirates, who have been abandoned on the ship by their crew, and realise that they're on a Lazer transporter, taking humans who have been contaminated with a virus to die on the colony of Terminus. Nyssa catches the disease, while the Doctor finds out that Terminus was responsible for the 'Big Bang' that started life in the universe, when a radioactive load was detonated. A second imminent detonation could reverse the effect and end everything. When he manages to avert this and get the Tardis back, Nyssa opts to stay and try and help the other Lazers, now that she is cured. . .

Episode One - (15/02/83)(7.0m)
Episode Two - (16/02/83)(7.5m)
Episode Three - (22/02/83)(6.5m)
Episode Four - (23/02/83)(7.4m)

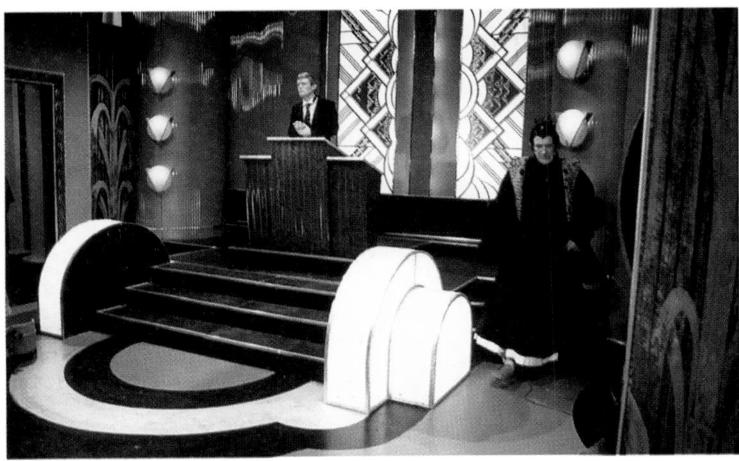

Kari . . . . Liza Goddard
Olvir . . . . Dominic Guard
Valgard . . . . Andrew Burt
Sigurd . . . . Tim Munro
Eirak . . . . Martin Potter
Bor . . . . Peter Benson
The Black Guardian . . . . Valentine Dyall
The Garm . . . . R. J. Bell
Director . . . . Mary Ridge
Designer . . . . Dick Coles
Visual Effects. . . . . Peter Pegrum
Costume Design . . . . Dee Robson

ENLIGHTENMENT (Serial 6H)
Written by Barbara Clegg (4 Episodes)
The Tardis materialises on what appears to be a Edwardian clipper ship, where the crew are strangely jolly and the officers somewhat distant. When the Doctor meets Captain Striker, he explains how they are part of a race for a glorious prize – Enlightenment. The ship is a space craft, and there are a whole fleet from different points in the Earth's history, sailing on the solar winds. One, a pirate woman called Captain Wrack, is an agent for the Black Guardian, and she is systematically destroying all of the competition. The Doctor overcomes Wrack, and is confronted by both the Black and the White Guardian. Turlough is offered Enlightenment by the Black Guardian, but he refuses and throws it at him, apparently destroying him, and showing loyalty to the Doctor. As the White Guardian leaves, he reminds the Doctor that the Black Guardian will always be after him for revenge. . . .

Episode One - (01/03/83)(6.6m)
Episode Two - (02/03/83)(7.2m)
Episode Three - (08/03/83)(6.2m)
Episode Four - (09/03/83)(7.3m)

Captain Striker . . . . Keith Barron
Captain Wrack. . . . . Lynda Barron
Marriner . . . . Christopher Brown
Jackson . . . . Tony Caunter
The White Guardian . . . . Cyril Luckham
The Black Guardian . . . . Valentine Dyall
Director. . . . . Fiona Cumming
Designer . . . . Colin Green
Visual Effects. . . . . Mike Kelt
Costume Design . . . . Dinah Collins

THE KING'S DEMONS (Serial 6J)
Written by Terence Dudley (2 Episodes)
King Richard is fighting the Crusades, whilst there are two King Johns in England. One is the true villain, whilst the other is Kamelion, a shape changing android under the control of the Master, who plans to use him to alter the course of history. Discovered by the Master of Xeriphas, the android is mind controlled, and after a battle of wills, the Doctor frees him from the Master and Kamelion joins the Tardis crew.

Episode One - (15/03/83)(5.8m)
Episode Two - (16/03/83)(7.2m)

The Master & Sir Giles . . . . Anthony Ainley
King John & The Voice of Kamelion . . Gerald Flood
Ranulf . . . . Frank Windsor
Isabella . . . . Isla Blair
Hugh . . . . Christopher Villiers
Sir Geoffrey . . . . Michael J. Jackson
Director. . . . . Tony Virgo
Designer. . . . . Ken Ledsham
Visual Effects. . . . . Tony Harding
Costume Design . . . . Colin Lavers

THE FIVE DOCTORS (Serial 6K)
Written by Terrance Dicks (One 90-Minute Episode)
The fifth Doctor begins to suffer from side-effects as somebody starts to take his past incarnations and companions out of time, and heads for Gallifrey. In the Death Zone, the remains of a game the Time Lords played in the Dark Times, pitting alien races against each other in mortal combat, the second Doctor, accompanied by the Brigadier, and the third Doctor, with Sarah Jane Smith, make their separate ways to the Tomb of Rassilon, encountering a Yeti and a troop of Cybermen along the way. The first Doctor, reunited with Susan Foreman, after battling a Dalek, finds his way to the Tardis, where he joins with Tegan to head to the tomb as well, while Turlough and Susan look after the Tardis. The fifth Doctor comes across the Master, sent into the Death Zone by the Inner Council of Time Lords to help the Doctor, with the incentive being a new cycle of regenerations if he succeeds. After an attack by the Cybermen, where the Doctor uses his transmat device to return to the capitol, the Master joins up with them and heads for the Dark Tower as well. Eventually, with the Cybermen destroyed and the Master held captive, the combined efforts of Doctors one, two, three and five (the fourth Doctor is trapped in time, cue SHADA footage) defeats the true villain, President Borusa, and everyone departs for their rightful places in time. . . .

Episode One - (25/11/83)(7.7m)

The second Doctor . . . . . Patrick Troughton
The third Doctor . . . . Jon Pertwee
The first Doctor. . . . . Richard Hurndall
The fourth Doctor . . . . Tom Baker
Susan Foreman . . . . Carole Anne Ford
Brigadier Lethbridge-Stewart . . . . Nicholas Courtney
Sarah Jane Smith. . . . . Elisabeth Sladen
Romana. . . . . Lalla Ward
The Master . . . . Anthony Ainley
Borusa . . . . Philip Latham
Chancellor Flavia. . . . . Dinah Sheridan
Castellan. . . . . Paul Jerricho
Jamie . . . . Frazer Hines
Zoe. . . . . Wendy Padbury
Liz Shaw . . . . Caroline John
Captain Yates. . . . . Richard Franklin
Cyberleader . . . . David Banks
Cyberlieutenant . . . . Mark Hardy
Cyberman . . . . William Kenton
Raston Warrior Robot . . . . . . Keith Hodiak
Dalek Voice by Roy Skelton
Voice of K9 by John Lesson
Director . . . . Peter Moffatt
Designer . . . . Malcolm Thornton
Visual Effects . . . . John Brace
Costume Design . . . . Colin Lavers

Season Twenty One

Regular Cast
The Doctor . . . Peter Davison (Serial 6L-6R)
The Doctor . . Colin Baker (Serial 6S onwards)
Tegan . . . . Janet Fielding (Serial 6L-6P)
Turlough . . . . Nicola Bryant (Serial 6Q onwards)

Regular Production Team
John Nathan-Turner . . . . Producer
Eric Saward. . . . . Script Editor

WARRIORS OF THE DEEP (Serial 6L)
Written by Johnny Byrne (4 Episodes)
The crew of an undersea base on Earth in the 21st century are continually on edge, due to the never-ending threat of nuclear attack by a rival power bloc. The Tardis arrives, and the Doctor not only has to overcome the problems caused by enemy spies trying to sabotage Sea Base Four, but also an invasion attempt by the combined forces of the Sea Devils and the Silurians. Their plan is to trigger a nuclear war, which would cleanse the Earth, and allow them to claim it as their own world once again. . . .

Episode One - (05/01/84)(7.6m)
Episode Two - (06/01/84)(7.5m)
Episode Three - (12/01/84)(7.3m)
Episode Four - (13/01/84)(6.6m)

Vorshak. . . . . Tom Adams
Nilson . . . . Ian McCulloch

Solow . . . . Ingrid Pitt
Karina. Nitza Saul
Bulic. . . . . Nigel Humphreys
Maddox . . . . Martin Neil
Preston . . . . Tara Ward
Sauvix. . . . . Christopher Farries
Icthar . . . . Norman Comer
Director . . . . Pennant Roberts
Designer. . . . . Tony Burrough
Visual Effects . . . . Mat Irvine
Costume Design. . . . . Judy Pepperdine

<u>THE AWAKENING</u> (Serial 6M)
Written by Eric Pringle (2 Episodes)
The Tardis lands in Little Hodcombe, where Tegan plans to visit her grandfather, but a local civil war war game is getting out of hand, with Sir George Hutchinson pushing the realism a little too far. The Doctor discovers that the local Church was built over a powerful alien creature, the Malus, which creates negative emotions and feeds off them. With the war games raging, enough power has been absorbed by the Malus to regain its strength, and the Doctor has to stop it before its influence can break free and devastate the Earth. . . .

Episode One - (19/01/84)(7.9m)
Episode Two - (20/01/84)(6.6m)

Sir George Hutchinson. . . . . Denis Lill
Jane Hampden . . . . Polly James
Colonel Wolsey . . . . Glyn Houston
Joseph Willow . . . . Jack Galloway
Will Chandler . . . . Keith Jayne
Director . . . . Michael Owen-Morris
Designer. . . . . Barry Newbery
Visual Effects. . . . . Tony Harding
Costume Design. . . . . Jackie Southern

<u>FRONTIOS</u> (Serial 6N)
Written by Christopher H. Bidmead (4 Episodes)
The Tardis lands on Frontios. One of the last surviving colonies from Earth crashed there years before, and the Doctor finds them fighting for survival against an unseen villain. Meteroite attacks and strange disappearances underground have gone without explanation, and the Doctor finds the humans are being manipulated by the powers of the Tractators, giant woodlouse-like creatures with extraordinary mental abilities to control gravity. The Gravs, the Tractator's leader, finds out about the Tardis, and disassembles it until the Doctor agrees to show him how to travel through time, but once the vessel is back together the creature becomes powerless and the Doctor abandons him on an

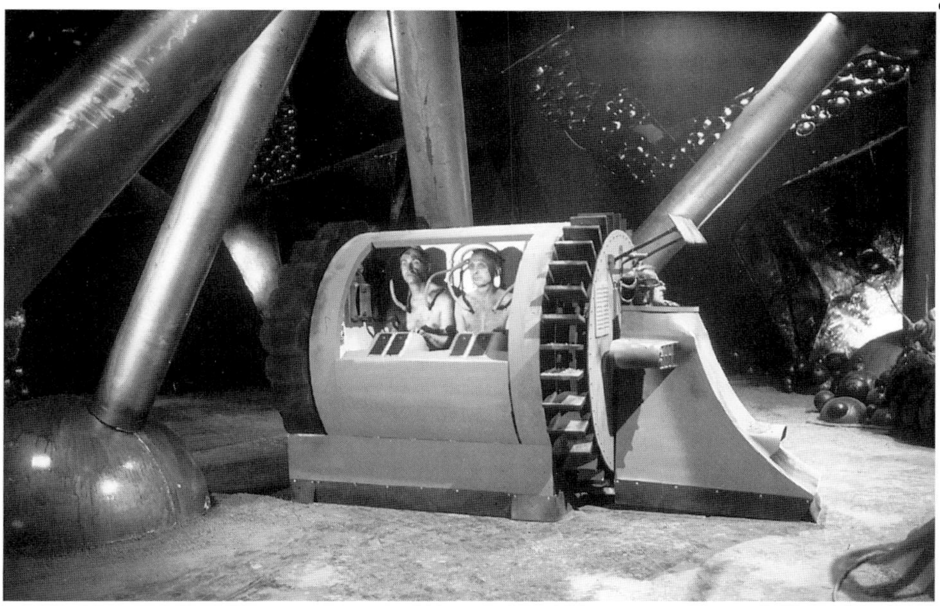

uninhabited planet, leaving the humans on Frontios in peace. . . .

Episode One - (26/01/84)(8.0m)
Episode Two - (27/01/84)(5.8m)
Episode Three - (02/02/84)(7.8m)
Episode Four - (03/02/84)(5.6m)

Mr Range . . . . William Lucas
Brazen . . . . Peter Gilmore
Plantagenet. . . . . Jeff Rawle
Norna . . . . Lesley Dunlop
Cockerill . . . . Maurice O'Connell
Gravs . . . . John Gillett
Director . . . . Ron Jones
Designer. . . . . David Buckingham
Visual Effects . . . . Dave Havard
Costume Design . . . . . . Anushia Nieradzik

<u>RESURRECTION OF THE DALEKS</u> (Serial 6P)
Written by Eric Saward (2 Episodes – 45 Mins Each)
Caught in a Time Corridor, the Tardis is dragged to Earth, where the Doctor joins forces with an escaped prisoner from the future called Stein, and follows the corridor back to its source – a Dalek battle cruiser which has rescued Davros from a space prison. Davros slowly begins to turn one Dalek after another onto his side, so he can destroy the Daleks who no longer follow his orders. The Daleks have made duplicates of all the Tardis crew, with the plan being to invade Gallifrey, and conquer time itself, and many lives are lost as the Doctor battles against them and eventually wins. Tegan is unable to cope with seeing so many deaths, and leaves the Tardis crew, remaining on modern Earth. . . .

Episode One - (08/02/84)(7.3m)
Episode Two - (15/02/84)(8.0m)

Commander Lytton . . . Maurice Colbourne
Stein . . . . Rodney Bewes
Colonel Archer . . . . Del Henney
Professor Laird . . . . Chloe Ashcroft
Davros . . . . Terry Molloy
Styles . . . . Rula Lenska
Kiston. . . . . Les Grantham
Director . . . . Matthew Robinson
Designer. . . . . John Anderson
Visual Effects . . . . Peter Wragg
Costume Design . . . . Janet Tharby

<u>PLANET OF FIRE</u> (Serial 6Q)
Written by Peter Grimwade (4 Episodes)
On Lanzarote, Turlough meets Peri Brown, a botany student from America, who is taken to Sarn as the Master regains control of Kamelion. On that planet, Turlough meets his brother, and realises that in amongst the primitive society are clues that could reveal his roots to him, as his true background has eluded him so far. The Master has been shrunken to only a few inches in height, and plans to use the numisation gases of the planet to regain his size, and increase his power. The Doctor realises that it will be impossible to defeat him if he gains such energy. In defeating the Master, Kamelion is destroyed, and the Doctor has to bid farewell to Turlough, who decides to stay with his people. Peri leaves with the Doctor, as a new companion on board the Tardis. . . .

Episode One - (23/02/84)(7.4m)
Episode Two - (24/02/84)(6.1m)
Episode Three - (01/03/84)(7.4m)
Episode Four - (02/03/84)(7.0m)

The Master . . . . Anthony Ainley

Timanov . . . . Peter Wyngarde
Malkon . . . . Edward Highmore
Sorasta. . . . . Barbara Shelley
Professor Howard Foster. . . . Dallas Adams
Amyand . . . . James Bate
Voice of Kamelion by Gerald Flood
Director. . . . . Fiona Cumming
Designer . . . . Malcolm Thornton
Visual Effects. . . . . Peter Logan
Costume Design . . . . John Peacock

THE CAVES OF ANDROZANI (Serial 6R)
Written by Robert Holmes (4 Episodes)

On the planet Androzani Minor, the Doctor and Peri become caught up in the conflict between the disfigured arms dealer-cum-renegade, Sharaz Jek, and his nemesis, Morgus, whom he longs to be able to destroy. They both fight for control of the supplies of a drug called Spectrox, which reduces the aging process and prolongs life. As the battle between the two factions rages, Jek becomes infatuated with Peri, who contracts Spectrox toxaemia, and slowly starts to die. The Doctor, who also has the disease, races to get the milk of the queen bat from the lower depths of the cave system, the only known cure for it, but as he gets Peri back to the Tardis, with both Jek and Morgus dead in the aftermath of a final confrontation, there is only enough of the antidote for her. As she recovers, she watches in amazement as the body of the fifth Doctor dies from the disease, and he starts to regenerate. . . .

Episode One - (08/03/84)(6.9m)
Episode Two - (09/03/84)(6.6m)
Episode Three - (15/03/84)(7.0m)
Episode Four - (16/03/84)(6.3m)

Sharaz Jek . . . . Christopher Gable
Stotz . . . . Maurice Roeves
Morgus. . . . . John Normington
Salateen . . . . Robert Glenister
Krelper. . . . . Martin Cochrane
President . . . . David Neal
Timmin . . . . Barbara Kinghorn
Director . . . . Graeme Harper
Designer . . . . John Hurst
Visual Effects. . . . . Jim Francis
Costume Design . . . . Andrew Rose

THE TWIN DILEMMA (Serial 6S)
Written by Eric Saward (4 Episodes)

The Sixth Doctor proves to be erratic and wildly unpredictable, with Peri suffering the main brunt of his explosive temper. The Tardis lands on a planet where the two of them find the wreckage of a space crash, and take the sole survivor on board, before

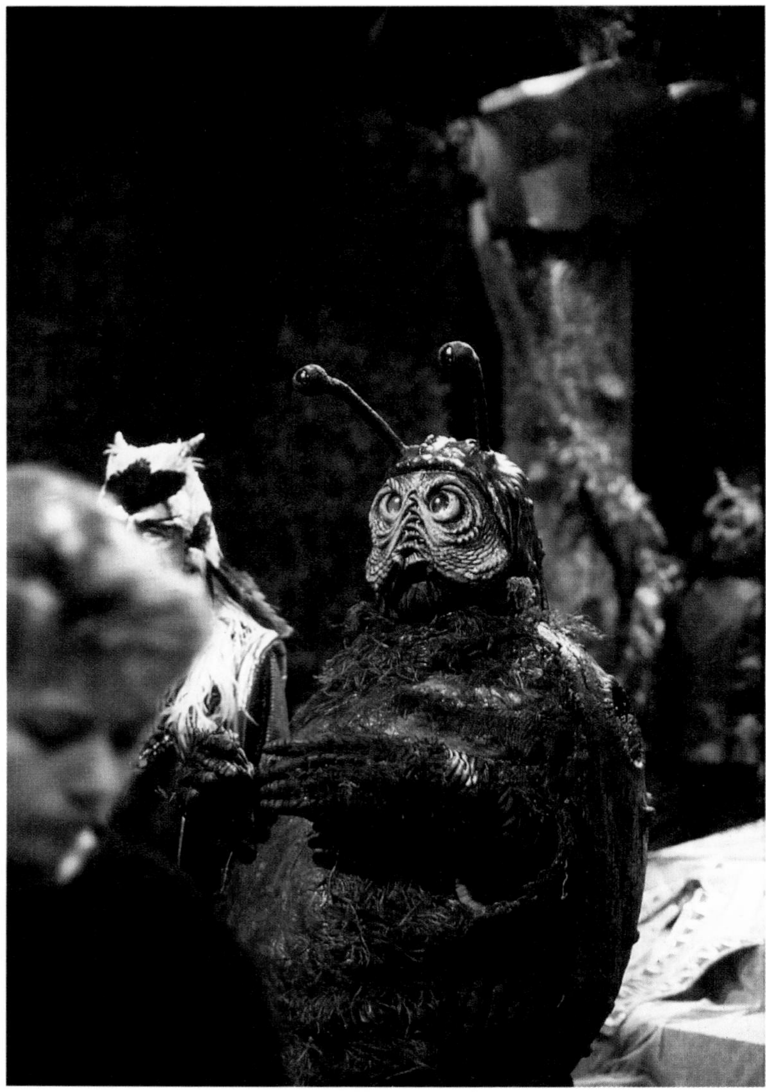

travelling to Jaconda, where the population has been enslaved by the slug-like Mestor and his Gastropods. An old friend of the Doctor's, Azmael, a retired Time Lord, has been forced to kidnap a pair of twins who are mathematical geniuses, so Mestor can use their calculations to throw Jaconda into its sun, with the resulting explosion being large enough to spread Gastropod eggs throughout the galaxy. . .

Episode One - (22/03/84)(7.6m)
Episode Two - (23/03/84)(7.4m)
Episode Three - (29/03/84)(7.0m)
Episode Four - (30/03/94)(6.3m)

Edgeworth/Azmael . . . . . Maurice Denham
Hugo. . . . . Kevin McNally
Mestor. . . . . Edwin Richfield
Drak . . . . Oliver Smith
Remus. . . . . Andrew Conrad
Romulus . . . . Gavin Conrad
Chancellor . . . . Seymour Green
Director. . . . . Peter Moffatt
Designer . . . . Valerie Warrender
Visual Effects . . . . Stuart Brisdon
Costume Design . . . . Pat Godfrey

Season Twenty Two

(Episodes 45-mins each)

Regular Cast

The Doctor . . . . Colin Baker
Peri . . . . Nicola Bryant

Regular Production Team

John Nathan-Turner . . . . Producer
Eric Saward. . . . . Script Editor

ATTACK OF THE CYBERMEN (Serial 6T)
Written by Paula Moore (2 Episodes)
With uncredited work by Eric Saward

The Cybermen have established a base in London's sewers in 1985, planning to divert Halley's Comet so that it destroys the Earth, and thus saves Mondas from being obliterated in 1986 (in THE TENTH

PLANET). The Doctor and Peri become involved with Commander Lytton (From RESURRECTION OF THE DALEKS), who is working for the Cryons on Telos, who were enslaved by the Cybermen and forced to build the Tombs there. On that planet, the Doctor once again encounters the Cybercontroller, and Lytton sacrifices his life to save the Cryons, much to the Doctor's surprise. . . .

Episode One - (05/01/85)(8.9m)
Episode Two - (12/01/85)(7.2m)

Lytton . . . . Maurice Colbourne
Griffiths. . . . . Brian Glover
Russell . . . . Terry Molloy
Stratton . . . . Jonathan David
Bates. . . . . Michael Attwell
Flast. . . . . Faith Brown
Varne . . . . Sarah Greene
Cybercontroller . . . . Michael Kilgarriff
Cyberleader . . . . David Banks
Director . . . . Matthew Robinson
Designer. . . . . Marjorie Pratt
Visual Effects . . . . Chris Lawson
Costume Design . . . . . . Anushia Nieradzik

VENGEANCE ON VAROS (Serial 6V)
Written by Philip Martin (2 Episodes)
While the population of Varos are kept subdued by a continual stream of executions and scenes of torture being broadcast directly into their homes, the Governor of the planet is fighting to save the economy, negotiating with the slug-like Galatron Mining delegate, Sil, over the price he is willing to pay for Zeiton Seven, an ore natural to the planet. The Doctor needs some of the same mineral to power the Tardis, and arrives on Varos to get some, but gets caught up with a band of rebels in the punishment dome and has to convince the Governor to take the upper hand in bartering for his planet's export materials. . . .

Episode One - (19/01/85)(7.3m)
Episode Two - (26/01/85)(7.0m)

The Governor . . . . Martin Jarvis
Security Chief . . . . Forbes Collins
Quillam . . . . Nicholas Chagrin
Jondar . . . . Jason Connery
Areta . . . . Geraldine Alexander
Sil Nabil Shaban
Arak . . . . Stephen Yardley
Etta. . . . . Sheila Reid
Director . . . . Ron Jones
Designer . . . . Tony Snoaden
Visual Effects . . . . Charles Jeanes
Costume Design . . . . Ann Harding

THE MARK OF THE RANI (Serial 6X)
Written by Pip & Jane Baker (2 Episodes)
During the industrial revolution, the workers at Lord Ravensworth's mines are staging increasingly violent luddite attacks. The Doctor discovers an old enemy from his academy days, the Rani, is tampering with the workers' minds so that they are unable to rest or sleep. When she joins forces with the Master, using her chemical skills to try and destroy the Doctor, the danger he faces has effectively been doubled. . . .

Episode One - (02/02/85)(6.8m)
Episode Two - (09/02/85)(7.3m)

The Rani . . . . Kate O'Mara
The Master . . . . Anthony Ainley
Lord Ravensworth. . . . . Terence Alexander
George Stephenson . . . . . . Gawn Grainger
Luke Ward. . . . . Gary Cady
Jack Ward . . . . Peter Childs
Tim Bass . . . . William Ilkley
Director. . . . . Sarah Hellings
Designer . . . . Paul Trerise
Visual Effects . . . . David Barton
Costume Design . . . . Dinah Collins

THE TWO DOCTORS (Serial 6W)
Written by Robert Holmes (3 Episodes)
The Time Lords are concerned about time experiments being carried out on the space station J7, by Professors Kartz and Reimer, and send the second Doctor, travelling with Jamie, to try and stop them. The head of the station, Dastari, has been augmenting the primitive Androgum slave, Chessene, with added intelligence, and she, in turn, has betrayed the station to the Sontarans, who invade and take the Doctor captive. The sixth Doctor arrives, and finds Jamie stranded there, having reverted to almost primitive instincts to survive. With Peri and his former companion, he traces Chessene and Dastari to Seville in Spain, where the Sontarans Stike and Varl are waiting for an operation to be carried out on the second Doctor, which will trace a vital chromosome that will enable them to use the Kartz/Reimer time machine, but he is augmented into an Androgum, and leaves on a good hunt with Shockeye, another one of the race from the space station. Both Doctors have to join forces to stop Chessene's schemes, as the Sontarans are betrayed and killed by her as well. . . .

Episode One - (16/02/85)6.6(m)
Episode Two - (23/02/85)(6.0m)
Episode Three - (02/03/85)(6.9m)

The second Doctor . . . . . Patrick Troughton
Jamie . . . . Frazer Hines
Dastari. . . . . Laurence Payne
Chessene . . . . Jacqueline Pearce
Shockeye. . . . . John Stratton
Oscar Botcherby. . . . . James Saxon
Stike. . . . . Clinton Greyn
Varl. Tim Raynham
Director. . . . . Peter Moffatt
Designer. . . . . Tony Burrough
Visual Effects . . . . Steven Drewett
Costume Design . . . . Jan Wright

TIMELASH (Serial 6Y)
Written by Glen McCoy (2 Episodes)
The Doctor last visited Karfel during his third incarnation, and found it to be a hospitable, friendly place. When he returns with Peri, the society is now ruled by the Borad, seemingly a benevolent elderly man, but in reality a hideous mutant cross between a human and a reptile. Anyone who crosses him is thrown into the Timelash, a device which either hurls you to some distant point in space or destroys you. The Doctor pursues Vena as she is thrown in and finds her on Earth in the early part of the 20th century, where she has met H. G. Wells. The Doctor takes him back to Karfel and enlists his help to defeat the Borad. . . .

Episode One - (09/03/85)(6.7m)
Episode Two - (16/03/85)(7.4m)

The Borad . . . . Robert Ashby
Elderly Man. . . . . Denis Carey
Tekker. . . . . Paul Darrow
Mykros . . . . Eric Deacon
Brunner . . . . Peter Robert Scott
Vena . . . . Jeananne Crowley
Sezon . . . . Dicken Ashworth
H. G. Wells . . . . David Chandler
Android . . . . Dean Hollingsworth
Director . . . . Pennant Roberts
Designer. . . . . Bob Cove
Visual Effects. . . . . Kevin Molloy
Costume Design . . . . Alan Hughes

REVELATION OF THE DALEKS (Serial 6Z)
Written by Eric Saward (2 Episodes)
On the planet Necros, Davros has set up a base in the cyrogenics centre where wealthy people pay to be frozen until a cure can be found for their various ailments. He is selling the bodies to Kara as a base protein, which she then sells to solve various famines at great profit, and also building up a new army of white Daleks at the same time. Kara sends two assassin, Orcini and Bostock, to kill Davros thinking that all that is left of him is a head in a life support machine, but Davros is exactly as

he always was, and promptly defeats the two men. The Doctor and Peri are caught in the middle of everything, as a rival faction of Daleks arrive, and all hell breaks loose as they try to capture Davros to take him back to Skaro to face trial. . . .

Episode One - (23/03/85)(7.4m)
Episode Two - (30/03/85)(7.7m)

Davros . . . . Terry Molloy
Kara . . . . Eleanor Bron
Vogel . . . . Hugh Walters
Orcini . . . . William Gaunt
Bostock . . . . John Ogwen
Jobel . . . . Clive Swift
Tasambeker . . . . Jenny Tomasin
Takis . . . . Trevor Cooper
Lilt. . . . . Colin Spaull
D.J. . . . . Alexei Sayle
Dalek Voices by Roy Skelton
Director . . . . Graeme Harper
Designer . . . . Alan Spaulding
Visual Effects . . . . John Brace
Costume Design . . . . Pat Godfrey

Season Twenty Three

Regular Cast

The Doctor . . . . Colin Baker
Peri . . . . Nicola Bryant (Serial 7A-7B)
Mel . . Bonnie Langford (Serial 7C onwards)
The Valeyard . . . . Michael Jayston
The Inquisitor . . . . Lynda Bellingham

Regular Production Team

John Nathan-Turner . . . . Producer
Eric Saward . . . . Script Editor
(Episodes 1-8 & 13)

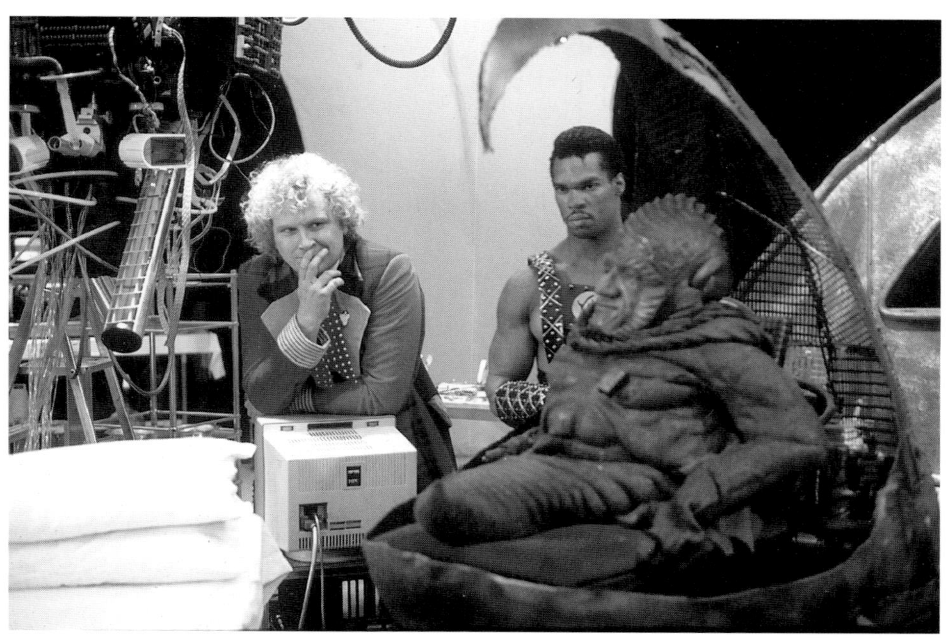

THE TRIAL OF A TIME LORD (Serial 7A-7C)
(14 Episodes)
Written by: Robert Holmes (Episodes 1-4) (Serial 7A); Philip Martin (Episodes 5-8) (Serial 7B); Pip & Jane Baker (Episodes 9-12 & 14) (Serial 7C); (Episode 13 by Robert Holmes)

Taken out of time, the Tardis is brought to a vast space station, where the Doctor faces a trial by the Time Lords for crimes of interference. The Inquisitor is effectively the Judge, whilst the Valeyard is the Prosecutor. The Doctor can only watch, with his memory of the immediate past prior to his arrival gone for the moment, as the Valeyard uses an incident from his past as the first part of his evidence, projected before the jury by the Matrix data bank.

(7A) On the planet Ravolox, the Doctor and Peri encounter Drathro, a huge robot, whose mission is to guard Time Lord secrets stolen by invaders from the Andromedan Galaxy years before, which have been placed in his care. A race of servile humans tend to the tunnels surrounding his base, and a group of primitives on the surface of the planet try to attack it every so often, but with little success. Two con men, Glitz and Dibber, arrive planning to steal the secrets, but Drathro is prepared to destroy everything to protect them, so the Doctor has to intervene. . . .

The Valeyard continues with his evidence, as he shows the events immediately prior to the Doctor's arrival at the space station. As the events unfold on the Matrix screen, the Doctor's memory slowly returns. . . .

(7B) On Sil's home planet, Thoros-Beta, a scientist has been employed to find a way of transferring the mind of the species head Mentor, Lord Kiv, into another body, but Crozier has yet to find the perfect host. Kiv's brain is expanding slowly, and the continual pain is stopping him from carrying out the all important commerce negotiations, with the inevitable profit that the Mentors thrive on. King Yrcanos, of the Krontep, is also on Thoros-Beta, held captive by the Mentors. The mighty warrior becomes infatuated with Peri, who becomes the ideal candidate to house Kiv's brain when both the King and Doctor's skulls prove unsatisfactory. The Doctor's behaviour becomes strange, as Time Lords start to manipulate him, and he is then taken out of time to leave Peri to her fate. Yrcanos is seen fighting his way towards Crozier's laboratory, where Kiv's transplant is now complete, and on seeing the dehumanised Peri, he seems to blast everyone in the room to death with a phaser. . . .

It is now the Doctor's turn to present his defence, and although still in shock from witnessing Peri's apparent death, he selects events from his future, which appear on the screen.

(7C) Something is murdering the passengers on the Hyperion III space liner. Three Botanists unwittingly unleash the deadly plant lifeforms, the Vervoids, who start to slaughter any humans they find, and the Doctor and his 'new' companion, Mel, have to fight off the creatures and stop the ship from being destroyed by entering a black hole.

The Valeyard accuses the Doctor of committing genocide by destroying the Vervoids, and the next stage of the trial is reached as some unexpected witnesses arrive; Mel and Glitz. The Master suddenly appears on the Matrix screen, who explains that the Valeyard is in league with the Gallifreyan High Council, in an attempt to frame the Doctor over the secrets he discovered on Ravolox. The Valeyard tries to escape into the Matrix, with the Doctor and Glitz in pursuit, where they track him down in a bizarre nightmare world which he has created. He fights for survival, but is eventually defeated, with the Doctor leaving Glitz to escape back to reality, after overcoming the Master as well.

The Valeyard was a future interim incarnation of the Doctor, and he deceived the court into believing that Peri was killed. She now lives with Yrcanos as his Queen.

Mel leaves with the Doctor in the Tardis, although she is actually a companion he has yet to meet. . . .

Episode One - (06/09/86)(4.9m)
Episode Two - (13/09/86)(4.9m)
Episode Three - (20/09/86)(3.9m)
Episode Four - (27/09/86)(3.7m)
Episode Five - (04/10/86)(4.8m)
Episode Six - (11/10/86)(4.6m)
Episode Seven - (18/10/86)(5.1m)
Episode Eight - (25/10/86)(5.0m)
Episode Nine - (01/11/86)(5.2m)
Episode Ten - (08/11/86)(4.6m)
Episode Eleven - (15/11/86)(5.3m)
Episode Twelve - (22/11/86)(5.2m)
Episode Thirteen - (29/11/86)(4.4m)
Episode Fourteen - (06/12/86)(5.6m)

Guest Cast 1-4
Katryca . . . . Joan Sims
Glitz . . . . Tony Selby
Dibber . . . . Glen Murphy
Humker . . . . Billy McColl
Tandrell . . . . Sion Tudor Owen
Merdeen . . . . Tom Chadbon
Broken Tooth . . . . David Rodigan
Drathro . . . . Roger Brierley
Operated Uncredited by Paul McGuiness
Guest Cast 5-8
King Yrcanos . . . . Brian Blessed
The Lukoser . . . . Thomas Branch
Sil Nabil Shaban
Lord Kiv . . . . Christopher Ryan
Crozier . . . . Patrick Ryecart
Matrona Kani . . . . Alibe Parsons
Frax . . . . Trevor Laird
Tuza . . . . Gordon Warnecke
Mentor . . . . Richard Stanley
Guest Cast 9-12
Professor Lasky . . . . Honor Blackman
Commodore . . . . Michael Craig
Rudge . . . . Denys Hawthorne
Janet . . . . Yolande Palfrey
Grenville & Enzu . . . . Tony Scoggo
Doland . . . . Malcolm Tierney
Bruchner . . . . David Allister
Kimber . . . . Arthur Hewlett
Guest Cast 13-14
The Master . . . . Anthony Ainley
The Keeper of the Matrix . . . . . James Bree
Glitz . . . . Tony Selby
Mister Popplewick . . . . . . Geoffrey Hughes
Directors . . . . (1-4) Nick Mallett
(5-8) Ron Jones
(9-14) Chris Clough
Designers . . . . (1-4) John Anderson
(5-8) Andrew Howe-Davies
(9-12) Dinah Walker
(13-14) Michael Trevor
Visual Effects . . . . (1-4) Mike Kelt
(5-8) Peter Wragg
(9-14) Kevin Molloy
Costume Design . . . . (1-4) Ken Trew
(5-8) Dorka Nieradzik
(9-14) Shaunna Harrison

Season Twenty Four

Regular Cast
The Doctor . . . . Sylvester McCoy
Mel . . . . . . Bonnie Langford (Serial 7D-7F)
Ace . . . Sophie Aldred (Serial 7G onwards)

Regular Production Team
John Nathan-Turner . . . . Producer
Andrew Cartmel . . . . Script Editor

TIME AND THE RANI (Serial 7D)
Written by Pip & Jane Baker (4 Episodes)
A power beam draws the Tardis towards Lakertya, where it lands heavily and induces a regeneration for the Doctor, who is taken captive by the Rani and her lead Tetrap, Urak, as they enter the craft. The Doctor is taken to the Rani's base, while Mel befriends Ikona, a Lakertyan, in the waste-land surrounding the Tardis landing site. The Rani has assembled many of the great thinkers from history, with her plan being to drain their minds and form one vast brain. This will be turned into a giant Time Manipulator when the missiles positioned on her base strike an asteroid of strange matter in the planet's orbit. The bewildered Doctor, who is fooled for a time into believing that the Rani is Mel, has to try and defeat her and come to terms with the shock of his regeneration. . . .

Episode One - (07/09/87)(5.1m)
Episode Two - (14/09/87)(4.2m)
Episode Three - (21/09/87)(4.3m)
Episode Four - (28/09/87)(4.9m)

The Rani . . . . Kate O'Mara
Beyus . . . . Donald Pickering
Faroon . . . . Wanda Ventham
Ikona . . . . Mark Greenstreet
Urak . . . . Richard Gauntlett
Sarn . . . . Karen Clegg
Director . . . . Andrew Morgan
Designer . . . . Geoff Powell
Visual Effects . . . . Colin Mapson
Costume Design . . . . Ken Trew

PARADISE TOWERS (Serial 7E)
Written by Stephen Wyatt (4 Episodes)
Paradise Towers was planned as the perfect residential home, but while a majority of the occupants are away fighting a war, the complex's Caretakers seem to have taken control. Groups of vandals, known as Kangs, roam the corridors with three gangs being designated by colour codes; Red, blue and yellow, although all the yellow Kangs have been killed. The Chief Caretaker is under the control of Kroagnon, the Great Architect, who designed Paradise Towers, and is imprisoned as a vast machine in the cellar. The cleaning robots feed humans they have killed to this machine – both Kangs and residents alike. When the Great Architect takes over the Chief Caretaker, the Doctor has to try and stop him from killing the few survivors left in the place. . . .

Episode One - (05/10/87)(4.5m)
Episode Two - (12/10/87)(5.2m)
Episode Three - (19/10/87)(5.0m)
Episode Four - (26/10/87)(5.0m)

Chief Caretaker . . . . Richard Briers
Deputy Chief Caretaker . . . . Clive Merrison
Tabby . . . . Elizabeth Spriggs
Tilda . . . . Brenda Bruce
Maddy . . . . Judy Cornwell
Bin Liner . . . . Annabel Yuresha
Fire Escape . . . . Julie Brennon
Pex . . . . Howard Cooke
Blue Kang Leader . . . . . . Catherine Cusack
Director . . . . Nick Mallett
Designer . . . . Martin Collins
Visual Effects . . . . Simon Tayler
Costume Design . . . . Janet Tharby

DELTA AND THE BANNERMEN (Serial 7F)
Written by Malcolm Kholl (3 Episodes)
The Bannermen are hunting the last of the Chimerons, a queen, after eradicating her entire race, and follow her as she joins a group of Navarino tourists. Disguised as humans, they are on their way to a holiday camp on Earth during the 1950s. The space travelling coach they're in crashlands in Wales outside the 'Shangri-La' camp, where they decide to stay while the Doctor helps Murray, the coach Driver, repair the damaged engines. The Bannermen arrive and kill the Navarinos, and the Doctor has to fight to save Delta and her new, rapidly growing daughter from them. . . .

Episode One - (02/11/87)(5.3m)
Episode Two - (09/11/87)(5.1m)
Episode Three - (16/11/87)(5.4m)

Delta . . . . Belinda Mayne
Gavrok . . . . Don Henderson
Weismuller . . . . Stubby Kaye
Hawke . . . . Morgan Deare
Billy . . . . David Kinder
Ray . . . . Sara Griffiths
Garonwy . . . . Hugh Lloyd

The Tollmaster . . . . Ken Dodd
Murray . . . . Johnny Dennis
Director . . . . Chris Clough
Designer . . . . John Asbridge
Visual Effects . . . . Andy McVean
Costume Design . . . . Richard Croft

DRAGONFIRE (Serial 7G)
Written by Ian Briggs (3 Episodes)
Iceworld is renowned as a huge shopping centre, and the Doctor and Mel meet Glitz there, who is embarking on a treasure hunt. They join him, along with a young girl called Ace. The treasure in question is also being sought by Kane, as it can release him from his prison, and takes the form of a crystal, which is revealed as being stored inside the head of a bio-mechanoid creature that roams the lower ice caverns of the planet. With Kane defeated, Mel decides to travel with Glitz and leave the Tardis, so Ace takes her place as the Doctor's companion. . . .

Episode One - (23/11/87)(5.5m)
Episode Two - (30/11/87)(5.0m)
Episode Three - (07/12/87)(4.7m)

Glitz . . . . Tony Selby
Kane. . . . . Edward Peel
Belazs . . . . Patricia Queen
Kracauer . . . . Tony Osoba
McLuhan . . . . Stephanie Fayerman
Bazin . . . . Stuart Organ
Zeo. . . . . Sean Blowers
Director . . . . Chris Clough
Designer . . . . John Asbridge
Visual Effects . . . . Andy McVean
Costume Design . . . . Richard Croft

Season Twenty-Five

Regular Cast
The Doctor. . . . . Sylvester McCoy
Ace. . . . . Sophie Aldred

Regular Production Team
John Nathan Turner . . . . Producer
Andrew Cartmel . . . . Script Editor

REMEMBRANCE OF THE DALEKS
(Serial 7H)
Written by Ben Aaronovitch (4 Episodes)
The Tardis travels back to the Winter of 1963, and lands near Coal Hill School, shortly after the original crew departed from Earth. The Doctor left the Hand of Omega behind, a sentient device with immense powers from Gallifrey, which two factions of Daleks are also searching for. The Doctor realises that there must be humans helping both sides, and he allows the device to be captured by the white Imperial Daleks, whose Emperor is revealed to be Davros, who thinks he now has the power for universal conquest . . .

Episode One - (05/10/88)(5.5m)
Episode Two - (12/10/88)(5.8m)
Episode Three - (19/10/88)(5.1m)
Episode Four - (26/10/88)(5.0m)

Captain Gilmore. . . . . Simon Williams
Ratcliffe . . . . George Sewell
Alison . . . . Karen Gledhill
Rachel . . . . Pamela Salem
Davros . . . . Terry Molloy
Mike Smith . . . . Dursley McLinden
Harry . . . . Harry Fowler
Headmaster. . . . . Michael Sheard
Dalek Voices by Roy Skelton, Royce Mills & Brian Miller
Dalek Battle Computer Voice by John Leeson
Director . . . . Andrew Morgan
Designer. . . . . Martin Collins
Visual Effects . . . . Stuart Brisdon
Costume Design . . . . Ken Trew

THE HAPPINESS PATROL (Serial 7L)
Written by Graeme Curry (3 Episodes)
On the Earth colony of Terr Alpha, if anybody fails to meet the dictate of their leader Helen A to be happy, they are executed by the Happiness Patrol. The Doctor and Ace arrive and become separated. Ace joinis up with an unhappy member of the patrol and retreating to the sewers, where they encounter the rodent-like Pipe People, and the Doctor helps an underground movement who believe in free emotion. His greatest problem, however, is to overcome the Kandy Man, a sugar-based robotic creation, with several lethal sugar-based forms of death he likes to inflict on humans. The Doctor is an ideal candidate.

Episode One - (02/11/88)(5.3m)
Episode Two - (09/11/88)(4.6m)
Episode Three - (16/11/88)(5.3m)

Helen A . . . . Sheila Hancock
Joseph C . . . . Ronald Fraser
Susan Q. . . . . Lesley Dunlop
Gilbert M . . . . Harold Innocent
Daisy K . . . . Georgina Hale
Trevor Sigma. . . . . John Normington
Earl Sigma . . . . Richard D. Sharp
Kandy Man . . . . David John Pope
Director . . . . Chris Clough
Designer . . . . John Asbridge
Visual Effects. . . . . Perry Braham
Costume Design . . . . Richard Croft

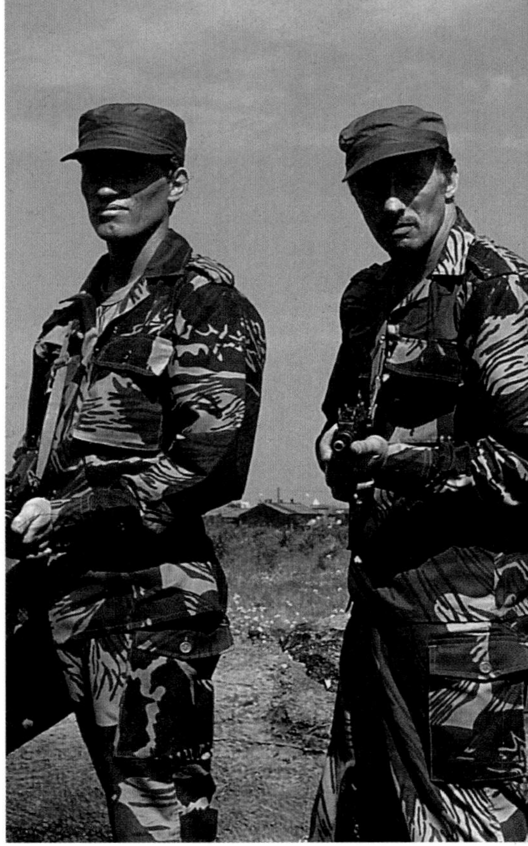

SILVER NEMESIS (Serial 7K)
Written by Kevin Clarke (3 Episodes)
When the Doctor and Ace are attacked, while they are quietly listening to some live jazz at a riverside Inn, they realise someone is controlling the men responsible. The mystery deepens as the Cybermen, the 17th century Lady Peinforte and her man servant Richard, and a group of modern-day Nazis, led by De Flores, all congregate in England, 1988, in search of the nemesis statue. The statue is a Validium based Gallifreyan artifact which is, in effect, a powerful living metal. The Doctor and Ace have to out manoeuvre all three parties to ensure the statue does not fall into the wrong hands. . . .

Episode One - (23/11/88)(6.1m)
Episode Two - (30/11/88)(5.2m)
Episode Three - (07/12/88)(5.2m)

De Flores . . . . Anton Differing
Lady Peinforte . . . . Fiona Walker
Richard. . . . . Gerard Murphy
Karl . . . . Metin Yenal
Mathematician. . . . . Leslie French
Mrs. Remington. . . . . Dolores Gray
Cyberleader . . . . David Banks
Cyberlieutenant . . . . Mark Hardy
Director . . . . Chris Clough
Designer . . . . John Asbridge
Visual Effects . . . . Perry Brahan
Costume Design . . . . Richard Croft

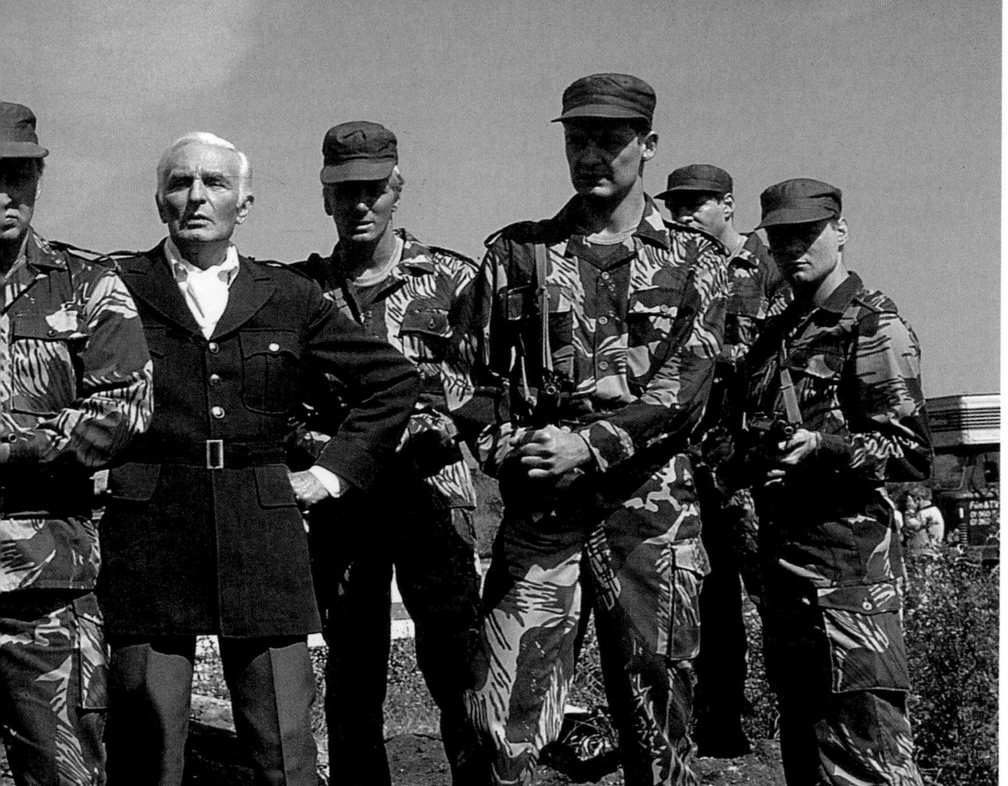

THE GREATEST SHOW IN THE GALAXY (Serial 7J)
Written by Stephen Wyatt (4 Episodes)
The Doctor and Ace arrive at the Psychic Circus on the planet Segonax, where various travellers arrive and take part in a talent contest in the main arena. A seemingly human family passes judgement, with a failure to entertain resulting in instant death. The Doctor realises they are really the Gods of Ragnarok, and that the clowns of the Circus are merely gathering more victims to amuse them or be destroyed. The Doctor's turn comes in the ring, while Ace races to get help. . . .

Episode One - (14/12/88)(5.0m)
Episode Two - (21/12/88)(5.3m)
Episode Three - (28/12/88)(4.8m)
Episode Four - (04/01/88)(6.6m)

Captain Cook . . . . T. P. McKenna
Mags . . . . Jessica Martin
Ringmaster . . . . Ricco Ross
Stallslady . . . . Peggy Mount
Chief Clown . . . . Ian Reddington
Bellboy . . . . Christopher Guard
Deadbeat/Kingpin . . . . Chris Jury
Nord. . . . . Daniel Peacock
Whizzkid . . . . Gian Sammarco
Director . . . . Alan Wareing
Designer . . . . David Laskey
Visual Effects . . . . Steve Bowman
Costume Design . . . . Ros Ebbutt

Season Twenty Six

Regular Cast
The Doctor. . . . . Sylvester McCoy
Ace . . . . Sophie Aldred

Regular Production Team
John Nathan Carter. . . . . Producer
Andrew Cartmel . . . . Script Editor

BATTLEFIELD (Serial 7N)
Written by Ben Aaronvitch (4 Episodes)
Two factions of Knights land on Earth, staging a fight in the middle of a UNIT convoy, transporting a nuclear missile across the countryside. Brigadier Lethbridge-Stewart comes out of retirement to work alongside the Doctor and Ace, as they take on the Morgaine, who seeks the legendary Excalibur, buried in the bottom of a lake with the body of King Arthur inside a space craft. If the Doctor does not comply, she threatens to unleash a dimension wrecking demon called the Destroyer, and it's Lethbridge-Stewart who bravely faces the creature as it prepared to eradicate mankind. . . .

Episode One - (06/09/89)(3.1m)
Episode Two - (13/09/89)(3.9m)
Episode Three - (20/09/89)(3.6m)
Episode Four - (27/09/89)(4.0m)

Brigadier Lethbridge-Stewart . . . . Nicholas Courtney
Morgaine . . . . Jean Marsh
Peter Warmsley . . . . James Ellis
Brigadier Bambera . . . . Angela Bruce
Mordred. . . . . Christopher Bowen
Ancelyn . . . . Marcus Gilbert
Doris Lethbridge-Stewart . . Angela Douglas
The Destroyer . . . . Marek Anton
Director . . . . Michael Kerrigan
Designer. . . . . Martin Collins
Visual Effects . . . . Dave Beskorawsjny
Costume Design . . . . . . Anushia Nieradzik

GHOST LIGHT (Serial 7Q)
Written by Marc Platt (3 Episodes)
In a mansion called Gabriel Chase in London, during the Victorian era, the Doctor and Ace become guests of Josiah Smith and his bizarre household; the austere Mrs Pritchard; his ward, Gwendoline; the deranged Redvers Fenn Cooper, convinced he is still an explorer; and Nimrod, a Neanderthal butler, who takes care of a strange creature locked away in the futuristic cellar. The basement is really a spaceship, which Light had been using as a base while he catalogued Earth's species, but one of them escaped, trapping Control and ensured Light remained inert while the creature evolved into Josiah. When the Doctor sets Light free, the almost ethereal being wants to know what went wrong with his survey, and is prepared to destroy everything to find out. . . .

Episode One - (04/10/89)(4.2m)
Episode Two - (11/10/89)(4.0m)
Episode Three - (18/10/89)(4.0m)

Josiah Smith . . . . Ian Hogg
Mrs. Pritchard . . . . Sylvia Syms
Redvers Fenn-Cooper . . . Michael Cochrane
Inspector McKenzie . . . . Frank Windsor
Control. . . . . Sharon Duce
Reverend Ernest Matthews . . John Nettleton
Gwendoline . . . . Catherine Schlesinger
Nimord . . . . Carl Forgione
Director . . . . Alan Wareing
Designer . . . . Nick Somerville
Visual Effects . . . . Malcolm James
Costume Design . . . . Ken Trew

THE CURSE OF FENRIC (Serial 7M)
Written by Ian Briggs (4 Episodes)
The Tardis lands at a naval base at the height of World War Two, where the crippled Doctor Judson is trying to decode the elaborate Viking inscription discovered on the walls of a local tomb. Commander Millington, who runs the base, has become obsessed with cracking the code, but there is a darker side to their work. The encryp-

tion machine Judson is working with has been booby-trapped, so that when a group of Russian Commandos in the area try to steal it, a lethal nerve gas will be released from within when they get it back to their base. Fenric, an ancient evil, causes the Heamovores, vampiric creatures from the depths of the sea, to rise and move in on the base, where he has manipulated the Doctor into arriving through time, influencing Ace ever since she joined him on the Tardis. The Doctor knows he has to destroy Fenric once and for all. . . .

Episode One - (25/10/89)(4.3m)
Episode Two - (01/11/89)(4.0m)
Episode Three - (08/01/89)(4.0m)
Episode Four - (15/01/89)(4.2m)

Doctor Judson . . . . Dinsdale Landen
Commander Millington . . . . . Alfred Lynch
Reverend Wainwright . . . Nicholas Parsons
Captain Soren . . . . Tomek Bork
Nurse Crane. . . . . Anne Reid
Jean . . . . Joanne Kenny
Phyllis. Joanne Bell
Vershinin . . . . Marek Anton
Kathleen Dudman . . . . Cory Pulman
Director. . . . . Nick Mallett
Designer . . . . David Laskey
Visual Effects. . . . . Graham Brown
Costume Design . . . . Ken Trew

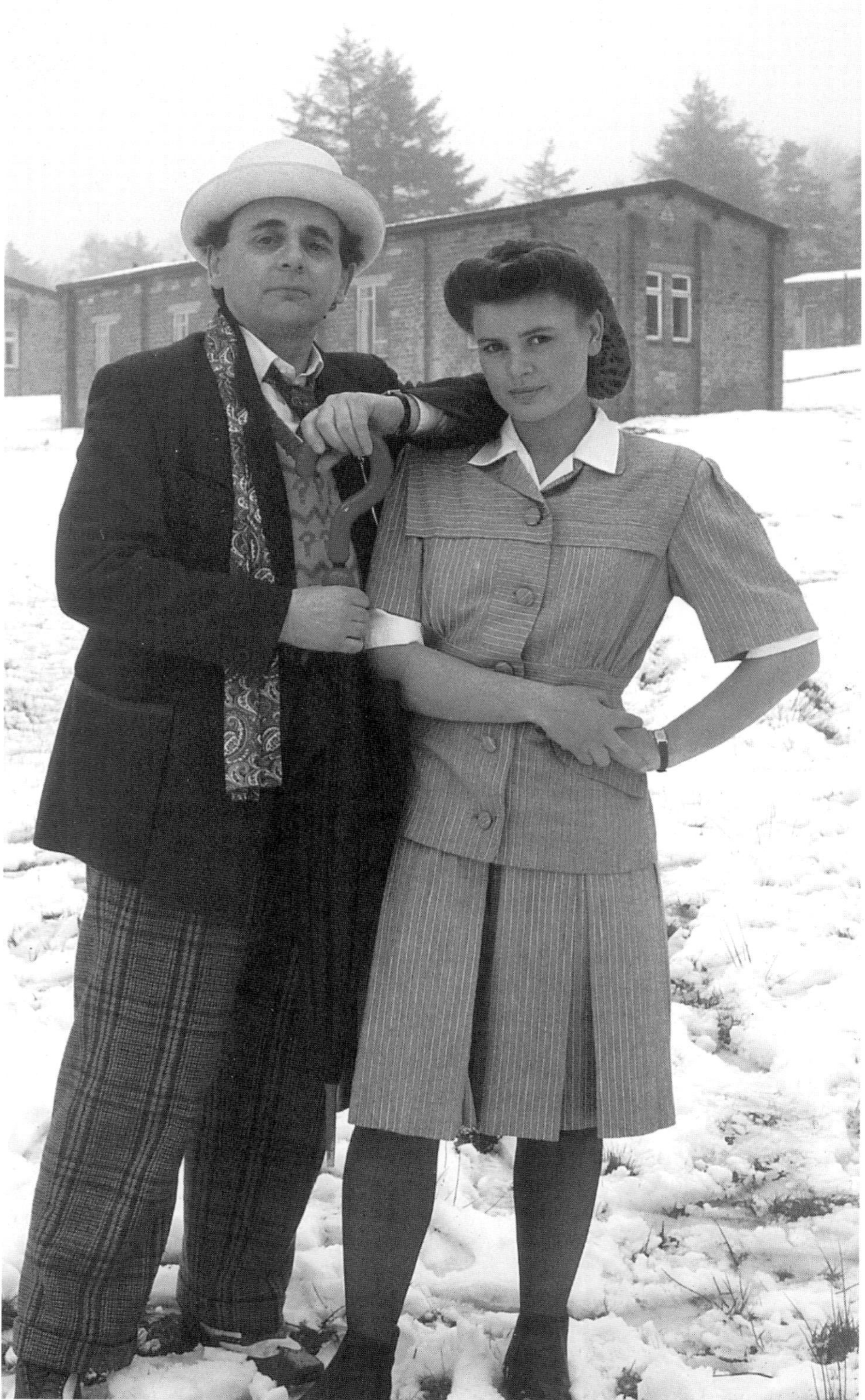

SURVIVAL (Serial 7P)
Written by Rona Munro (3 Episodes)

The Tardis arrives back in Ace's old home of Perivale, and all of her old friends seem to have disappeared. A strange Cheetah-like creature appears from nowhere and pursues her on horseback, transporting her to its home planet as it catches her. Humans are being transported there, where the Cheetah People hunt them down for sport, and the Doctor finds that the Master is controlling them. The longer you stay on the world, the more feline and savage you become, and with the Master and Ace already showing signs, the Doctor has to race to get the humans back to Earth as he begins to become affected as well. At the end, with everything back as it should be, the Doctor and Ace head off towards the Tardis, and on to new adventures . . . perhaps?

Episode One - (22/11/89)(5.0m)
Episode Two - (29/11/89)(4.8m)
Episode Three - (06/12/89)(5.0m)

The Master . . . . Anthony Ainley
Paterson . . . . Julian Holloway
Karra . . . . Lisa Bowerman
Midge. . . . . William Barton
Shreela. . . . . Sakuntala Ramanee
Harvey . . . . Gareth Hale
Len . . . . Norman Pace
Squeak. . . . . Adele Silva
Director . . . . Alan Wareing
Designer . . . . Nick Somerville
Visual Effects . . . . Malcolm James
Costume Design . . . . Ken Trew